'This book is an excellent collection of psychological insights into people's perception, understanding and reactions to the SARS-CoV-2 pandemic. The scholarly analysis of individual, group and societal dynamics deals with emotions, risk perception and decision making, trust in experts and institutions, adaptation processes and the fight against restrictions to regain the lost freedom...a must-read for everybody trying to understand the crisis and a valuable source for students and researchers in the field of psychology and behavioral sciences.'

Prof. Erich Kirchler, *University of Vienna, Austria*

'In the course of the COVID-19 pandemic, an extraordinary number of people turned overnight into specialists in individual psychology, social psychology, and sociology. Peremptory statements about how people feel, individually and collectively, circulated widely and irresponsibly. This book represents a timely and successful effort to counter such epistemic trespassing, by laying out what is known in the relevant fields. Warmly recommended.'

Prof. David Leiser, *Ben Gurion University of the Negev, Israel*

'How Social Psychology contributes to facing the crisis related to the pandemic is the topic of this book. It covers individual and group perspectives, as well as society's, with a focus on the role of institutions' trust, and the influence of social capital in terms of compliance. The importance of cultural differences, with the examples of Islam and Hinduism, is well shown. The last chapter is particularly interesting as it describes how little scientific evidence is taken into account in public policy responses to the pandemic, and how psychology can contribute to facilitating adaptation to a prolonged pandemic. It is a must!'

Prof. Christine Roland-Lévy, *President – International Association of Applied Psychology (IAAP), University of Reims Champagne Ardenne, France*

'The COVID-19 pandemic has taken lives of millions worldwide and put our world into chaos. As the pandemic unfolded, it became clear that understanding and mitigating the process requires the collective work of various specialists, including virologists, medical doctors, mathematicians, but also representatives of the social sciences. The pandemic changed our behaviour and daily routines; it affected our mental health and increased the prevalence of psychiatric disorders. Interestingly, our behaviour also affects the pandemic, as the occurrence of "waves" largely reflect our habits, and to a lesser extent, the seasonality of the virus. Strikingly, social sciences, in some cases, appear to be more relevant in controlling the pandemic than medicine and biology. However, the importance of these studies is not reflected by the funding and attention they deserve. The book *Human Behaviour in Pandemics* addresses a lot of these issues, critically discussing the problem of the pandemic on the level of a single person, a group, and a society. It discusses communication and miscommunication and confronts us with many unobvious aspects of the pandemic. I highly recommend the book. It is one of the first positions that comprehensively address the topic. While it refers to the COVID-19 pandemic, the messages are universal. Important to read now, but also worth considering before the next crisis.'

Krzysztof Pyrć, *Ph.D., D.Sc. Full professor in virology, Jagiellonian University, member of the European Group of Experts on SARS-CoV-2 Variants*

Human Behaviour in Pandemics

This timely interdisciplinary book brings together a wide spectrum of theoretical concepts and their empirical applications in relation to the COVID-19 pandemic, informing our understanding of the social and psychological bases of a global crisis.

Written by an author team of psychologists and sociologists, the volume provides comprehensive coverage of phenomena such as fear, risk, judgement and decision making, threat and uncertainty, group identity and cohesion, social and institutional trust, and communication in the context of an international health emergency. The topics have been grouped into four main chapters, focusing on the individual, group, social, and communication perspectives of the issues affecting or being affected by the pandemic, based on over 740 classic and current references of peer-reviewed research and contextualized with an epidemiological perspective discussed in the introduction. The volume finishes with two special sections, with a chapter on cultural specificity of the social impact of pandemics, focusing specifically on both Islam and Hinduism, and a chapter on the cross-national differences in policy responses to the current health crisis.

Providing not just a reference for academic research, but also short-term and long-term policy solutions based on successful strategies to combat adverse social, cognitive, and emotional consequences, this is the ideal resource for academics and policymakers interested in social and psychological determinants of individual reactions to pandemics, as well as in fields such as economics, management, politics, and medical care.

Małgorzata Kossowska, full professor in psychology, head of the Social Psychology Unit and Center for Social Cognitive Studies in the Institute of Psychology at Jagiellonian University.

Natalia Letki, associate professor at the Faculty of Political Science and International Studies and Centre for Excellence in Social Sciences, University of Warsaw.

Tomasz Zaleskiewicz, full professor in psychology, head of the Center for Research in Economic Behavior at SWPS University of Social Sciences and Humanities, Wroclaw, Poland.

Szymon Wichary, associate professor at the Institute of Psychology, Jagiellonian University, Krakow.

Human Behaviour in Pandemics

Social and Psychological Determinants in a Global Health Crisis

Małgorzata Kossowska,
Natalia Letki,
Tomasz Zaleskiewicz,
and Szymon Wichary

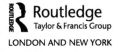

LONDON AND NEW YORK

Cover image: Getty Images

First published in English 2022 by Routledge
by Routledge
4 Park Square, Milton Park, Abingdon, Oxon OX14 4RN

and by Routledge
605 Third Avenue, New York, NY 10158

Routledge is an imprint of the Taylor & Francis Group, an informa business

© 2022 Małgorzata Kossowska, Natalia Letki, Tomasz Zaleskiewicz and Szymon Wichary

The right of Małgorzata Kossowska, Natalia Letki, Tomasz Zaleskiewicz and Szymon Wichary to be identified as authors of this work has been asserted in accordance with sections 77 and 78 of the Copyright, Designs and Patents Act 1988.

All rights reserved. No part of this book may be reprinted or reproduced or utilised in any form or by any electronic, mechanical, or other means, now known or hereafter invented, including photocopying and recording, or in any information storage or retrieval system, without permission in writing from the publishers.

Trademark notice: Product or corporate names may be trademarks or registered trademarks, and are used only for identification and explanation without intent to infringe.

Published in Polish by Smak Słowa 2021

British Library Cataloguing-in-Publication Data
A catalogue record for this book is available from the British Library

Library of Congress Cataloging-in-Publication Data
A catalog record has been requested for this book

ISBN: 9781032183534 (hbk)
ISBN: 9781032183527 (pbk)
ISBN: 9781003254133 (ebk)

DOI: 10.4324/9781003254133

Typeset in Bembo
by codeMantra

Contents

List of figures	ix
List of tables	xi
List of contributors	xiii

PART 1
Individuals, groups, and society in times of pandemics   1
Małgorzata Kossowska, Natalia Letki, Tomasz Zaleskiewicz, and Szymon Wichary

Introduction   3
Małgorzata Kossowska, Natalia Letki, Tomasz Zaleskiewicz, and Szymon Wichary

1   Individual perspective   7
Małgorzata Kossowska, Natalia Letki, Tomasz Zaleskiewicz, and Szymon Wichary

2   Group perspective   49
Małgorzata Kossowska, Natalia Letki, Tomasz Zaleskiewicz, and Szymon Wichary

3   Societal level   65
Małgorzata Kossowska, Natalia Letki, Tomasz Zaleskiewicz, and Szymon Wichary

4   Communication in times of pandemic   85
Małgorzata Kossowska, Natalia Letki, Tomasz Zaleskiewicz, and Szymon Wichary

viii *Contents*

5 Summary 97
Małgorzata Kossowska, Natalia Letki, Tomasz Zaleskiewicz,
and Szymon Wichary

References 109

PART 2
Culture and policy in times of pandemics: case studies 151
Edited by: Małgorzata Kossowska, Natalia Letki, Tomasz
Zaleskiewicz, and Szymon Wichary

6 The COVID-19 epidemic in Poland, as of summer 2021 153
Jerzy Duszyński

7 Pandemic and cultural differences: examples from Islam
and Hinduism 161
Piotr Kłodkowski and Anna Siewierska-Chmaj

8 Public policy responses to the pandemic: a comparative
perspective 177
Jarosław Górniak, Seweryn Krupnik, and Maciej Koniewski

References 197

Index 201

Figures

6.1	Comparison of Poland's and Germany's daily confirmed cases per 1 million habitants, 7-day moving average	157
6.2	Comparison of Poland's and Germany's daily deaths per 1 million habitants, 7-day moving average	157
8.1	Country clusters and intervention categories	194
8.2	The numbers of interventions within ten categories (Airport restrictions, Border restrictions, Closure of educational institutions, Mass gathering cancellation, National lockdown, Small gathering cancellation, Public transport restrictions, Quarantine, Individual movement restrictions, Mandatory use of masks) introduced by the OECD countries in the following weeks of 2020	195

Tables

8.1 Different intervention categories and the related assumptions about target groups' behaviours — 182

8.2 OECD countries included in the dataset by Desvars–Larrive et al. (2020), grouped in quartiles based on the geometrical mean of daily changes in new cases during six months from the day when the first 100 COVID-19 cases were reported in each country — 192

Contributors

Jerzy Duszyński Professor at the Nencki Institute of Experimental Biology and President of the Polish Academy of Sciences (PAS).

Jarosław Górniak Professor of social sciences at the Jagiellonian University in Krakow, specializing in the field of social research methods, methodology of evaluation and analysis of public policy, and sociology of economy and education. Vice-rector of the Jagiellonian University in Krakow. President of the Council of the National Congress of Science (2016–2018), the advisory body focused on designing the reform of higher education and research in Poland.

Piotr Kłodkowski Professor at the Centre for Comparative Studies of Civilisations of the Jagiellonian University in Krakow. A visiting professor at the University of Rochester, New York. Former Ambassador of Poland to India (2009–2014). A member of the Advisory Board of "Muslim Perspectives", published by Muslim Institute (Islamabad, Pakistan).

Maciej Koniewski Assistant professor at the Jagiellonian University, Krakow, Poland.

Małgorzata Kossowska Full professor in psychology, head of the Social Psychology Unit and Center for Social Cognitive Studies in the Institute of Psychology at Jagiellonian University.

Seweryn Krupnik Assistant professor at the Jagiellonian University, Krakow, Poland. He is also a project manager and researcher at the Center for Evaluation and Analysis of Public Policies (CEAPP) at Jagiellonian University. His major research interests are innovation policy and qualitative comparative analysis.

Natalia Letki Associate professor at the Faculty of Political Science and International Studies and Centre for Excellence in Social Sciences, University of Warsaw.

xiv *Contributors*

Anna Siewierska-Chmaj Associate professor at the University of Rzeszow and a political scientist. Author of publications on, inter alia, the anthropology of politics and psychology of politics, and the language of politics and migration policy.

Szymon Wichary Associate professor at the Institute of Psychology, Jagiellonian University in Krakow.

Tomasz Zaleskiewicz Full professor in psychology, head of the Center for Research in Economic Behavior at SWPS University of Social Sciences and Humanities, Wroclaw, Poland.

PART 1

Individuals, groups, and society in times of pandemics

Małgorzata Kossowska, Natalia Letki, Tomasz Zaleskiewicz, and Szymon Wichary

INTRODUCTION[1]

Małgorzata Kossowska, Natalia Letki, Tomasz Zaleskiewicz, and Szymon Wichary

The pandemic we are currently facing is considered to be the gravest crisis of its kind since World War II. It has mustered and intensified a herculean joint effort by scientists representing diverse disciplines to understand how the SARS-CoV-2 virus infects and propagates, to refine diagnostic tests, and find effective drugs. However, how the development of the disease itself, COVID-19, has unfolded is markedly influenced by psychological and social factors. In other words, people's beliefs and behaviours play a prominent role in how the disease spreads, who becomes infected, how many people succumb to the disease, and what preventive measures are undertaken. The search for more effective vaccines and drugs is ongoing, but in the meantime, and in parallel, successful containment of the disease, in order to safeguard the health and wellbeing of entire societies, largely depends on decisions made by a range of decision makers as well as the willingness of individuals to adhere to the guidelines and recommendations arising from those decisions.

Uncertainty is inherent in people's decision making and behaviours as they endeavour to cope with this dire predicament. The official decision makers themselves seem to have scant and/or partial knowledge of the disease, and the available information is often of poor quality, fragmented, and/or contradictory (Ioannidis, 2020). In these circumstances, decision making is contingent on the decision makers' willingness and ability to predict people's behaviour, on the values and beliefs they rely on when assessing the quality of available evidence and expert opinions, and on their approaches to resolving moral dilemmas (e.g., choosing who receives access to a ventilator) and value conflicts (such as safety versus civil liberties). Whether the populace is willing to comply with any rules and recommendations emerging from this decision-making process, in turn, largely hinges on their level of trust in decision makers: their competence, sincerity, and good intentions.

Both the apparent uncertainty among decision makers and people's concern about whether their decisions are right feed pandemic-related anxiety, which spreads much like a virus, affecting various aspects of our lives. Worry centres on not only our own health and that of loved ones but also on the number of restrictions imposed on everyday life, the manner in which the labour market is subject to seismic shifts, and how the economy or education

DOI: 10.4324/9781003254133-2

4 *Individuals, Groups, and Society in Pandemics*

will function as the pandemic ensues. Expectations of an economic recession and thoughts of preparing for the worst instill fear, anxiety, and uncertainty, and when experienced over extended periods of time, lead to a deterioration in people's health, a diminishment in their ability to act effectively, and the potential for developing damaging defensive behaviours. Coping with such negative feelings poses enormous challenges during a pandemic (Taylor, 2019).

The current pandemic should be seen as more than just a health crisis. It has knocked people out of their daily routines, altering both behaviour and the social and economic rules that organize behaviour. It has placed everyone in a situation that is not only threatening (people are actually contracting the disease and dying in worrying numbers) and novel (if forced to undertake remote work or distance learning) but also unpredictable (the prevalence and longevity of the viral threat is unclear). One might even go so far as to say that the pandemic has utterly dismantled the world we knew, or has at least caused a sea-change. We must learn to live anew – change our ways, learn new behaviours, and turn them into habits.

There is no doubt the pandemic has led to a crisis experienced on multiple levels. A crisis, however, does not necessarily lead to calamity. Used properly, it may even facilitate positive change. Wise-headed decisions and the behaviours that support them are a key to success. It is therefore essential to understand the mechanisms underlying the behaviours of individuals, groups, and societies, both during the pandemic and when it finally ends. These mechanisms, in turn, may be described in terms of individual factors (cognitive, emotional, and behavioural), social factors (group and intergroup), and institutional factors (those referring to state–citizen relations and to the laws that regulate them). These factors are not isolated from each other. On the contrary, they are closely linked and dynamically interrelated. Therefore, our review makes an attempt at including all three levels of analysis and, whenever possible, reveals their interconnections.

We focus on the role of psychological and social factors, since these two categories, though typically ignored by decision makers (who prefer to rely on their intuitions), play a key role in effective crisis management. During the current pandemic, we have all observed tremendous efforts and resources being expended in the provision of medical help for COVID-19 patients, while the needs of entire social groups that have been affected by the pandemic in other ways have been neglected (e.g., groups suffering from mental health problems, such as anxiety and depressive disorders, panic attacks, or stress; groups displaying behavioral problems, such as non-compliance with COVID-19 restrictions and medical guidelines, risky behaviour, and stigmatization; and those experiencing domestic violence). The neglect also extends to those who have lost their livelihoods or have no access to healthcare services (the underprivileged, those experiencing homelessness, and immigrants). Serious consequences may follow as a result in the near and longer-term future.

We realize this monograph does not exhaust the subject of psychological and social behaviours during the current pandemic. In fact, we set out to answer just two questions: (1) How ought we prepare people for the social and economic crises related to the pandemic? (2) What constitutes the major risks that may contribute to the crisis persisting unduly? Since one of the most serious risks, in our view, is the uncontrolled spread of the disease, we devote a great deal of attention to preventive measures aimed at reducing the spread of the coronavirus disease (such as hygiene practices, obeying government-imposed rules, etc.), and how these could be communicated effectively to the public. These two questions turn out to be very broad, so each section of this book may serve as a starting point for separate in-depth analyses. We focus on those aspects of the problem that (1) we consider essential for gaining a holistic understanding of people's behaviour during a pandemic, (2) have a sufficient body of reliable evidence relevant to the issues, and (3) can be used as the basis for developing recommendations for decision makers. Aiming as we do to offer a comprehensive account of this complex problem, we have inspected it from different behavioural and social science perspectives: cognitive and social psychology, behavioural economics, sociology, and political science. In this way, we are in line with the best practices recommended to researchers during a pandemic (see Hahn et al., 2020), fully aware that no social problem can be accurately described from the perspective of just one discipline. This approach, however, requires the marrying of different research and methodological perspectives and a certain unification of the language of description. Integrating advances in various scientific disciplines is far from being an easy task. What exacerbates the difficulty is the fact that the behavioural and social sciences are often contextual, that is, the effects they describe depend on the place, a particular moment in history, public moods, and the contemporary social and political discourse. Hence, the task of distinguishing between the universal and the specific is not always easily accomplished from existing data.

This book's inception dates from May 2020, at a time when the pandemic appeared to be more under control and social life was slowly returning to normal. The initial shock sparked by the large number of cases was subsiding, the unprecedented restrictions were being loosened, and lockdown was gradually being lifted. By July 2020, once the book was ready, people's minds in Poland were occupied with the presidential election, summer holidays, and some rumblings about another possible wave of the pandemic in the fall. There were also reports that a vaccine for COVID-19 was ready. At the same time, on July 18, 2020, the World Health Organization (WHO) reported the biggest daily increase in the number of new COVID-19 cases since the start of the pandemic (260,000; BBC, 2020). A couple of weeks earlier, economists at the World Bank forecast that the economic recession caused by the pandemic would be the deepest since 1970 (World Bank, 2020). Given all this, it is hard to believe the health crisis is over. What we know with certainty, though, is that a social and economic crisis is yet to come. Therefore, regardless of the

6 *Individuals, Groups, and Society in Pandemics*

further dynamics of the COVID-19 pandemic around the world, the analyses presented in this book will remain valid for the foreseeable future. Most of the effects and mechanisms discussed here, especially those related to anxiety and uncertainty, are universal. We encounter them in any situation perceived as a crisis; that is, in any emergency situation that threatens human life, health, resources, and the environment, that prevents normal functioning, and that requires extraordinary measures to be overcome. In this book, we emphasize, as much as possible, both the mechanisms specific to a pandemic (such as the fear of becoming infected and its consequences) and those that are universal, typical of any crisis (e.g., helplessness and low perceived control of one's environment).

Finally, bearing in mind the weaknesses of social and behavioural sciences (or, more generally, basic sciences) as an instrument for policy making (IJzerman et al., 2020), we must concede that our analyses can only demonstrate what we know, or what we think, is probable. At the same time, we are clear about what we lack evidence for when it comes to people's behaviour in a crisis situation. What sets this review in line with other publications that have been developed in response to the challenges related to the epidemic crisis is its commitment to collecting high-quality scientific evidence and translating it into the language of practice (see Van Bavel et al., 2020; Lunn et al., 2020; Haslam et al., 2020). Possible recommendations for public policy, which also serve as a succinct summary of the scientific review, are provided at the end of Part 1 of this book. We hope this reader-friendly summary, inevitably somewhat simplified, will prove useful, especially to those most concerned with the practical applications of the evidence-based scientific knowledge presented in this work, such as decision makers at different levels of management, both in business organizations and in the public or government sector.

The main part of this book is complemented by the scientific argument, with a commentary demonstrating how important it is to incorporate the cultural perspective when understanding people's behaviour during an epidemic. The closing chapter showcases a variety of state or government responses to the pandemic and discusses how systematized databases of public interventions may support the processes of public policy making and crisis management.

Note

1 In this part of the book, we use the report "Covid 19: Social Sciences in the fight against the pandemic", prepared by Małgorzata Kossowska, Natalia Letki, Tomasz Zaleskiewicz, Szymon Wichary, and Jarosław Górniak, and commissioned by the Małopolska School of Public Administration, University of Economics in Krakow, July 2020.

1 INDIVIDUAL PERSPECTIVE

Małgorzata Kossowska, Natalia Letki,
Tomasz Zaleskiewicz, and Szymon Wichary

1.1 HUMAN AS PROBLEM OR HUMAN AS SOLUTION

Approaches to managing a crisis pivot on one's view of humanity. According to Haslam and colleagues (2020; see also https://www.youtube.com/watch?v=Hmokdb11b7w), there are two such conflicting perspectives in science. The first says that, in a crisis, it is the human being who is the problem, seeing people as both sensitive and self-centered, as prone to breakdown, driven by emotions, reliant on heuristics, and eager to lay blame outside themselves. Therefore, based on this stance, humans are in need of clear guidance, a paternalistic government with full knowledge of the best path forward for people, and a strong leader capable of imposing these solutions. This perspective seems to be prevalent among decision makers but is especially ubiquitous in the media, where we are told humans lack the self-discipline to follow rules concerning masking and social distancing. Media commentators predict people will soon tire of complying with restrictions and return to their old habits, flying in the face of warnings and common sense.

This approach has practical implications, the worst of which include waiting too long to make decisions based on medical recommendations, for example delaying the decision on lockdown; the doling out of harsh penalties to individuals walking their dogs, strolling, or cycling; and collective deprivations in the form of locking down parks and forests. Contrary to this worldview, studies of people's behaviour in many countries show that individuals followed pandemic-related restrictions to a larger extent than expected by governments (whose representatives, by the way, frequently disregarded their own rules; Reicher, 2021). Interestingly, there were a variety of reasons underlying this civil obedience, but in most cases, the primary factor was trust – in scientists (as in Sweden) or in the government (as in Germany). Several analyses, including studies conducted in Poland, showed that relatively few people intentionally violated the restrictions, and their infringements were minor compared to the disproportionately harsh punitive measures inflicted upon them (Wiadomości Onet, 2020; *Gazeta Prawna,*

DOI: 10.4324/9781003254133-3

2020). Conversely, in Poland, it was a profound *distrust* in the healthcare system (perceived as totally inefficient) that was associated with adherence to restrictions (Biliński, 2020). Global research also shows that when COVID-19 restrictions were not observed, it had little to do with insubordination or a lack of motivation but rather resulted from pragmatic difficulties. Not everyone could work from home; people employed in healthcare, transportation, and other services had to attend workplaces every morning. Some needed space more than others, for example because of poor housing conditions. Researchers note that any crisis, including the current one, hits the poor and disadvantaged, and that the virus itself, though the cause of illness regardless of a sufferer's status, is by no means egalitarian, since not everyone can take adequate precautions to prevent infection. Therefore, it is important to understand the reasons why people break rules and, where appropriate, to offer them support instead of sanctions. We know punitive approaches can corrode people's willingness to obey rules and, in consequence, lead to violations, disobedience, and disorder (Łętowska and Sobczak, 2012).

The "human-as-problem" approach is not the only option, though. There is a considerable body of evidence suggesting that, in times of crisis, it is humans themselves who are the solution (Haslam et al., 2020; Van Bavel et al., 2020; Reicher, 2021). Human energy and motivation can be easily harnessed to transform what is damaging and dysfunctional into a new quality. Taking this perspective brings with it several advantages, the most significant one being the prospect of enhancing such positive phenomena as solidarity, helpfulness, and cooperation. Hence, this perspective also will be the focus of further analysis in this book.

1.2 PSYCHOLOGICAL EXPERIENCE OF PANDEMIC: ANXIETY AND UNCERTAINTY

Anxiety is one of the most common emotional responses to a pandemic (Ahorsu et al., 2020; Harper et al., 2020). It could be defined as a generalized feeling of danger from an "object" that cannot be precisely located, and is often accompanied by feelings of uncertainty or insecurity associated with a lack of clear rules on how to avoid the threat or survive unscathed (Kossowska et al., 2018). Humans, like other species, are equipped with special defenses for coping with threats (LeDoux, 2012) but while some survival strategies may be successful in dealing with a threat, they may also increase people's vulnerability to additional stressors. For example, while it is adaptive to seek information about the pandemic, share this information, and join online discussion groups on the subject, these activities may also evoke further the feeling of threat; though better informed, fears may be fueled as the strategy itself becomes a source of anxiety. Paradoxically, the result is that the feeling of anxiety itself is not reduced but instead is further aggravated.

Basic anxiety is worsened by our dearth of knowledge concerning the numbers infected, the real effectiveness of government measures and precautions (such as social distancing or lockdown), and the effects these measures might have on the economy and the health of individuals, groups, and societies on the whole. What's more, it is frequently apparent that scientists and decision makers are not fully apprised of all the facts, either. Consider the recommendation to wear face masks in public places. Whether this precaution is effective is not known (WHO recommends using face masks but, at the same, admits there is no scientific evidence for their effectiveness; in Poland, the Minister of Health changed his mind on mask-wearing several times). We know with certainty, however, that the effectiveness of face masks depends not only on whether people use them or not, but also on how masks are worn and what people do with them after use (Greenhalgh et al., 2020). There is also a psychological aspect that may be a source of additional anxiety: we can assume that wearing face masks, even properly, is likely to have negative effects for individuals and groups, prompting us to ask questions such as, "Could it contribute to dehumanization and social isolation?" and "Is it a signal of risk or rather a symbol of being a good group member, and concerned about the health of others?". It is difficult to provide definitive answers to these questions, given the available data. What we know for certain, however, is that the feeling of threat will linger.

The psychological mechanisms related to uncertainty and threat, and the responses to them, are universal, regardless of the causal factor (the pandemic or the resulting social and economic crisis, and the subsequent change in behaviours forced by the crisis). These mechanisms must be well-understood to facilitate properly targeted interventions to reduce individual and public anxiety. We already know that pandemic-related anxiety can aggravate clinical symptoms of phobias, social anxiety, depression, and other mental disorders (Li et al., 2020; Taylor, 2019). Anxiety leads to behaviours that are harmful both individually, such as self-harm and substance abuse, and on the social level, for instance, violence and aggression (Satchell et al., 2018). It also contributes to wider social conflict and tension (Kossowska et al., 2018). Not accidentally, David Murphy, President of the British Psychological Society, pointed to fear and anxiety as the key issues people (citizens and decision makers) are compelled to deal with during a pandemic (Murphy, 2020).

What about when the pandemic is over? Anxiety directly related to COVID-19 may decrease, but anxiety caused by other stressors will remain. This has been demonstrated in research – on the 2014–2015 Ebola virus epidemic in Africa and the SARS pandemic in 2003 – which shows that the psychological effects of a pandemic may be much more serious and enduring than its direct medical consequences (e.g., Desclaux et al., 2017; Washer, 2004). It is therefore important that efforts to reduce these effects are not limited to the present situation. Instead, we should also develop long-term strategies to promote wellbeing in the future.

1.2.1 HEALTH AND DEATH ANXIETY: SPECIFIC TYPES OF ANXIETY IN TIMES OF PANDEMIC

Maladaptive responses of individuals facing the epidemic risk may be a result of their experience of health anxiety. This type of anxiety refers to being "alarmed by illness-related stimuli, including but not limited to, illness related to infectious diseases" (Taylor, 2019, p. 49). Note that health anxiety is a variable with a wide range of values: from extremely low (a very weak or even inappropriately weak response to signals of the risk of becoming infected) to extremely high (a very strong or inappropriately strong response to these signals). Individuals with low levels of health anxiety may ignore preventive recommendations (for example, to wear masks or avoid human gatherings) because they simply do not feel the need to protect themselves (Goodwin et al., 2009; Williams et al., 2015). Similarly, someone who is unafraid of insects will be unlikely to flee on sight. On the other hand, people with extremely high health anxiety can show unreasonably strong reactions to any information about the possibility of getting infected. This may take the form of excess healthcare utilization (Bobevski et al., 2016; Hagger et al., 2017) or cyberchondria, characterized by intense online searching for medical information (Mathes et al., 2018). In this context, Peters (2020) reports a study in which over 1,200 Americans were asked about how frequently they spent time reading information about the coronavirus on the internet. Nearly 50% of the respondents said they did so daily, leading Peters to label them "statistics stalkers". This subgroup was characterized by increased anxiety (38% reported worrying about the coronavirus, compared to 18% of non-stalkers) and a stronger belief they were likely to get the coronavirus (14% of statistics stalkers said they were likely to become infected, while just 5% of non-stalkers did). Similar results were obtained in studies conducted in Poland (Sobkow et al., 2020). Although the findings reported, both by Peters and by Sobkow and colleagues, should be seen as preliminary and requiring confirmation, they admittedly fit within the broader context of the psychological phenomenon referred to as health anxiety.

Intriguingly, high health anxiety is associated not only with taking particular protective measures but also with a specific way of perceiving reality. For example, individuals with high levels of anxiety tend to overestimate the likelihood of developing a serious disease (Wheaton et al., 2010). They may also show aversive responses to photos of people depicting symptoms of varying severity. One study (Hedman et al., 2016) found that the level of health anxiety was positively related to the subjects' ratings of such pictures in terms of disgust, contagiousness, and anxiety, and negatively related to ratings of attractiveness and willingness to socialize. This clearly negative perception of ailing people by respondents with high health anxiety may explain at least some of the attacks against individuals known to be infected with SARS-CoV-2 (a possible occurrence of such behaviour has already been mentioned in this book).

Individual Perspective 11

In his work, Taylor (2019) lists several factors that seem to be related to health anxiety. These include:

- Misinterpretation of health-related stimuli – bodily sensations that actually do not signal infection (e.g., muscle aches) are subjectively interpreted as signs of illness, and other people's behaviours (such as coughing) are seen as evidence that cases of the disease in question (e.g., COVID-19) are common.
- Specific beliefs about health and disease – selective retrieval of memories about previous illnesses and their own biased interpretations ("In the past, whenever I was feeling physically weak, it turned out I had the flu") or sharing some common but scientifically unsupported beliefs ("Chest pain is always a sign of a heart attack").
- Focus of attention – hypervigilance to any physiological symptoms that may signal illness (e.g., paying attention to every single cough or feeling of dyspnea during the coronavirus pandemic), careful monitoring of one's bodily responses, or even recording them.
- Maladaptive coping – a tendency to engage in or avoid behaviours that seem to prevent or facilitate infection (e.g., avoiding any contact with physicians during the pandemic, guided by a belief that every physician is likely to be a virus carrier, or unreasonably frequent, or even compulsive, handwashing and sanitizing).

Reports on a serious threat to life and health, pervasive during the pandemic, provoke thoughts of death and, consequently, may lead to existential anxiety (Greenberg et al., 1986). Psychology has developed a substantial understanding of the effects of death anxiety. Until recently, only its negative consequences were typically demonstrated: how it affects individual and group wellbeing (Edmondson et al., 2008; Routledge et al., 2010), leads to anxiety disorders (Strachan et al., 2007), and impairs self-regulation (Gailliot et al., 2006; Pyszczynski and Kesebir, 2011; Routledge and Juhl, 2010; Strachan et al., 2007). It is also known that death anxiety may be reduced by enhanced self-esteem and stronger ingroup identification, which leads to negative attitudes and behaviours toward outgroups (from prejudice and aggression to supporting war and terror; see a review in Greenberg et al., 2008).

More recently, however, some positive effects of death anxiety have also been noted, related to engagement in positive health behaviours and helping behaviour (Vail et al., 2012; Zaleskiewicz et al., 2015). An awareness of mortality is linked to the activation of prosocial motivations or the desire to minimize harm to self and others while engaging in behaviours that promote physical, social, and psychological wellbeing. Moreover, the effects of thinking about one's own mortality vary depending on whether such thoughts are conscious (i.e., we are thinking about death deliberately, considering its different variants and scenarios) or whether we are influenced by these notions without even realizing it (Pyszczynski et al., 1999). The latter occurs when we see or learn about another person's death but our mind is engaged by something else. Thus, thoughts around death do not centrally occupy our attention but are accessible according to the principle of deep cognitive activation (Wegner and Smart, 1997). Thoughts regarding death brought into our conscious awareness motivate us to make an effort to eliminate their cause. We may consider means of preventing death or delaying it as best we might. Research shows that the activation of death-related thoughts makes people more likely to go to the gym and engage in physical activity (Arndt et al., 2003), reduce smoking (Arndt et al., 2013), and apply sunscreen when sunbathing (Routledge et al., 2004). Still, the occurrence of such health-promoting behaviours, does require a pre-existing belief that they are effective (Cooper et al., 2010) and will bring about the desired outcome (Arndt et al., 2006). During a pandemic, thoughts about death may occur frequently, causing us to contemplate partaking in health behaviours that could protect us from infection. The easier it is to come up with such behaviours, the more we will be likely to engage in them. It is therefore extremely important to publish clear and reliable guidance and recommendations on what to do to maintain good health.

Another potential positive effect of having conscious thoughts about death involves a re-evaluation of our goal hierarchy. Situations that trigger death-related thoughts are often described as turning points in our lives (a reality check or awakening experience; Heidegger, 1982; Yalom, 1980). Death makes people think about what really matters in life and – as demonstrated by research – trivialize goals which are commonly regarded as important, such as wealth, fame, and physical attractiveness, and shift toward goals related to personal growth or strengthening relationships with others (Kosloff and Greenberg, 2009; Lykins et al., 2007; Heflick et al., 2011). Anecdotally, these kinds of shift were commonly observed during the COVID-19 pandemic; we all know people who took the time to re-evaluate their lives and their potential for change (TVN24, 2020).

Thoughts of mortality outside of conscious awareness, occurring incidentally as a result of an excess of information about the subject in question, tend to activate standards of evaluation, norms, and values which, if present, may be beneficial for the individual and the group (Vail et al., 2012). If culturally shared standards of value promote personal and social wellbeing, rather than a focus on hierarchy, divisions, and telling right from wrong, death-related uncertainty may lead people toward positive solutions, such as health promotion, helping those in need, or leaning on positive relationships with others. For example, Routledge, Arndt, and Goldenberg (2004) demonstrated that subjects experiencing death anxiety showed more interest in tanning (considered to be a risky behaviour), but only when they associated their own physical attractiveness with tanned skin. When, however, their self-esteem depended on living up to the standard of being healthy, anxiety motivated them to engage in positive health behaviours (such as a healthy diet or increased physical activity). Other studies show that if people see themselves as environmentalists, they will be more likely to engage in conservation behaviour (Brook, 2005), whereas when there is no association between conservation behaviour and self-esteem, people tend to accept the exploitation of the natural environment (Kasser and Sheldon, 2000). The same is true for self-esteem being associated with financial success (e.g., Gasiorowska et al., 2018; Goldenberg et al., 2000; Koole and Van den Berg, 2004; Zaleskiewicz et al., 2013). These and many other studies suggest an important aspect of promoting positive health behaviours: if we want expert opinion to reach the public following the activation of thoughts of death, then their arguments should be strongly linked to self-esteem standards. By conveying that being a decent person who cares about other people's safety (especially those most vulnerable) is desired and respected by significant others, we will make these messages heard in times of uncertainty. Obviously, peer groups have a role to play in suggesting what is important for self-esteem. Today, these groups are mainly found on social media, but also within the school and the community. Apart from self-esteem standards, which are facilitated by unconscious thoughts of death, these group norms and values are also easily activated. Greenberg and colleagues (1992) demonstrated that thoughts of death fostered tolerance, empathy, and forgiveness; Gailliot et al. (2008) – helping behaviour; Vail et al. (2009) – compassion; and Jonas et al. (2008) – norms of pacifism. It was also shown that after the September 11 attacks, there was an increase in such values as gratefulness, hope, optimism, kindness, and team work (Peterson and Seligman, 2003). Thus, it can be expected that in the throes of a pandemic, when death anxiety is triggered spontaneously, almost incidentally, as a result of being immersed in a discourse about the potential threats and actual effects of the pandemic, it is relatively easy to activate deeply hidden regulatory standards: prosocial values, group-strengthening norms, or images of self and others as decent, good people who work for the common good.

A review by Vail and colleagues (2012) shows that thoughts of death – and the accompanying anxiety – may foster innovation, creativity, and flexibility (Arndt et al., 2009; Wisman and Koole, 2003). This is consistent with research by Kossowska and colleagues (2018) on the positive effects of uncertainty, which found that under specific conditions (such as clear, unambiguous instructions, unavailability of the most obvious solutions, or decreased confidence in one's own judgement) uncertainty may also lead to open-mindedness. During a pandemic, when it is important to look for non-standard solutions, existential anxiety may, paradoxically, become our ally.

Appropriate conditions must be met for this to happen, though. First, the people experiencing anxiety must be accustomed to facing challenges. Of course, positive strategies of coping with stress are worked out throughout our lives, but this type of personal development becomes even more urgent during a pandemic. What can further this aim is various means of psycho-education, or provision of information about how to live through the pandemic and how to manage stress. An impressive recent example of this is an initiative by the Jagiellonian University's Institute of Psychology, which launched a special website offering pandemic-related advice to faculty members, students, and anyone in need of help and support (http://psychologia. uj.edu.pl/kwarantanna/nie-jestes-sam-a). Second, the social environment must be open to non-standard ideas. A notable example here is the response of the Stockholm University authorities in the first months of the pandemic; they encouraged staff members to use that time for themselves and their families, to spend it in nature and build up their reserves of strength before returning to their everyday reality.

1.2.2 ANXIETY SENSITIVITY AND INDIVIDUAL DIFFERENCES IN HOW ANXIETY IS EXPERIENCED[1]

Some groups may be more vulnerable to the psychosocial effects of the pandemic than others. These include, in particular, infected people; high-risk individuals (such as the elderly, people with impaired immune function, and those in nursing homes and other residential care facilities); and persons with pre-existing medical conditions, psychiatric problems, or substance abuse (Armitage and Nellums, 2020). Young people are a particularly vulnerable group. Although they are less likely to develop the disease, and even if they do, experience milder symptoms (Liu et al., 2020), they suffer from a destabilized family life, isolation from peers, and having to change their daily routines, often without any help or support from their loved ones (e.g., Ford et al., 2020). Pandemic-related stress adds to the stress associated with developmental issues. Therefore, young people should be provided with special (often professional) care in the time of a pandemic (see the statement of the COVID-19 Advisory Team to the President of the Polish Academy of Sciences).[2]

Healthcare workers are another group exposed to heightened stress levels (Lai et al., 2020; Collishaw, 2015). These frontline workers brave the perils of becoming infected through potential or actual exposure to the disease. Additionally, they are highly concerned about the possibility of infecting those in their immediate circle, frustrated by the shortages (or lack) of personal protective equipment (PPE), stressed out (if not burnt out) by having to work longer hours, and distressed by their involvement in making decisions about resource allocation, which are heavily charged both emotionally and ethically. Moreover, healthcare professionals are often attacked (verbally and physically) by individuals who fear infection. Other groups in need of special care include minorities and other socially stigmatized and excluded groups who experience societal prejudice and hostility (Kirby, 2020). These vulnerable groups should have constant access to professional care services, including both psychological support and appropriate treatment. Research shows that an excellent tool for providing support for those in need is the use of remote interventions (telehealth and telepsychology; Miner et al., 2020; Lattie et al., 2020; Duan and Zhu, 2020).

The feeling of threat aroused by the spread of disease may cause stress – the body's mobilization to avoid the threat or cope with it in another way (O'Connor et al., 2020) – the immediate emotional symptoms of which include the feelings of anxiety and uncertainty, as mentioned above. We should remember, however, that as an intense, chronic response of the whole body, stress may also have lasting effects. One of these negative long-term consequences of stress is the increased risk of developing depression.

"Depression" is a broad and ambiguous term. Most often it is defined as marked mood disruptions persisting for at least two weeks (low mood, loss of joy and energy), frequently accompanied by reduced activity, sleep and appetite disturbances, negative self-esteem, and suicidal ideation. Depression is one of the most common disorders in today's world, affecting about 264 million people worldwide. Every year, close to 800,000 people die due to depression-related suicide (James et al., 2018). There are many different determinants and types of depression, which is always a result of multiple interacting factors, but one of the basic criteria for classifying depression encompasses its causes, which may be internal (biological, genetic, or biochemical) in endogenous depression or external (environmental conditions, traumatic events, or stress) in exogenous depression.

Extensive reviews of research on the effects of stress – both acute, traumatic stress and chronic stress – have found a clear causal relationship between stress and exogenous depression. These studies show that patients diagnosed with depression are 2.5 times more likely to have a history of episodes involving severe stress than healthy control subjects. In population studies, 80% of all identified cases of depression are preceded by stressful life events. These studies also show that stressors related to loss or potential loss (e.g., of life, health, a loved one, or a job) have the most severe effect in terms of increasing the risk of depression. Furthermore, chronic stress – as opposed to short-term stress – is very strongly related to the risk of developing depression (Mazure, 1998; Hammen, 2005).

Certainly, one should remember that, just as with other psychological effects, there are large individual differences in terms of resilience to stress and susceptibility to stress-related depression. Most studies on the relationship between stress and depression have been conducted on female samples, primarily because depression is more likely to be diagnosed in women than in men. In part, regardless of their gender, people also differ in terms of their genetically determined susceptibility to developing depression. Nonetheless, the relationship between depression and stress should be regarded as a real, well-documented phenomenon (Hammen, 2005).

One of the traditional explanations of this effect, offered by psychology, was an increased feeling of helplessness related to ineffective attempts to cope with a threat (Seligman and Maier, 1967). According to this theory, learned helplessness occurs when the coping strategy used by an individual does not reduce the threat (or when it is not known if it does). In other words, dealing with threats, which is always emotionally and physically costly, aims to achieve the desired effect, to change the situation the individual has found themselves in. When coping strategies are used over a longer period without achieving the desired effect (or when it is not known whether they bring about any positive result), this may lead to exhaustion and is associated with an increased risk of developing depression. However, new research in neuroscience has brought an unexpected reversal in how this phenomenon is interpreted by showing that passivity is an automatic, default response to a prolonged threat, while active ways of coping are a result of learning effective strategies (Maier and Seligman, 2016).

Notably, one of the key protective factors against the negative effects of chronic stress is self-efficacy (Luszczynska et al., 2005; Shoji et al., 2016), or the individual's feeling that the strategies they use to cope with a threat are appropriate and effective. This feeling can be modified. For example, by demonstrating the effectiveness of specific ways of reducing the threat, or by assuring people that they are able to cope with the situation.

Changes in lifestyle related to working remotely (or loss of a job), reduced social interactions, and the need to reorganize family life (home schooling), force people to change habits that have helped them to maintain somatic and mental health. Consequently, they cause stress and anxiety in all of us. People, however, differ in terms of their susceptibility to anxiety and insecurity. This helps us understand why, during a pandemic, we can see a whole range of emotional responses – from indifference, to avoidance and denial, to strong fear (Honigsbaum, 2009; Pettigrew, 1983; Wheaton et al., 2012). These varied responses lead to different attitudes to health recommendations: Some people, concerned about their health, take repeated tests, avoid any contact with others (in many cases, even with animals), refuse to go to work or to send their children to school, and take desperate, ineffective, often harmful measures to protect themselves and their loved ones (such as drinking chloride, eating ginger and garlic, or sanitizing banknotes in the microwave; e.g., Cheng, 2004; Saxena, 2018). Conversely, others ignore all recommendations and thus put themselves and other people at risk. The psychological characteristics underlying these differences include temperament and personality traits (for example, impulsiveness, sensation seeking, openness to new experiences and extroversion, neuroticism and agreeableness, tolerance of uncertainty, and fearfulness or anxiety sensitivity, i.e., fear of bodily sensations associated with the experience of arousal or anxiety), as well as cognitive styles (for example, a tendency to persistently watch for cues indicating risks to one's health, or avoiding any threatening information and downplaying its significance, showing unrealistic optimism etc.).

Given the existence of several risk groups and individual differences in responses to threats, individualized ways of providing help and support in the pandemic situation should be tailored to the recipient (Holmes et al., 2020). During this kind of supportive work, it is necessary to identify and monitor: (1) any factors that increase the effect of COVID-19-related stressors (such as being exposed to contact with infected persons, having infected

Individual Perspective 17

family members, losing one's loved ones, or being in quarantine); (2) any side effects of pandemic-related stress (such as economic loss or relationship breakdowns); (3) any psychosocial effects (such as depression, generalized anxiety, health anxiety, insomnia, increased substance use, and domestic violence); and (4) any indicators of vulnerability (such as pre-existing physical or psychological conditions that increase sensitivity to stress). Importantly, close collaboration is needed between the medical field and researchers in behavioural and social sciences. What plays a crucial role in alleviating fears and anxiety in those who cope well with the pandemic is communication (which will be discussed in more detail further in the book) and psychoeducation, i.e., providing information about how to live through the pandemic and how best to cope with stress.

1.2.3 STRATEGIES OF COPING WITH FEAR AND UNCERTAINTY[3]

People develop different ways of coping with uncertainty and fear. For some, it is enough to engage in activities experienced as pleasurable, such as eating, drinking alcohol, using recreational drugs, having sex, or purchasing goods (McGregor et al., 2010; McGregor et al., 2013). These work to suppress negative thoughts and sensations related to situations of uncertainty. Although enjoyable and rewarding, they are not effective in the long run because they stop working as soon as the rewarding stimulus is removed. They are also ineffective because they lead to other problems, such as obesity or addiction. Unfortunately, it is these strategies we are most likely to hear about in the media during the pandemic.

Another strategy is to increase one's sense of control in areas unrelated to the original uncertainty, when it is impossible to regain control in the area where it has been lost. This type of strategy is exemplified by the situation of many people who have lost their jobs and have not been able to secure new employment for long stretches of time. During the pandemic, this strategy has taken the form of sewing face masks, engaging in collective efforts, or volunteering, and it has been chosen by many people (for example, in Western Europe the number of volunteers willing to provide help for those in need has grown significantly; see Gardner, 2020).

When faced with uncertainty, people are also more effective in carrying out their personal projects, for example in learning various skills (McGregor et al., 2010). Being successful in important areas of life leads to increased perceived control and reduces uncertainty. Of course, uncertainty may sometimes engender rash decisions, gambling, or dangerous but rewarding behaviours, such as risky sex (Cavallo et al., 2009; Nash et al., 2013). The choices we make usually depend on personality characteristics (e.g., stimulation seeking or fearfulness), on what is valued by a group which we feel is important to us, and also on the availability of meaningful personal projects.

18   *Individuals, Groups, and Society in Pandemics*

On the social level, coping strategies typically manifest as an increased need to affiliate with others. The feeling of connection in close relationships is what works best, but in times of high uncertainty, comfort and relief can be provided by contact with any person, regardless of the quality of inter-action (Florian and Mikulincer, 1998; Mikulincer et al., 2003). When faced with uncertainty, people show an increased tendency to seek and experience connection with their significant others. They are more likely to remember their parents, and positive (but not negative) aspects of their relationship with them. They also report a stronger desire to become parents themselves and are more likely to see strangers as resembling their own parents. Positive feelings associated with interpersonal contact are effective in reducing negative arousal caused by uncertainty. Moreover, affiliation gives individuals access to other people's skills and resources, which may be helpful in dealing with their own situation. This strategy of reducing anxiety – the most obvious one for many people – was confounded by the requirements of quarantine, isolation, and social distancing, even if this was partly mitigated by online interactions.

Other social strategies involve the area of values and beliefs. For example, when under the influence of uncertainty, people tend to see themselves in a more positive light, believe they have greater power, and prefer products that attest to their high status (see Pyszczynski et al., 2004). Indeed, beauty sup-ply stores earned record revenues during the pandemic. Importantly, when faced with uncertainty, people identify themselves with groups perceived as independent, cohesive, intentional, and having agency (McGregor et al., 2008; Brewer et al., 2004). Such groups promise effective action, so collective thinking and acting as part of a group, in terms of "us" instead of "me", re-store a sense of personal control. It should be emphasized again, however, that when experiencing uncertainty and fear – feelings aroused by a pandemic – people habitually choose coping strategies that are available, which they have used before, and which are considered effective. This means people will be most likely to use strategies recommended during the pandemic when these strategies are built on what is familiar and commonly accepted, and if they have proven effective in the past.

Effective risk reduction strategies during a health crisis are (or at least should be) informed by medical and scientific knowledge, and developed by health institutions such as WHO on the international level, and the Ministry of Health (or the sanitary authorities) on the national level. One important question arising during a prolonged pandemic is whether, and to what extent, people will adhere to these recommendations. A related question concerns factors that contribute to people complying with them.

One of the main theories helpful in answering these questions is the Self-Regulatory Model (SRM; Leventhal et al., 1992), according to which people form a subjective opinion about a disease, and then use it to inform their decisions on whether to follow recommendations concerning the disease. Their representation of the disease comprises five dimensions: (1) symptoms associated with the disease; (2) causes (personal opinions about the etiology); (3) timeline (duration); (4) consequences; and (5) beliefs about the possibility of controlling and curing the disease. Research shows that these subjective beliefs are related to what extent individuals follow recommendations concerning the disease in question (Byer and Myers, 2000; Myers, 2020). Consequently, from the perspective of institutions that issue COVID-19 guidelines and recommendations, it is absolutely paramount to ensure that subjective beliefs about the disease, which are formed in potential patients' minds, are as close as possible to the views shared by experts.

Research on people's adherence to medical advice and, more broadly, compliance with legal regulations and social norms, has found that one of the key factors influencing adherence to norms and regulations is other people, especially those who we see as significant to us. This is termed social proof or the influence of authority (Cialdini, 2009). By copying the actions of the majority of the people around us or the behaviours of those who are significant to us, we feel that the actions (and the norms behind them) are appropriate for the circumstances and beneficial, thus increasing our motivation to engage in this behaviour. Of course, people differ in terms of their tendency to be influenced by the majority, authorities, and norms, and these differences are associated with such personality traits as agreeableness and conscientiousness (e.g., Xie et al., 2020). Despite us knowing this, it is of little use in pandemic management, as these personality traits are essentially unmodifiable in the context of the COVID-19 pandemic. What is more important is consistent adherence to medical recommendations demonstrated by significant group members, and promoting these recommendations as a valid social norm.

Turning now to cognitive factors, the first research findings are now available on how these factors are related to people's adherence to medical recommendations during the COVID-19 pandemic. As discussed elsewhere in this book, the human mind has a limited capacity, which influences the use of complex decision-making rules. Certainly, there are individual differences in the capacities of cognitive systems, and, as demonstrated by the latest research conducted during the ongoing pandemic, these are related to adherence to medical recommendations. Xie and colleagues (2020) found that in the American population, compliance with the social distancing guidelines was associated with a relatively high capacity of short-term memory but was unrelated to variables such as the socio-economic status or the main personality traits: extraversion and neuroticism. In their discussion of the results of the study, the authors argue that when social distancing is just recommended (rather than mandatory) and the social norm to maintain social distance is not well-established in the population, high working memory capacity allows the individual to perform a complex analysis of the costs and benefits that accrue from following the recommendation. Conversely, in the same social situation, low working memory capacity prevents the individual from carrying out such a complex cost–benefit analysis, which may lead to non-compliance with the guidelines. This problem may be solved by (1) imposing and enforcing orders rather than simply issuing recommendations, or (2) making social distancing a well-established, automatically applied norm in the population.

1.3 EMOTIONAL MECHANISMS RELATED TO THREAT

Emotions are a key component of the complex system of human psychology. Studies of neurological patients, in whom brain damage has severely impaired the ability to process emotions, have found that they were unable to function well in the social world and struggled to make even the simplest decisions. For example, they accepted an unreasonably high risk and ignored the possibility of losing (Bechara et al., 2005; Damasio, 2011; Poppa and Bechara, 2018; Weller et al., 2009). In contrast, people characterized by high emotional intelligence do far better in many areas of life than those who lack the skills of emotional recognition and control (Brackett et al., 2016). A positive relationship was also found between effective emotional processing and good mental and somatic health (Kubzansky and Winning, 2016).

The emotional network in the human brain was shaped by evolution (Plutchik, 2002), so it must serve important adaptive functions: Experiencing emotions and responding to stimuli based on these experiences both serve to increase our chances of survival in uncertain environments. Strong emotions have an effect at early stages of information processing: They determine which information is picked out as essential from the multitude of incoming stimuli. The effects of emotion on perception and attention have been long known. These involve paying selective attention to stimuli that are congruent with our emotional state (Koster et al., 2005; Yiend, 2010). For instance, individuals experiencing anxiety will primarily attend to negative, threatening information while ignoring positive signals. The same is true for positive emotions – when in a positive mood (or under the influence of positive emotions), people are likely to attend to positive events but disregard threatening ones (Becker and Leinenger, 2011). Studies of the effects of emotion on long-term memory and retrieval lead to a similar conclusion: Externally generated emotions – and more diffuse states known as moods – facilitate retrieval of information congruent with the experienced mood or emotion (Gaddy and Ingram, 2014). This means that individuals experiencing fear and anxiety tend to recall negative events in their lives and, more generally, negative material. Again, this effect is also true for positive emotions – when in a positive mood (or under the influence of positive emotions), people are more likely to bring to mind past positive events (Matt et al., 1992).

Many years of research into the effects of high arousal emotions (such as anxiety, fear, or disgust) on information processing have demonstrated that these affective states lead to attention narrowing and to reduced working memory capacity, thus impairing the ability to process several bits of information at the same time. This conclusion is strongly supported by various literature reviews (e.g., Arnsten, 2009; Moran, 2016; Unsworth and Robison, 2017). Under the influence of such emotional states, people are only capable of processing one bit of information at a time. This means that in a situation generating anxiety, fear, and disgust – such as a pandemic – people tend to process information very selectively and fail to integrate information from a range of different sources, compounding the difficulty, for instance, in understanding complex messages, recommendations, or regulations. This selective processing is biased toward emotion-congruent information. So, when experiencing anxiety, an individual will attend to messages, recommendations, and regulations related to threat severity and reduction. Conversely, one should bear in mind that, under the influence of positive emotions, such as relief or elation, people will be inclined to ignore negative information concerning the hazards associated with the pandemic.

Emotions serve many valuable functions. The very experience of feeling certain emotions is a clear signal that the individual has encountered a challenge in the environment, which then produces a specific motivational response (Frederickson, 1998; Frijda, 1986; Schwarz, 2001). To exemplify this, we know that the feeling of anxiety is a signal of threat, and motivates the individual to withdraw or prepare for self-defense, whereas experiencing sadness is a signal of loss and activates behaviours needed to cope with it successfully (Lazarus, 1991). The informative function of emotions is extremely important in the context of analyzing human behaviour during a pandemic. Anxiety, as experienced by most people aware of the epidemic risk (Kanadiya and Sallar, 2011; Rubin et al., 2009), motivates them to engage in protective behaviours, and as such, has a mobilizing function (LaBar, 2016; LeDoux, 2012a, 2020). If anxiety is too low or absent (for example, as a result of certain brain dysfunctions; Feinstein et al., 2011), the individual's motivation to take protective measures (such as wearing a face mask or using hand sanitizer) will also be low, leading to an increased risk of infection, or even death.

Apart from the self-regulatory functions of emotion (feeling anxiety – engaging in protective behaviour), there are functions that come into play in social interactions (Fischer and Manstead, 2016). Emotions are used to communicate messages to other people; specific emotional expressions inform us that someone has made us feel wretched or violated our values (Keltner et al., 2016). One instance of an emotion carrying out an important communicative function is anger, which is responsible for supporting the process of goal pursuit (Harmon-Jones and Harmon-Jones, 2016). During a pandemic, the goal we are all pursuing is to avoid infection, illness, and death. Notwithstanding this, the effectiveness of efforts focused on reducing the risk of infection depends not only on the individual but also on the behaviour of other members of the community. In light of the experts' emphasis of the fact that face masks are only effective when worn by everyone (not just by some), individuals who strictly follow hygiene rules may respond with anger against those who ignore or violate them (by refusing to wear masks, not disinfecting their hands when entering a premises, or flouting the rules of self-isolation). The external expression of anger is very obvious as it comprises immediately noticeable features, such as lowered eyebrows, an ominous look in the eye, flared nostrils, and clenched teeth (Izard, 1977). As such, it is likely to elicit a quick response from the interacting partner. In other words, expressing anger is an effective way to make others comply with safety measures. Disgust is

22 *Individuals, Groups, and Society in Pandemics*

another emotion that serves significant adaptive functions, of particular importance during a pandemic. This emotion evolved as part of our behavioural immune system (BIS; Neuberg et al., 2011) – a set of evolutionarily ancient psychological mechanisms that protect us from pathogen-related threats. Like anger, disgust is accompanied by a clear facial expression, which performs a communicative function: The face of a person experiencing disgust tells others that the situation presents a pathogen threat.

Emotions have social effects, too. For example, a number of studies suggest that threat-related emotional states lead to preference potentiation, that is, in high arousal situations, decision makers are more determined to choose their preferred options and devote less attention to considering alternative choices (Yu, 2016). To put it another way, when under stress, people are more likely to make habitual choices and less likely to choose what is new or less preferred. According to the risk-as-feelings hypothesis (Loewenstein et al., 2001), emotional states and risk taking are closely related to each other. More specifically, it proposes that experiencing anxiety leads to reduced risk taking – an idea supported by numerous studies (Traczyk et al., 2015; Traczyk and Zaleskiewicz, 2015; Sobkow et al., 2016). This means that when people experience increased anxiety, they are less likely to take risks compared to when high levels of anxiety are absent.

The influence of strong emotions is associated with the effect of disgust on our moral judgements and evaluations of other people's behaviour (Schnall et al., 2008). Apart from fear and anxiety, the emotions of disgust and revulsion are prevalent in times of pandemic. Recent meta-analyses (e.g., Landy and Goodwin, 2015) show that disgust can amplify moral judgements, i.e., under the influence of disgust (related to toxin or pathogen threats) people are more likely to categorize others' behaviour as violating moral norms and to condemn such behaviour. Literature reviews show that the activation of these mechanisms leads to increased prejudice, especially against people whose appearance may indicate health issues and, more generally, those deviating from locally accepted norms (Schaller, 2016). Another fascinating effect of activating the behavioural immune system is an increased preference for physically attractive leaders (political or social ones) and a decreased preference for those who are less physically attractive, especially when their appearance may signal health issues.

Trust and cooperation are influenced by affective states according to a number of studies. In general, positive emotions increase cooperation (DeSteno et al., 2010; Tabibnia and Lieberman, 2007), while stress and negative emotions tend to decrease it (Lee et al., 2011; von Dawans et al., 2018). Having said this, it is also worth bearing in mind the paradoxical effects of existential anxiety noted earlier in this book.

Experiencing emotions, occasionally disproportionately strong ones, in the context of the epidemic threat may also stem from a tendency to develop vivid images of the negative consequences of the threat (Sobkow et al., 2016; Traczyk et al., 2015; Zaleskiewicz and Traczyk, 2020). Imagining the future is a natural mental activity (Kosslyn et al., 2001; Moulton and Kosslyn 2009; Suddendorf and Corbalis, 2007), and numerous studies show that clear-cut, vivid mental images are associated with the experience of intense emotions (Holmes and Mathews, 2005, 2010; Holmes et al., 2006; Holmes et al., 2008; Ji et al., 2016). As emphasized by Hirsch and Holmes (2007), strong and negative retrospective images appear in the minds of individuals affected by post-traumatic stress (a specific stress response to trauma that an individual cannot cope with on their own). The same authors cite research suggesting that mental images play a part in aggravating social phobia (a strong fear of all, or selected, social situations; for example, interactions with others). People affected by this disorder conjure up mental images of themselves performing poorly in interactions with others, which leads to increased social anxiety. Likewise, it stands to reason that vivid images depicting the scale of the pandemic, and its long-term consequences, may prompt increased health anxiety. Certainly, the media (especially those using visual communication) contribute greatly to the creation of such striking images. Evidence from randomized controlled trials in clinical psychology shows that cognitive behavioural therapy (CBT) is effective in managing unreasonably strong health anxiety (Cooper et al., 2017; Taylor et al., 2005).

The abovementioned characteristics of emotion appear to contribute to perceptions of and responses to a pandemic that may activate appropriate behaviour (e.g., protective measures). However, emotion may also motivate individuals to use inappropriate regulation strategies (Barrett, 2013). Experiencing anger facilitates goal attainment but may also lead to uncontrolled aggressive outbursts (Holtzworth-Munroe and Clements, 2007). There have been repeated media reports about violent attacks against people suspected by their neighbours of being infected with COVID-19. Fear mobilizes the body and activates defensive behaviour, but it may also lead to widespread panic when affective responses are transferred from person to person (an effect known as emotional contagion; Kramer et al., 2014). Naturally, social media represents a powerful force in the rapid transfer of all sorts of information and images (both true and false) concerning pandemic-related risks and the collective panic response (Van Bavel et al., 2020).

1.4 COGNITIVE MECHANISMS RELATED TO THREAT

The COVID-19 pandemic has dramatically changed societies' functioning by forcing individuals and groups to limit or at least significantly change their habits and routines over sizeable periods of time. Behavioural science may be helpful in understanding people's behaviour in these circumstances, in terms of their adherence to social norms and legal regulations, economic decisions, or health behaviours. The conclusions presented in this section are based on evidence from psychology and neuroscience, especially cognitive psychology and neuroscience, the psychology of decision making and neuroeconomics, and the psychology of individual differences. The main conclusion from cognitive psychology is that the human mind is characterized by very limited information processing capacity. This property has far-reaching consequences for how people understand messages and social norms, how they comply with legal regulations, and what views and attitudes spread in social groups. This section discusses current scientific knowledge in selected areas around people's behaviour during long-term change associated with a pandemic.

A pandemic caused by a new pathogen for which there is no effective drug places people in an alarming situation, which generates (1) anxiety, or a generalized feeling of threat from an object that cannot be precisely located; (2) uncertainty, or anxiety related to a lack of clear rules suggesting what behaviour would allow us to avoid the threat and survive the situation intact; and (3) disgust, which serves the adaptive function of pathogen avoidance (Neuberg et al., 2011). As mentioned earlier, the human mind has limited processing capacity. Evidence supporting this idea has been collected by cognitive psychology since at least the 1950s. Recent literature reviews summarize these findings, suggesting one to four items as the typical capacity of human short-term memory (e.g., Oberauer et al., 2016). Threat-related affective states characterized by high arousal (such as anxiety, fear, or disgust) additionally reduce this capacity, thus increasing the tendency for selective information processing.

Strong emotions guide human cognition toward seeking information congruent with the current emotional state as well as pre-existing knowledge (thus causing us to be resistant to information inconsistent with what we already know). This type of cognition, referred to as motivated cognition, may result in decision making based on information that is incomplete, and often inaccurate, but consistent with our beliefs (Kunda, 1990; Kahan, 2017). This means that even if we systematically follow reports about the unfolding of the pandemic, we are likely to focus on a selective portion of the information, making our resultant knowledge biased. To make matters worse, when under threat, the knowledge we have gleaned becomes consolidated and resistant to change in the face of new data. In the midst of the COVID-19 pandemic, the more negative the emotions, the more likely people are to seek negative information and consider it valuable and trustworthy, and, as a consequence, to reach decisions on the basis of this information. In addition, the process will be intensified, as the negative effects of the pandemic persist or perhaps even worsen over time. Once formed, beliefs about the pandemic are quite impervious to change, despite new information being made available.

In a wider sense, a feeling of threat casts a pall over our perceptions of reality, our judgement, and predictions about the future. It is well documented that in threatening situations, under the influence of anxiety and other negative emotions, people tend to ignore important data, which may lead to mistakes in estimating the probability of future events (e.g., Gray, 1999; Keinan, 1987). Two types of cognitive biases are at play here. On the one hand, people may overestimate pandemic-related risks while, on the other, some underestimate them (unrealistic optimism; e.g., Klein and Helweg-Larsen, 2002; Dolinski et al., 2020), with both biases potentially producing disastrous outcomes. The former bias leads to increased anxiety and, consequently, has negative effects on somatic and mental health (psychosomatic disorders, depression, suicide, and aggression) and generates considerable social or public costs (mood radicalization, approval of radical and authoritarian policies, and exploitation of the weak and vulnerable); the latter bias is associated with non-compliance with medical recommendations, such as isolation, hygiene rules, etc., and thus leads to behaviours that may harm others. (The related topics of positive illusions and risk perception will be discussed later on in this book.)

Still, it would be wrong to assume fear and uncertainty always impair our cognitive functions by making information processing overly simplified. Some studies reveal that, in response to the feeling of uncertainty, individuals may attempt to reduce uncertainty by looking for additional information (Han et al., 2007; Kossowska et al., 2018). Nevertheless, due to their limited memory capacity, individuals demonstrate a reduced ability to integrate what they have learned, which in itself is a highly aversive state, and may lead to limited information seeking. When it comes to working memory capacity, positive emotions have the opposite effect to that of their negative counterparts: they increase working memory capacity, or at least prevent its reduction under stress and information overload (Ashby and Isen, 1999). In other words, when threatened by an epidemic, people may seek additional information about the threat, but the limited capacity of their cognitive system will impede their proper utilization of this knowledge, especially when there is a surfeit of information, and/or when its content changes from day to day. On those occasions when people seek out information and, in doing so, encounter difficulties when attempting to process it, information overload is experienced, which, as a type of stress, has cognitive effects not dissimilar to those of strong emotions. Findings from the aforementioned studies also suggest that complicated legal rules and regulations, which change over time and are communicated in a nebulous and/or equivocal fashion, may be poorly or improperly understood and, as a result, virtually ignored. The same can be said about health behaviours, which, according to government officials, should be regulated by laws and guidelines. However, if they turn out to be overly complex and constantly subject to change, the predictable outcome will be that people will fail to process them (and, accordingly, will comprehend or retain them inadequately), which, in turn, could lead to non-compliance. Similarly, it can be also assumed that given the high complexity and dynamic nature of the economic environment during the pandemic, entrepreneurs are liable to disregard complicated legal regulations, adhere to them selectively, or apply them erroneously.

1.5 OPTIMISM

Forming predictions and expectations about the future is a key function of the human cognitive system. People endeavour to estimate the odds of attaining personally important goals (for example, securing a job after graduation, overcoming a disease, completing a project on time, etc.), avoiding adverse events (such as a relationship breakdown or incurring a loss on a financial investment), establishing good social relationships, etc. These expectations can be generalized, i.e., take the form of a general belief that the individual will do well or poorly in life; or they can be specific, i.e., pertain to specific, local goals. The higher the uncertainty, the more vital it becomes to form predictions, as there are few, if any, clear indicators to inform us about how the situation is about to unfold (Tetlock and Gardner, 2015). This also holds true for the current pandemic, which generates extraordinarily high levels of uncertainty. Attempts are made to forecast when the risk to one's health will be completely or at least partly eliminated, when a vaccine or an effective drug will be available, how effective the preventive measures (such as mask wearing and social distancing) actually are, and how strongly the pandemic is having an impact on the economy and one's personal finances. The manner in which these predictions are made, and the extent to which they are optimistic, can play a crucial role in the development of people's motivations to take protective measures and follow hygiene recommendations. This will be the topic under consideration in more detail further on in this chapter.

1.5.1 THE ROLE OF OPTIMISM IN SELF-REGULATION AND SOCIAL RELATIONSHIPS UNDER THREAT

Optimism (or pessimism) is intimately involved in the process of forming expectations and, more generally, in pondering the future. The definition of optimism in psychological science is surprisingly consistent with the lay understanding of the term: Optimists are people who expect good things to happen to them, while pessimists expect negative outcomes in their lives (Carver and Scheier, 2014; Carver et al., 2010). Compared to pessimists, optimists have a tendency to create more positive images of the future (Blackwell et al., 2013). Although optimism and pessimism are often seen as black and white, dichotomous categories, we should keep in mind that optimism is a continuous variable, which means there are few extreme optimists and extreme pessimists, and thus most of us fall somewhere between the two extremes. Even so, research shows people are more likely to have optimistic rather than pessimistic attitudes (Carver et al., 2010).[4] Optimists and pessimists are different in many ways, for example in how they solve problems, in their responses to failure, in the emotions they usually experience, in their perceptions of their own skills and resources, and in how they form and modify interpersonal relationships. Differences between the two groups involve not only psychological resources, but also somatic health: Optimists are on average healthier (Rasmussen et al., 2009) and have a higher socio-economic status (Robb et al., 2009; Schutte et al., 1996; Segerstrom, 2007) than pessimists. Obviously, these associations are a consequence of how these two groups function in daily life, what self-regulation mechanisms they use, and how they build their relationships with others.

Optimism, by definition, is the opposite of helplessness. When it comes to self-regulatory aspects, empirical evidence shows that compared to pessimists, optimists are more certain they are able to achieve a personally important goal and more persistent in pursuing it patiently and consistently. Crucially, these are generalized attributes, which is to say, they pertain to a broad range of behaviours rather than any specific situation (Scheier and Carver, 1992). Differences between optimists and pessimists become especially clear when it comes to coping with difficulty, adversity, and failure. A meta-analysis of studies with an overall number of nearly 12,000 subjects (Nes and Segerstrom, 2006) shows that dispositional (i.e., relatively stable) optimism is: (1) positively related to approach coping strategies, which aim to actively change, reduce, or remove stressors; and (2) negatively related to avoidance (defensive) strategies, which involve withdrawing from difficult situations, seeking to eliminate unpleasant emotions, or simply ignoring, or even denying, risks and obstacles. In other words, optimists are focused on solving the problems they have encountered; they show "fighting spirit" (Carver et al., 2010).

When facing obstacles, optimists tend to seek information that may be helpful in overcoming them. This may involve efforts to obtain accurate knowledge about the threat facing them and to identify the dimensions and level of risk (Radcliffe and Klein, 2002). Active coping with problems, based on accurate knowledge and verified information, an attribute which is typical of optimists, is reflected in specific behaviours that hold great significance for health. It has been found that individuals with high levels of optimism spend more time exercising, eat more healthily, and are less likely to engage in substance use (such as smoking or drinking). They are also more conscientious when participating in rehabilitation programmes, and they are less likely to engage in casual sex, thus reducing the risk of contracting HIV (Carver and Scheier, 2014; Carver et al., 2010; Lopez and Leffingwell, 2020). So, optimism is not a matter of adopting a "things will work out one way or another" attitude and passively waiting for problems to vanish on their own, but rather about actively engaging in specific efforts to reduce, or even eliminate, obstacles.

It seems obvious that the abovementioned characteristics of the optimistic approach will come into play in the midst of a pandemic (Taylor, 2019). The epidemic threat is an obstacle or a problem each of us has had to deal with. It is associated with an increased risk of losing one's health, or even one's life. This desperate plight is made worse when coupled with mandatory isolation, the thwarting of personal goals, and new obligations to conform to ever-changing legal, economic, and medical regulations. In these adverse and trying circumstances, the literature suggests that, in comparison to pessimists, optimists will not only enjoy greater levels of certainty that things will return to normal over time, and that effective ways of coping with the threat will be discovered, but will also engage in more rational behaviour, both in the realm of health (e.g., wearing face masks, regular hand disinfection, or social distancing) and in the economic sphere (e.g., refraining from impulsive financial decisions, developing a rational survival plan for the company, or taking advantage of the various opportunities offered by

28 *Individuals, Groups, and Society in Pandemics*

pandemic relief packages). Optimists can also be expected to make decisions based on verified data and substantiated information while disregarding all kinds of conspiracy theories, panic stories, and fake news. All the available research evidence seems to support these hypotheses. For example, individuals with high levels of fearfulness and threat avoidance – characteristics strongly linked to pessimism – tend to overestimate the negative consequences of a risky situation and, paralyzed by negative emotions, fail to engage in reasonable coping behaviours (Taylor, 2019). One study (Lai and Cheng, 2004) found that adolescents who scored higher on an optimism scale reported themselves to be more willing to take a vaccine in the face of a hypothetical epidemic.

As we explore the connection between optimism and a tendency to engage in rational behaviour in response to threats to our health or wellbeing, we should also consider the social aspects of the trait. It has already been stated that optimists have a wider network of interpersonal relationships than pessimists, so they can count on more social support (Srivastava et al., 2006; Vollmann et al., 2011). Several reasons for this are suggested in the literature (Carver et al., 2010). First, optimists are more appealing than pessimists as companions – they are more accepted and seen as people one wishes to be in the company of; hence, it is naturally easier for them to develop social connections. Second, optimists find it easier to handle problems in a relationship, which makes them altogether more satisfied with their relationships. Pessimists, by contrast, are more likely to end a relationship when problems emerge, instead of working hard to fix it. Third, optimists tend to hold firmer beliefs about the importance of their relationships and be more committed to them, which is consistent with their general style. The positive effects of optimism on social relationships appear to be critical in the context of the current pandemic. The uncertainty and difficulties we are all struggling with become less distressing when others provide us with support – both material (for example, given that a significant increase in unemployment is one of the economic effects of the epidemic, they may lend support by helping us find a new means of employment after the loss of our previous one) and symbolic or affective (for example, when forced isolation limits social contact, it is of benefit to have people one can invariably rely on to be in contact with, and can converse with).

1.5.2 UNREALISTIC OPTIMISM AND POSITIVE ILLUSIONS

Our discussion so far would seem to suggest that optimism is an indisputably positive phenomenon, but that would not paint the complete picture: Optimism can potentially have its darker side, too. This is the case when optimism is no longer just a belief that things are likely to turn out well but rather leads people to see the world in an unrealistically positive way, unverified by objective indicators (Weinstein, 1980; Weinstein and Klein,

1996), taking the form of the optimism bias or positive illusion (Makridakis and Moleskis, 2015; Sharot, 2011; Taylor and Brown, 1988). People may be called unrealistic optimists when they believe that their current outcomes are better and more favourable in comparison to those indicated by an objective standard, or to their own average outcomes in the past (unrealistic absolute optimism), or in comparison to the average outcomes of their peers (unrealistic comparative optimism; Shepperd et al., 2015). An example of unrealistic absolute optimism is when an individual significantly underestimates their personal risk of contracting a disease (e.g., COVID-19) compared to the level or risk indicated by statistical data. One example of unrealistic comparative optimism is when an individual can believe they are less likely to contract the disease in question than an average member of their peer group. Numerous studies in business psychology have demonstrated that entrepreneurs show very high levels of unrealistic comparative optimism: They believe that they are more likely to succeed in the market than other businesses and that the probability of failure and loss is much higher for their competitors (Coelho, 2010; Zaleskiewicz, 2006; Zaleskiewicz, Bernardy, and Traczyk, 2020). Summing up, the essence of unrealistic optimism is an individual's prediction that good things are more likely to happen to them than to other people, whereas bad things are less likely to happen to them than to others (Weinstein, 1980; Weinstein and Klein, 1996). Remarkably, unrealistic optimism is quite common. Empirical evidence suggests that this motivational and cognitive phenomenon not only exists, but also constitutes the social norm (Coelho, 2010).

Interpreting the reality through the lens of unrealistic optimism may have serious consequences, such as excessive risk taking (Shepperd et al., 2016; Weinstein, 1989). Using a business example, overly optimistic entrepreneurs will not only overestimate their chances of success, but also choose inappropriate business strategies, take on projects requiring skills they do not have (rather than rely on other people's expertise), and focus on positive feedback, ignoring any negative information (Coelho, 2010). Since individuals fostering positive illusions underestimate their personal risk, their attention to risk information is relatively low (Radcliffe and Klein, 2002). As a result, their tendency to take risks is increased (Dillard et al., 2009) while their willingness to take precautions is reduced (O'Brien et al., 1995). For example, research shows that smokers who have unrealistically optimistic expectations report to be less likely to plan to quit smoking than individuals in a comparison group (Dillard et al., 2006), which may result from their unjustified belief that they can quit smoking any time, once they decide to do so (Weinstein, 2001). Similarly, college students who were overly optimistic about unchecked alcohol consumption experienced more problems related to alcohol abuse, such as missing classes or getting into fights with their peers (Dillard et al., 2009). Yet another example involves high-risk sexual behaviours. Findings from recent studies suggest that one of the causes of such negative outcomes as contracting HIV or unintended pregnancies

30   *Individuals, Groups, and Society in Pandemics*

among young people may be their unrealistically optimistic belief that they are unlikely to engage in numerous casual sexual encounters while under the influence of alcohol (Lopez and Leffingwell, 2020).

Being prone to unrealistic optimism or positive illusions has an effect on the likelihood of engaging in certain behaviours during a pandemic (Taylor, 2019). Individuals demonstrating very high levels of unrealistic optimism seem to believe that they are completely immune to infection and that the risks do not apply to them (Ji et al., 2004), which in turn makes them far less willing to get vaccinated when compared to those who have more realistic perceptions (Taha et al., 2013). These high levels of unrealistic optimism are accompanied by thinking along the lines of: "Why should I take a vaccine if I'm very unlikely to get the disease?" Kim and Niederdeppe (2013) studied the relationship between harbouring positive illusions and engaging in flu-prevention behaviours. The authors found that unrealistic optimists (i.e., individuals convinced that their chances of getting infected were lower compared to an average person in their reference group) were less willing to engage in frequent hand-washing and sanitizing to reduce the risk of contracting H1N1 (a subtype of influenza A virus) than subjects categorized as realists or pessimists.

Another interesting question concerns the cognitive and affective effects of a situation where an individual's outcomes (*ex post*) are inconsistent with their overly optimistic expectations (*ex ante*). In other words, what happens when illusory predictions undergo a reality check? The answer can be found in the results of a study that looked at employees' predictions about how quickly they would receive a job promotion (Ngan and Tze-Ngai Vong, 2018). First of all, it turned out that employees' expectations were optimistically biased, as suggested by the comparison of their promotion expectations and the company's statistics (unrealistic absolute optimism). Secondly, when their unrealistically optimistic expectations were not met, employees reported decreased job satisfaction and a higher level of intent to seek a new job. These findings suggest that when people come to realize their expectations are biased, they experience frustration and negative emotions, which makes them more likely to engage in contesting behaviours. An obvious analogy with people's behaviour during a pandemic comes to mind. If the public health situation unfolds more negatively than they expected (for example, there are more cases of the disease, more deaths, and more preventive restrictions than expected), people are more likely to experience dissatisfaction, and thus to increasingly oppose restrictions imposed by health and administrative authorities.

On the whole, in the context of a pandemic, it would seem more advisable to be optimistic, that is, to believe one can play an active role in avoiding infection and to expect that things will work out well (for example, to trust that given the current level of scientific progress, it will not take long to develop a vaccine and discover an effective drug to treat the infection). Efforts to foster and augment this kind of optimism are definitely worthwhile.

Based on our literature review, we can see that people who display optimism with regards to the pandemic may be expected to have a higher motivation to follow safety rules and consistently engage in protective behaviours (such as wearing face masks, sanitizing their hands, social distancing, or washing food products). Moreover, even though under certain circumstances optimism may lead to unrealistic perceptions of the situation, it improves psychological wellbeing and increases life satisfaction (Baumeister, 1989; Taylor and Brown, 1988, 1994), which may, in turn, protect individuals from the build-up of negative emotions, especially at the outset of a crisis (epidemic or economic), when uncertainty is tremendously high.

On the other hand, it is important to remember that people have a natural tendency to make overly optimistic predictions about the future, which will gradually distort their perceptions of the situation and reduce their willingness to engage in rational protective behaviours (Baumeister, 1989). Keeping this in mind, let us tackle the question of how optimism can be prevented from taking this overblown, unrealistic, and illusory form. What we know about the determinants of unrealistic optimism can provide helpful clues here. According to researchers, these can be categorized as either motivational or cognitive factors (Coelho, 2010; Hoorens, 1993; Weinstein, 1980). The motivational category includes: (1) developing and maintaining high self-esteem; (2) projecting a positive social image (self-presentation); and (3) protecting the ego from threats and fear. The cognitive category includes: (1) the need for control; (2) biases in estimating probability; and (3) a lack of personal experience with respect to the event in question. Unrealistic optimism can be reduced by influencing both categories of determinants. For example, we may provide people with relevant knowledge by presenting accounts of those who have experienced the event, or we may cause them to come to the realization that they are unable to actively influence the course of events in order to reduce the probability of negative outcomes.

1.6 PERCEPTION OF RISK

When people experience increased uncertainty and are faced with a variety of threats (to their health, life, or financial stability), it is particularly important to understand how risk is perceived and assessed, that is, the process of risk perception, which is assumed to be associated with people's tendency to engage in preventive behaviours. For example, when, during an epidemic, an individual believes the risk of becoming infected is very high, they will be more likely to strictly follow guidelines such as social distancing, mask wearing, or frequent hand washing.

In social science, when we consider risk perception, we mean a specific combination of cognitive and motivational factors, which determines whether risk is subjectively perceived as high or low. In other words, we investigate what people think and how they feel about risk (Parrott, 2017; Renner et al., 2015; Slovic, 2000; Weber, 2017). The cognitive aspect

32   *Individuals, Groups, and Society in Pandemics*

(thinking about risk) involves conscious consideration of the probability of experiencing negative consequences (for example, contracting a disease in a health-threatening situation; or financial loss due to a market collapse, when it comes to economic threats) and the severity of these consequences. Feeling a sense of risk, in turn, refers to conscious or non-conscious affective factors related mainly to the experience of fear and anxiety. Later on in this chapter, we will discuss (1) the psychological determinants of risk perception (factors determining whether an individual perceives the level of risk as high or low), and (2) the relationship between risk perception and people's intent to engage in protective behaviours to prevent the negative consequences of a threat (including the threat of an epidemic). Since the social effects of a pandemic involve not only health matters but also the economic conditions, our next discussion will broach both areas.

1.6.1 ASSESSING RISK

As mentioned earlier, the two main aspects of cognitive risk assessment involve estimating the probability and severity of negative consequences (health-related, economic, or both). Obviously, the higher the probability of contracting a disease and the more severe its potential consequences (e.g., impaired health or death), the higher the risk. When it comes to finance, what is estimated is the probability of incurring a financial loss, and the size of any loss (for example, losing one's job or income necessary for stable functioning). Years of research in the field of cognitive psychology have provided evidence that people have enormous difficulty in processing probabilistic information (Benjamin, 2019; Gigerenzer et al., 2007; Gilovich et al., 2002), which may then lead to biased risk assessments (either underestimating or overestimating risk). A classic example of a bias in estimating probability is insensitivity to sample size (Tversky and Kahneman, 1974). Risk assessment based on a small number of observations is wholly unreliable, due to the fact that tiny samples tend to have higher levels of variance than large ones. Still, despite being problematic, people generally find such assessments extremely convincing (for example, the risk of becoming ill seems higher when there are 4 cases of the disease in a group of 6 people, than in a situation when there are 120 cases in a group of 200, even though the reliability of the first observation is much diminished by the miniscule sample size). People's tendency to disregard the sample size has been confirmed by recent replication studies: Decision makers are insensitive to whether their assessments are based on a sample of 10, 1,000, or 1,000,000 observations, and this cognitive bias is not neutralized when subjects receive monetary rewards for providing correct answers (Benjamin, 2019).

Another source of problems with probabilistic risk assessment is the fact that such assessments can be absolute or relative (Gigerenzer, 2015; Renner et al., 2015). Gigerenzer (2015) describes how British women were warned that oral contraceptive pills increased the risk of thrombosis twofold, that is, by 100% (the relative risk increase). The news influenced risk perception and led to a decrease in the use of oral contraceptives, which later contributed to a higher number of teen pregnancies and abortions. However, when you look at the data in absolute terms (i.e., what exactly the risk is and how great it was a month before, without reporting the relative change), you will find that thrombosis was diagnosed in 1 out of 7,000 women, so a twofold risk increase was actually a change from 1 in 7,000 to 2 in 7,000. Presented in this way, the change elicits a very different response on the part of decision makers. A similar effect may occur when we consider the risk of dying from SARS-CoV-2. The perception of changes in the risk level will depend on whether they are reported in relative terms (by what percentage the risk has grown recently) or in absolute terms (what exactly the risk is now and how high it was a month previously, without reporting the relative change).

Biases in processing probabilities are accompanied by distorted predictions about the severity or value of negative consequences, as these values are assigned subjective weights, referred to as utilities (Kahneman and Thaler, 2006). The utility of an outcome may change depending on whether the outcome is considered on its own or juxtaposed with another outcome (Hsee, 2000). For example, the risk of contracting SARS-CoV-2 will be interpreted differently depending on whether it can be compared to another type of virus (such as an influenza virus) or not. Moreover, when assessing the utility of an experience, people use a psychological heuristic referred to as the peak-end rule (Read, 2007; Redelmeier et al., 2003; Schreiber and Kahneman, 2000). For instance, when trying to evaluate the discomfort or painfulness of a medical procedure, we tend to focus on the intensity of pain at the worst and final moments of the procedure. When assessing the current economic risk caused by the pandemic, people may recall their previous experiences (such as the financial crisis of 2008). Their assessments of the current level of risk will be based on the severity of the worst financial consequences they experienced during the previous crisis (at its peak) and their losses at the final stage of the recession (at the end).

When considering cognitive biases in quantitative risk assessment, a question that naturally comes to mind is whether, and to what extent, these biases can be minimized. Research in cognitive psychology proves that biases in probabilistic assessments can be reduced by using the right format for reporting information about probabilities. It turns out it is better to present such data using frequency formats (e.g., out of 100 people infected with SARS-CoV-2, two will die) rather than numerical formats (e.g., the probability of dying from the SARS-CoV-2 infection is 0.02 or 2%; Gigerenzer, 2015; Gigerenzer et al., 2007; Petrova and Garcia-Retamero, 2018; Witteman et al., 2015). To further support effective processing of probabilistic data, it is helpful to use visual aids (such as an icon array representing all people at risk of infection as dots, with those who will actually contract the disease represented with a different colour dot; Garcia-Retamero and Cokely, 2013, 2017; Galesic and Garcia-Retamero, 2011; Okan et al., 2012). Using the frequency format to communicate probabilities (risk) seems particularly

34 *Individuals, Groups, and Society in Pandemics*

useful when reporting conditional probabilities (for example, the probability that an individual will have a positive SARS-CoV-2 test result, given that they are actually infected). Gigerenzer and colleagues (2007) presented the following scenario to a group of physicians: "The probability that a woman has breast cancer is 1%. If a woman has breast cancer, the probability that she tests positive is 90%. If a woman does not have breast cancer, the probability that she nevertheless tests positive is 9%. A woman tests positive, so what is the probability that she has cancer?" After reading the scenario, only 21% of the physicians gave the correct answer (out of a number of choices provided), that is, that out of 10 women with a positive mammogram, only 1 actually has breast cancer (the exact probability is 9.2%). However, when the format of data presentation was changed into natural frequencies, the proportion of correct answers grew to 87%, i.e., four times greater. Here is the same information presented in a frequency format: "10 out of every 1,000 women have breast cancer. Of these 10 women with breast cancer, 9 test positive. Of the 990 women without cancer, 89 nevertheless test positive". Disturbingly, the majority of doctors who were presented the probability information in the traditional (numerical or percentage) format, answered that the probability of cancer was 81% or 90%, grossly overestimating the actual risk.

1.6.2 *DUAL-PROCESS MODEL OF RISK PERCEPTION: THE ROLE OF EMOTIONAL AND COGNITIVE FACTORS*

To summarize our discussion so far, we can see that, on the whole, people are somewhat inept at quantitative risk assessment, primarily due to biases in estimating probabilities and a tendency to assign subjective weights to outcomes. However, the need to evaluate risk is inherent in our lives (for example, doctors expect their patients to estimate the risk of a surgery and come to a decision about whether to agree to it or not; financial advisors leave it to their clients to choose between financial products, recommending them to consider the level of risk they are willing to tolerate). So, the question then arises as to how people handle this exacting task. Psychology has been on the hunt for an answer since the 1970s, when it was observed that people strongly opposed nuclear power plants while accepting the risks incurred by everyday behaviours, such as smoking or cycling. These observations led to the development of the psychometric paradigm (Fischoff et al., 1978; Slovic, 1987; Slovic et al., 1986; Visschers and Siegrist, 2018), which was later successfully applied to interpreting perceptions of risk from cigarette smoking (Popova et al., 2018; Slovic, 2001) or a financial crisis (Michel-Kerjan and Slovic, 2010).

According to the psychometric paradigm, people evaluate risk using a set of psychological criteria, which can be divided into two general categories. The first one involves knowledge and familiarity (unknown risk), and the other, emotions (dread risk; Marris et al., 1997; Siegrist et al., 2005; Slovic, 1987; Zaleskiewicz et al., 2002). The first category relates to cognitive factors; risk is perceived as higher when an individual's personal knowledge about it is limited, when their trust in knowledge sourced from experts about the threat is low, when the threat seems atypical (i.e., the individual is not familiar with this type of risk), and when its potential consequences are delayed. In the second category, the affective factor, risk is assessed as higher when people have low perceived control, when potential consequences seem catastrophic, when the act of facing the threat triggers strong fear responses, when the threat may also affect future generations, and when the individual feels exposed to risk involuntarily.

Now let us consider how these characteristics might be seen to apply to the current pandemic: People know little about it; it is a new situation (the vast majority of people have not had personal experience of an epidemic in their lifetime); experts explicitly admit their knowledge is uncertain; it is not clear whether engaging in protective behaviours will bring the desired outcomes, which decreases perceived control; its negative consequences appear to be massive and catastrophic (hundreds of thousands of deaths over a short period of time); and exposure to risk is obviously involuntary ("I'm protecting myself, but other people I have contact with behave irresponsibly and can pass the virus to me").

One early study used the psychometric approach to analyze the determinants of perceptions of health and financial risks (Holtgrave and Weber, 1993). It found that health risk perceptions were significantly predicted by factors such as voluntariness, dread, novelty, catastrophic potential, and an inequitable distribution of risks and benefits. Perceptions of financial risk were determined by factors including perceived control, dread, and catastrophic potential. In recent years, the psychometric paradigm has been used for the analysis of risk perceptions in the context of people's low concern about environmental threats and their apparent tendency to significantly underestimate the risk of climate change (van der Linden, 2017; Weber and Stern, 2011). The negative consequences of climate change are delayed ("the negative effects of smog are chronic"); poorly observable ("we haven't seen any droughts yet"); they seem controllable ("we can stop coal mining at any time"); and are far from being novel ("this subject has been talked about for decades"). As a result, people do not engage in the behaviours they should be undertaking if their perceptions of the climate change risk were consistent with objective indicators (for example, saving energy and water, sorting waste, avoiding burning coal for heat, reducing travel etc.). In light of this, similar psychological mechanisms for estimating risk can be expected in the context of the pandemic. The negative consequences of the pandemic are delayed ("we get infected today, but we will develop serious disease later"); poorly observable ("you can't see the virus; you can only see the effects of decision makers' responses"); they seem controllable ("scientists are working on treatments and vaccines"); and they are not novel ("it is not the first pandemic in the world"). The risk of developing the disease seems low, so why comply with restrictions?

1.6.3 SPECIFIC EFFECTS OF ANXIETY AND KNOWLEDGE IN RISK PERCEPTION

The dual-process, cognitive-affective model of risk perception offered by the psychometric paradigm emphasizes the role of two factors: levels of knowledge and dread (or anxiety). The importance of both of these in risk perception is supported by research conducted outside this paradigm (e.g., Zaleskiewicz, Bernady, and Traczyk, 2020). Lerner and Keltner (2000, 2001) suggest that the effects of anxiety on risk perception could be interpreted in the context of experiencing uncertainty. Facing risk is associated with uncertainty about the outcomes of our actions (Grupe and Nitschke, 2013). Uncertainty leads to anxiety, and anxiety increases the feeling of uncertainty, so that the two factors feed off each other. Lerner and Keltner (2001) demonstrated that individuals experiencing experimentally induced fear (as opposed to induced anger) reported higher uncertainty and lower perceived control, and made more pessimistic risk estimates. What is more, perceived control mediated the relationship between fear and risk perception, that is, increased fear was associated with lower perceived control, which in turn was linked to higher risk estimates.

According to various models describing the role of emotions in risk assessment and risk taking (Bechara and Damasio, 2005; Lempert and Phelps, 2013; Loewenstein et al., 2001; Lerner et al., 2015; Mohr et al., 2010; Parrott, 2017; Pfister and Böhm, 2008; Zaleskiewicz and Traczyk, 2020), there is a bidirectional relationship between emotions and cognitive risk assessment, meaning that experiencing strong affect may contribute to biases in estimating probabilities and the severity of consequences. For example, people experiencing strong pandemic-induced anxiety may show inappropriate responses to information about the objective level of risk. Indeed, studies conducted in the past dozen years have demonstrated that sensitivity to changes in probability is decreased when individuals experience strong anxiety (Pachur et al., 2014; Petrova and Garcia-Retamero, 2018; Rottenstreich and Hsee, 2001). Rottenstreich and Hsee (2001) found that people were willing to pay similar amounts of money to avoid an aversive, fear-inducing stimulus, regardless of whether the probability of its occurrence was 99% or 1%. However, when the aversive stimulus did not trigger intense emotions, the amount people were willing to pay to avoid it was significantly higher when the chance it would occur was 99% (compared to the low probability condition), that is, the subjects' responses were more rational than in the intense fear condition. According to Petrova, Garcia-Retamero, Catena and van der Pligt (2016), when experiencing strong emotions, we seem to rely on the "prevention is always good" heuristic, which means, however, that sometimes risk is overestimated and preventive behaviour takes the form of a false alarm. Applying this example to the epidemic threat, we may say that even if the objective risk is quite low, if it causes intense fear then disproportionate preventive measures are likely to be taken (such as complete isolation), which can result in dire economic and social outcomes.

Another psychological support for the process of risk perception is the cognitive pillar of knowledge. The less we know about something, the less we understand it; and the less knowledge we gained about it in the past, the more risky it appears (March, 1997; Sjöberg, 2000, 2001; Van der Linden, 2015). If we have no previous experience with the risks of an epidemic and know little about it (which is actually quite common), we will perceive it as all the more dangerous. When it comes to risk assessment, however, what matters is not only our general knowledge about a subject (such as health, the natural environment, or the economy) but also numeracy and financial literacy. Numeracy is defined as the ability to correctly understand numerical and probabilistic concepts and operations (Cokely et al., 2012; Lipkus et al., 2001; Peters and Bjalkebring, 2015). Financial literacy is the ability to understand basic financial concepts and financial risks we are faced with in the market (Hung et al., 2009; Huston, 2010; Klapper et al., 2015). Empirical data from various countries shows that people, on average, score low on both types of skills. When it comes to numeracy, just over 50% of all subjects (N = 2,379, 14 countries on three continents) had scores in the first and second quartiles (Cokely et al., 2012). Lusardi and Mitchell (2013) reported that only one third of their sample were able to provide correct answers to three questions measuring financial literacy. Of the three tasks, the subjects had the most difficulty understanding that the lower diversification of investments, the higher the financial risk. Hence, it is easy to predict that during a financial crisis or an economic recession, consumers will have problems estimating risks accurately, and deciding what steps they ought to take.

1.6.4 RISK PERCEPTION AND ENGAGING IN PREVENTIVE BEHAVIOURS

It would seem obvious to state that risk perception should be associated with engaging in specific preventive behaviours, or failing to do so. It can be expected that when perceived risk increases, people will make efforts to protect themselves (for example, when the perceived risk of price rises becomes higher during an epidemic, people start hoarding supplies), and when perceived risk declines, such preventive steps seem less necessary (for example, when the perceived risk of infection decreases, people will be less likely to wear face masks and sanitize their hands). A study by Ferrer and colleagues (2018) explored whether perceptions of health risks were related to people's motivation to engage in preventive behaviours. It was found that there was a significant positive relationship between motivation and perceptions of risk, in both emotional and probabilistic terms. The more the subjects believed the threat was highly probable, the more likely they were to invest their resources and effort in prevention.

Although research evidence seems to support the relationship between estimating risk and motivation, it has long been known in psychology that attitudes or intentions are not always closely correlated with actual behaviours (e.g., Sheeran and Webb, 2016). Even when people themselves perceive risk as high, they may fail to take preventive steps because others are not doing so, which means that a range of social factors (such as conformity) play a role in the relationship between intentions and behaviour. Therefore, it is important to determine if there is a relationship between risk perception and the likelihood to engage in preventive behaviours (and if so, how strong the relationship between them is). This question seems to be of particular significance in the context of perceiving health-related risks and engaging in protective behaviours during a pandemic (e.g., perceptions of health-related risks and the willingness to get vaccinated; Ferrer and Klein, 2015).

Although there are a substantial number of studies on the relationship between perceptions of risks (especially health-related risks) and engaging in protective behaviours, their results have been inconclusive. Therefore, it is helpful to refer to meta-analyses, in which conclusions are based on a larger number of studies. One of these explored the relationship between health risk perceptions and taking preventive action, i.e., vaccination behaviour (Brewer et al., 2007). Based on 34 studies with a total sample of nearly 16,000 participants, the analyses found that (1) individuals who perceived the risk of infection to be higher were more likely to get vaccinated; (2) individuals who perceived themselves as more susceptible to an illness were more likely to be vaccinated; and (3) those who perceived the severity of illness to be higher were also more likely to take a vaccine.

Studies on the relationship between risk perception and behaviour are usually correlational, so they cannot be interpreted in terms of causality. Hence, it would be of interest to discover whether interventions aimed at changing the perceptions of risk can influence protective behaviours. For example, is it possible to change the behaviour of those who do not follow safety rules during an epidemic by increasing their perceptions of risk? A meta-analysis attempting to answer these questions was conducted by Sheeran, Harris, and Epton (2014). It included studies published in 208 articles and it found that raising people's awareness about their own susceptibility to a health risk had a positive effect both on intentions and on behaviour. Interestingly, the effect of an intervention was stronger when it addressed not only assessments of risk but also people's emotions, something which is consistent with the dual-process, cognitive-emotional model of risk (see also Slovic and Peters, 2006). The strongest effects were found for interventions that involved not only raising people's awareness about the level of risk but also improving their self-efficacy. Thus, decision makers appear to be most likely to behave reasonably (for example adhere to social distancing rules, wear face masks, and follow sanitizing procedures during an epidemic) when they believe the risk is high and can clearly see the effectiveness of their behaviours.

1.7 DECISION MAKING UNDER RISK

The impact of affective states on elementary cognitive processes extends to more complex cognitive processes, such as judgement and decision making. A basic

Individual Perspective 39

normative model of judgement and decision making is the multi-attribute utility theory (Keeney et al., 1993), which proposes that rational judgements and decisions are those made based on all the available information, and that each bit of information contributes to the final judgement or decision in proportion to its weight. However, in the presence of the previously discussed factors (such as fear, uncertainty, etc.), which all lead to highly selective cognitive processing, this manner of making judgements and decisions is impeded. Research shows that when under threat, and thus experiencing anxiety, people use simplified rules of decision making: In anxiety-provoking situations, they fail to take all the alternatives into consideration, instead making use of just a few highly relevant cues (Keinan, 1987; Lewinsohn and Mano, 1993; Mano, 1992; Wichary et al., 2016). Their time perspective is also shortened: People make decisions focusing on a more limited time horizon. For example, they prefer smaller immediate gains over larger but delayed ones (Gray, 1999; Lempert and Phelps, 2016). This means that, when feeling at risk under pandemic conditions, people's behaviour will focus on obtaining short-term benefits and achieving a sense of security in the here-and-now rather than in the future. So, for example, people will be more liable to spend their savings on buying a recreational lot than to set their money aside for their retirement. Their decisions will also be based on a selective cue analysis, which can lead to errors and post-decisional regret, but at the same time, helps to reduce emotional distress related to the task of processing excess information.

Having said this, we ought to bear in mind the significant individual differences in decision making – characteristics such as age, sex, personality, and motivational and affective factors – which modify general effects and make it so that the same phenomena occur to a higher degree in some people than in others. The predominant factor that influences decision-making processes and modifies their effects is sex, which results from links between sex and emotional regulation (van den Bos et al., 2013). Numerous studies have shown that in the general population, men are more inclined to take risks than women (Byrnes et al., 1999), and literature reviews (e.g., van den Bos et al., 2013) also support this finding. This relationship can be seen in laboratory studies and also in prison statistics (Guerino et al., 2011). Some research suggests that sex moderates the effect of stress on risk taking. For example, Lighthall and colleagues (2009) demonstrated that stress increased risk taking in men and decreased it among women. The tendency to simplify decision-making strategies under stress and intense emotions can also be moderated by sex: Some studies show that the relationship between arousal and the use of simple decision-making strategies is stronger in men than in women (Wichary et al., 2016). In general, these findings would suggest that among men the pandemic threat may be associated with increased risk taking and simplified decision making, whereas in women it will lead to decreased risk taking, without affecting the complexity of decision-making processes.

Age also plays a role in decision making. Since cognitive functions decline with age (Salthouse, 2011), elderly people are more prone to using simple

40   *Individuals, Groups, and Society in Pandemics*

decision-making heuristics than younger people (Keane and Thorp, 2016; Mata et al., 2007). Even though these effects may be compensated for by knowledge acquired over time, this is only the case for certain areas – those in which an individual's knowledge grows. Risk taking also decreases with age (Josef et al., 2016; Mata et al., 2011, 2016), so elderly people tend to take fewer risks than younger people. Moreover, age moderates the effect of stress on risk taking (Mather et al., 2009), that is, stress decreases risk taking in elderly people but increases it in younger ones. During a pandemic, this should make young people more likely to ignore medical recommendations than the elderly. An increase in the level of risk (e.g., a larger number of cases or another epidemic wave) would go further in reinforcing this tendency. At the same time, Czarnek and colleagues (2019, 2020) have found that the elderly can cope much better than the young in cognitively complex situations (despite the obvious decline in cognitive functioning in this group), but only when they are directly involved. This may suggest that during a pandemic, elderly people, who are at a higher risk than younger ones, will be more likely to use optimal decision-making strategies.

Sex and age are easily detectable demographic variables, giving them an advantage over other moderators (e.g., modifying factors that have to be gauged with special instruments). In other words, these factors can be used to predict behaviour without having to measure any hidden psychological variables; for example, they can be used to better calibrate large-scale models of epidemic spread.

Cognitive and decision-making processes are also influenced by temperamental and personality factors, which moderate the effects of risk on these processes. A comprehensive meta-analysis by Lauriola and colleagues (2014) found that impulsivity and sensation seeking were positively related to risk taking. Similarly, in their review article, Josef and colleagues (2016) demonstrate that risk taking is positively related to openness to experience and extraversion, and negatively related to neuroticism and agreeableness. Simply put, individuals who are impulsive, sociable, and thrill-seekers are more likely to take risks, whereas those who are agreeable and prone to experiencing fear and anxiety are much less likely to partake in risky behaviours.

Motivational factors are also associated with cognitive and decision-making processes. A special role is played by epistemic motivation, or the desire to gain a certain degree of knowledge and understanding about the situation, manifested as the need for cognitive closure (Kruglanski and Webster, 1996; Kossowska, 2005; Webster and Kruglanski, 1994). Individuals with high levels of epistemic motivation have a tendency to simplify decision-making processes (Wichary et al., 2008; Senderecka et al., 2018) and are less inclined to take risks (Schumpe et al., 2017). Under increased uncertainty, however, some paradoxical effects of this motivation/need may occur (Kossowska et al., 2018a): Individuals who typically choose simplified cognitive strategies become likely to engage in strenuous cognitive activity and complex information processing. Other motivational factors (such as physiological needs or the need for safety) may moderate cognitive and decision-making processes by changing the level of arousal, which has the same effect as strong affective states (e.g., fear, anxiety, or disgust).

These findings suggest we should not expect uniform responses to threats across individuals. However, certain subpopulations – such as young men versus elderly women – can be expected to react very differently to information concerning risk. The former will, in all likelihood, show an increased tendency toward violating legal regulations or ignoring medical guidelines, a tendency which will become even stronger as the risk grows. On the other hand, this group can also be expected to show increased innovation and readiness to invest in risky economic projects when under threat.

1.7.1 TRADE-OFFS IN DECISION MAKING

Decision makers sometimes have to make comparisons and trade-offs between differing values, which may end up producing conflict in decision making (Weber et al., 2001). The problem is not emotionally taxing when such comparisons are made within the same value category – for example, when a consumer chooses between a cheaper product in larger packaging, and a more expensive product in smaller packaging. Psychological complications occur when people have to weigh values that are hard to compare, such as money and a sense of security – for example, when a consumer attempts to decide whether to buy insurance and thus pay more to feel safe, or to choose a cheaper alternative, without insurance, at the cost of feeling insecure (Frances et al., 1999; Luce et al., 2001; Luce et al., 1999). Research shows that when faced with such dilemmas, people do their best to condense the differing values into a single common currency, that is, emotions (Peters et al., 2006; Zaleskiewicz and Traczyk, 2020). Decision makers can first ask themselves how much positive or negative feeling they experience at the thought of losing money, time, or control, and only then make a trade-off calculation.

When the values involved seem completely incomparable, such as health and finances, it can be particularly difficult to reach a decision (Tinghög and Västfjäll, 2018). Unfortunately, during a pandemic, people are repeatedly faced with such quandaries (Sokolowska and Zaleskiewicz, 2020). For example, should we close businesses (to ensure isolation) at the cost of higher unemployment and pay cuts? Should we block imports of cheap products from countries affected by the epidemic, thereby inviting inevitable price increases? Should we shut down schools and universities to slow the spread of the virus, at the cost of lowering the quality of teaching and making education inaccessible to a subgroup of students? Similar dilemmas between material and health values are faced by decision makers at the organizational level (for example governments) and also by individuals (Should I quit a job where the manager forces employees to come to work despite the high epidemic-related risk?).

Beattie and Barlas (2001) summarized studies on conflict in decision making and suggested a list of factors that predict difficulties in trade-off decision making: (1) the level of uncertainty; (2) levels of concern over the outcome (the more a decision maker cares about the outcome, the harder the trade-off is); (3) the similarity of the alternatives (trade-offs are particularly tricky when the values to be compared represent different categories, such as health and the economy); (4) the presence of moral factors (trade-offs are tougher when they involve morality, for example: Should we abandon the purchase of a large number of expensive ventilators when we are not sure whether they will still be needed after the pandemic?); (5) the material or non-material nature of the options (commodities versus non-commodities; trade-offs are much more challenging and emotionally burdening when they require the comparison of material and non-material values, such as friendship, or freedom, versus money).

The most extreme cases, where people display deep reluctance to make trade-offs, are those where several of the abovementioned factors are all present at the same time, or where a decision maker believes that some prized values (such as life, health, or freedom) cannot be compared to, or traded for, anything else. In social science, these are referred to as sacred values (Tetlock, 2003). Making any attempt to weigh them up is treated as a taboo violation (Chorus et al., 2018; Daw et al., 2015; Fiske and Tetlock, 1997; Harel and Porat, 2011; Tetlock et al., 2000) or as a repugnant transaction (Leuker et al., 2020; Roth, 2007, 2015). During the COVID-19 pandemic, strong emotions, in the form of moral outrage, were triggered by media reports that, in some countries, politicians had decided not to introduce strict lockdowns (thus increasing the probability of infection and death among the most vulnerable, such as the elderly) in order to promote herd immunity among younger people or, even worse (in the eyes of some), to protect some material values (for example, to avoid a dramatic rise in unemployment).

In a recent empirical study on the psychology of repugnant transactions, Leuker and colleagues (2020) have demonstrated that the repugnance of certain trade-offs (transactions) is associated with five factors: (1) moral outrage (witnessing repugnant transactions causes disgust, and dampens empathy for those involved in the transaction); (2) the need for regulation (aversion to transactions that are not properly regulated by law, which exposes one of the parties to extreme risk); (3) perceived incommensurability (the feeling that some values cannot be translated into other – e.g. monetary – values, and that the scales on which these values are expressed are incompatible – for example, you just cannot set a price for the marriage of a woman); (4) exploitation (the feeling that making trade-offs between dissimilar values will objectify one of the parties); and (5) unknown risk (when it is not clear whether or not the transaction may cause long-term consequences to ensue for future generations). The authors found that transactions or trade-offs between values were most strongly opposed in the following five cases: gun trade, child labour, selling voting rights, bride prices, and selling the right to hunt endangered animals. This repugnance of trade-offs probably represents one of the reasons why some decisions reached during the pandemic were so strongly opposed by the public.

It is also intriguing to consider behavioural, not just cognitive and emotional, consequences of placing people in a situation where they are compelled to make unwanted or (as they see it) unacceptable trade-offs (ones that still need to be made when under threat). Both earlier and more recent studies (Beattie et al., 1994; Gordon-Hecker et al., 2017) demonstrate that, in such circumstances, people are likely to show decision aversion and strive to avoid making any decision on the matter (for example, they procrastinate or attempt to shift the responsibility for the decision onto someone else). Another tactic is to make all sorts of rationalizations, for example, doing what they can to denigrate one of the values in the trade-off – a strategy which was commonly used by the Nazis during World War II when they questioned the value of Jewish lives (Arendt, 2006). Gordon-Hecker and colleagues (2017) found that when people felt their choice would violate equities in resource distribution, they would rather destroy a resource than accept such a violation, an act which seems completely irrational from the normative perspective.

Decisions that require trade-offs between different values are obviously inevitable during a pandemic, which makes it even more important for decision makers to be aware of the public perception of any trade-off and the mechanisms underlying them. A crucial skill, in this day and age, is the ability to describe these trade-offs, to issue statements about them to the public in appropriate ways, and to reduce public resistance to these decisions.

1.8 TRUST IN EXPERTS

When making decisions, people turn to external sources of information in two cases: (1) when there is too much information, so they are not able to process it all properly; and (2) when there is too little information or when they do not understand the information they already have (Payne and Bettman, 2004). In the current context of the pandemic, there is definitely a dearth of information, and many gaps in understanding prevail. For most people (including experts), it is still unclear what mechanisms are behind the clear and present danger of the disease, and what long-term consequences it might have. This is true both for the medical aspects (for example, the full spectrum of symptoms is not yet well understood), and for the economic or financial realm (the long-term effects of the pandemic on unemployment or inflation are difficult to predict). Expert knowledge is one source of information used by decision makers (Bonaccio and Dalal, 2006; Shanteau, 1992; Sniezek et al., 2004; Soll and Larrick, 2009; Yaniv, 2004). To obtain information about risks related to SARS-CoV-2, one may turn to epidemiologists and physicians, while information about the economic consequences of the pandemic can be expected from economists and financial analysts. However, individuals lacking the appropriate educational background may encounter a serious challenge, asking themselves the question: How can I determine who really is an expert, and who is not? In the era of widespread internet access, myriad types of information are accessible at any time (Googling "coronavirus" yields almost 3 million search results as of June 12, 2020), but we are often at a loss as to how we could possibly assess its credibility.

In his theory of lay epistemics, Kruglanski (1989a, 2012) argues that, when making decisions, individuals will only rely on advice from experts whom they perceive as reliable and trustworthy. Therefore, understanding factors that determine an expert's perceived reliability would seem to be of utmost importance. Because our judgements are often guided by intuition and gut feelings rather than a systematic analysis (Gigerenzer, 2008b; Gilovich et al., 2002; Kahneman, 2003), we are susceptible to making errors, affecting the quality of our decision making. In this context, these will stem from biases in assessing the reliability of expert advice, and in discriminating between sources of expertise and sources of fake knowledge, or fake science (Hopf et al., 2019).

One of the biases in evaluating expert authority is associated with the fact that lay people want to confirm their existing beliefs and opinions (Lord et al., 1979; Vallone et al., 1985), which leads to confirmation bias (Baron, 2006; Nickerson, 1998) or to egocentric advice discounting – filtering information through one's personal beliefs (Yaniv, 2004; Yaniv and Kleinberger, 2000; Yaniv and Milyavsky, 2007). Generally, these biases can be described as motivated reasoning, or selective processing of information, to make the evaluation consistent with one's goals (Haidt, 2012; Kunda, 1987, 1990; Lundgren and Prislin, 1998; Mercier and Sperber, 2011; Molden and Higgins, 2005). It has been empirically demonstrated that arguments inconsistent with one's belief system take longer to process, are analyzed more deeply, and perceived as weaker than arguments compatible with our beliefs (Ditto and Lopez, 1992). Thus, it can be expected that expert arguments will be assessed differently depending on whether they are consistent with an individual's personal beliefs or not. In other words, people will be likely to attribute more reliability to experts who confirm their pre-existing beliefs, which, of course, can lead to strong biases in decision making (Raviv et al., 1993; Zaleskiewicz and Gasiorowska, 2018, 2021; Zaleskiewicz et al., 2016). If an individual believes that the risks associated with the epidemic are extremely high, and will have serious social consequences, they will be more likely to trust experts who express similar opinions and, at the same time, discount advice from those claiming that the risk of infection is low. On the other hand, when an individual believes the risk is not very real, they will reject expert opinions that seek to express the idea that the risk of infection is high, and will be unlikely to adhere to hygiene recommendations.

Somewhat analogous peculiarities in the processing of expert knowledge may apply to assessments made in the realm of economics. Zaleskiewicz and Gasiorowska (2018, 2021) conducted a series of experimental studies to find out how the psychological mechanisms discussed earlier apply to financial advisors' opinions. Using data collected in Poland, the US, and the UK, and by analyzing decisions centered on various financial products (such as investment and insurance), it was found that evaluations of expert authority were strongly biased toward consistency between expert advice and the decision makers' pre-existing opinions. For example, the more strongly the subjects believed that investing their savings in the stock market was rational and profitable, the higher they evaluated advisors who recommended doing so. These findings support the notion that motivated reasoning and the desire to confirm one's own beliefs are highly involved in assessing any expert's reliability. Moreover, Zaleskiewicz and Gasiorowska (2021) have gone further by demonstrating that the effect of motivated reasoning on the perception of expert advice can be explained by three psychological phenomena: the desire to maintain self-esteem (Greenberg et al., 1986; Hewitt, 2009); seeing biases in experts who express uncomfortable opinions (Pronin et al., 2004; Scopelliti et al., 2015); and the tendency to trust more in more easily processed messages (Alter and Oppenheimer, 2009; Schwarz et al., 1991).

In a series of studies conducted in Poland between February and July 2020, Kossowska and colleagues (2021) demonstrated that, although trust in experts and scientists increased during the pandemic (compared to the levels before the crisis), this effect only occurred among people with left-wing or liberal views. Individuals with right-wing or conservative beliefs actually showed *decreased* levels of trust in scientists, an effect resulting from scientists being perceived as representing members of "the elite". In addition, increased trust in scientists was associated with more positive attitudes toward vaccination, and more positive evaluations of the vaccination policy. The studies show the damaging effects of "elite replacement" slogans, and of presenting experts as representatives of corrupt groups driven by self-interest rather than by a wish for the common good. These findings are consistent with those obtained in the US, but with the difference being that, in the States, the line of the political divide is not drawn between the elites and "ordinary people", but rather is linked to the perception of scientists as liberals working for institutions fostering liberal values (Confas et al., 2018).

By now applying this knowledge to the cognitive and social effects associated with how people go about interpreting the epidemic risk, we may conclude that individuals are more inclined to trust in medical and economic experts whose opinions are consistent with their own beliefs because: (a) information inconsistent with one's beliefs is threatening to one's self-esteem, and people are automatically inclined to protect their self-esteem; (b) people are naïve realists, which means that descriptions of the world inconsistent with their views seem unreliable to them; (c) information contradicting one's viewpoint is hard to process, which makes the individual dramatically less likely to trust it; and finally, (d) ideological self-identification is an important epistemic cue. Given all this, in order to correctly predict whether people are going to respond positively to expert recommendations during a pandemic or not (for instance, those concerning self-isolation, mask wearing, closing businesses that provide face-to-face services to their clients, or the avoidance of social gatherings and family reunions), we have to learn and understand what people's prior stances on them are. In other words, what matters is not

1.9 VACCINATION AS A WAY TO MANAGE THE PANDEMIC[5]

The subject of vaccination cannot be set aside in a discussion on the means of managing the COVID-19 pandemic. The invention of vaccines was one of the crowning achievements of medical science, making it possible to eliminate or reduce a large number of diseases that had long decimated the human population. Today, one of the toughest challenges has been to develop an effective and safe vaccine against SARS-CoV-2.

The race for a coronavirus vaccine was run at a breakneck speed. According to the World Health Organization, 176 potential vaccines are currently (i.e., at the time we are writing this book – in the summer of 2020) being developed worldwide. More than 30 of them are undergoing human trials. Over 200 academic and commercial research centres are engaged in this work (*The New York Times* mentions 37 of them; Corum et al., 2020). Will a vaccine help to manage the pandemic? Given the growing anti-vaccine movement, we have reason to be skeptical (Hussain et al., 2018; de Figueiredo et al., 2016). For the past few years, researchers have striven to understand the reasons for these anti-vaccine sentiments. The issue has become even more pressing now, since it has been proven beyond doubt that low acceptance of immunization programmes leads to an increased risk of infection, decreased population immunity, and the looming menace that the epidemic will go on to be concentrated in less developed countries. If vaccination programmes are taken up en masse by the public, the knowledge gained about the positive effects of high levels of immunization among the populace will facilitate future medical interventions, and thus serve to prevent the next epidemic. Stoffels (2020) noted that opposition to vaccination – in this case, a vaccine against SARS-CoV-2,[6] the virus causing COVID-19 – could intensify disease outbreaks, as was the case with measles in 2019 (see also Taylor, 2019; Lambert, 2019). As a reminder, anti-vaccination movements managed to persuade many parents across Europe to believe in the myth of the (alleged) harmfulness of the combined vaccine against measles, mumps, and rubella (MMR). Following a decrease in the number of vaccinated children, the three diseases returned, particularly measles, which is extremely infectious. It was for this reason that the WHO (2019) listed the reluctance or refusal to vaccinate oneself or one's children among the ten top threats to global health in modern times.

The question arises as to why widespread doubt about the effectiveness of vaccines has suddenly manifested itself. In fact, debates worldwide have shown how complex the answer to this question is (Larson et al., 2014). First off, people seem to know very little about the subject, and the current state of knowledge around the process of vaccination, types of vaccines, and their possible combinations is immensely complicated and highly specialized. At times, even experts may scratch their heads in bewilderment when sifting through all the data. Therefore, what is needed is a public education campaign with a solid, simple message supported by the authority of science (see CDC recommendations, 2018). It turns out, however, that information questioning vaccine safety may sometimes come from the medical field itself. A well-known example was an article by Andrew Wakefield and colleagues, published in 1998 in *The Lancet*, a reputable medical journal, demonstrating a relationship between the MMR vaccine and autism. The paper which, as was soon discovered, presented false data and conclusions, was later retracted, but the information it provided has sparked heated discussion on vaccination harmfulness ever since. Misconceptions of this kind endure despite irrefutable research evidence, and efforts to debunk them end up being futile, if not counterproductive. Instead of reducing the number of people who sustain such myths, they lead to a heightened polarization of public opinion (e.g., Attwell and Freeman, 2015; Daley et al., 2018). In other words, although increasing numbers of people are well-informed, the number of those who actively reject this factual knowledge is also on the rise. What's more, even the most solid and reliable of knowledge to do with vaccinations is often grossly distorted, misinterpreted, or deliberately falsified. Misinformation spreads like wildfire on social media, and has a greater reach than accurate information (Chiou and Tucker, 2018). Given all this, no wonder it can be so easy to begin doubting vaccine legitimacy and, above all, vaccine safety (Larson et al., 2011). More worryingly, we are also now witness to the alarming tendency of growing anti-vaccine sentiment among healthcare workers, despite their being the ones most exposed to diseases (Maltezou et al., 2018).

Numerous factors have been identified as causes of negative attitudes toward vaccination. We know, for instance, that people can refuse to be vaccinated for religious, scientific, and political reasons (Czarnek et al., 2020; Kahan, 2017; Lewandowsky et al., 2015; Ruthjens et al., 2018). Negative vaccine attitudes are reinforced by people's belief in conspiracy theories (Hornsey et al., 2018), low levels of trust in health services and science (Yaqub et al., 2014; Kossowska et al., 2021), as well as health anxiety, disgust with blood and needles, and strong fears of medical procedures such as injections (Clay, 2017; Clifford and Wendell, 2016; Hornsey et al., 2018). Other beliefs that may engender a negative stance include the notion that vaccines threaten people's autonomy and freedom of choice (Hornsey et al., 2018).

Many researchers maintain that it may be too daunting a challenge to endeavour to alter vaccine attitudes among those who are convinced that vaccinations are more threatening to life and limb than the diseases they are meant to prevent; however, they do hold out hope for a change of heart among one group that deserves special attention: vaccine-hesitant individuals (Larson et al., 2014). These hesitant people may refuse some vaccines but agree to others; they delay taking the vaccinations, but then they often eventually accept them, and agree to vaccinate their children, even if they are

48   *Individuals, Groups, and Society in Pandemics*

unsure of their decision (Opel et al., 2011; Benin et al., 2006). A number of factors are responsible for vaccine hesitancy: (1) low confidence (people do not trust the vaccine and its provider); (2) complacency (they do not perceive the need for a vaccine, i.e., do not value the vaccine); and (3) convenience (accessibility and affordability of vaccines; Larson et al., 2014). In March 2012, the SAGE Working Group on Vaccine Hesitancy was established to identify what contributes to vaccine hesitancy (www.who.int/immunization/sage/sage_wg_vaccine_hesitancy_apr12/en/), as the phenomenon appeared to be determined by a variety of factors. For instance, in Greece, insufficient or delayed vaccination of children was predicted by socioeconomic factors, such as the number of siblings or paternal education (Danis et al., 2010), whereas parental attitudes and beliefs about vaccines turned out to be insignificant. In Nigeria, the main reasons for non-immunization included maternal absence (women are more likely to vaccinate their children) and low awareness among mothers of the importance of immunization (Babalola, 2011). UK studies on parental decisions about combined MMR (measles, mumps, rubella) vaccinations showed it was difficult to identify a single pattern because decisions to vaccinate or not to vaccinate one's child were influenced by different factors, depending on the precise MMR dose history (Brown et al., 2011). According to SAGE, three categories of factors need to be considered in order to understand the reasons for vaccine hesitancy: (1) contextual influences – historical, socio-cultural, environmental, health system/institutional, economic, and political factors; (2) individual and group influences, arising from personal beliefs about vaccination or influences arising from the social and peer environment; and (3) vaccine and vaccination specific issues, which are directly related to the characteristics of the vaccine or the vaccination process. According to experts, efforts to promote vaccinations need to be carefully tailored to the target group, taking into account the whole range of the group's social characteristics.

Notes

1 This section was developed for the report by Duszyński et al. (2020), *Understanding COVID-19*, Warsaw: PAN.
2 https://institution.pan.pl/index.php/653-position-statement-no-10-of-the-covid-19-advisory-team-to-the-president-of-the-polish-academy-of-sciences-implications-of-the-covid-19-pandemic-for-the-mental-health-and-education-of-children-and-adolescents
3 Parts of this section come from the book by Kossowska, Szumowska, and Szwed (2020), *The Psychology of Tolerance in Times of Uncertainty*, and were quoted here with the authors' and the publisher's permission.
4 Later on in this book, we use the terms "optimists" and "pessimists", which, of course, are a simplification. By optimists and pessimists we mean individuals who obtain either high or low scores respectively on scales of trait optimism.
5 Paulina Szwed has contributed to this section.
6 Medical aspects of the COVID-19 vaccine and the progress of work on its development, are discussed in Duszyński et al. (2020), *Understanding COVID-19*. Warsaw: PAN. See also https://institution.pan.pl/index.php/covid-19-advisory-team

2 GROUP PERSPECTIVE

Małgorzata Kossowska, Natalia Letki,
Tomasz Zaleskiewicz, and Szymon Wichary

2.1 GROUPS MATTER IN CRISIS

Humans are a social species – they live and act in groups. How they see themselves in relationships with others determines their social behaviour. As a matter of course, each of us defines ourselves as a person with a unique set of attributes and characteristics (e.g., tall, intelligent, and proficient in foreign languages). In many contexts, however, we perceive ourselves as social beings, belonging to different groups, and sharing a variety of characteristics with other members of these groups (e.g., women, marathon runners; Tajfel and Turner, 1979). The first way of thinking, in terms of the individual self, focusses us on our distinctive qualities in contrast to others. Hence, we are motivated to seek out information that allows us to see ourselves as, for instance, taller, more intelligent, and more linguistically talented than others. This tendency inevitably leads to a common phenomenon known as the above average effect. The second approach to perceiving ourselves, as our social self, causes us to look out for similarities between ourselves and other members of our in-group, or a group we identify with (Turner, 1982), and to make efforts to find differences between ourselves and those not belonging to our group, known as the outgroup (Turner et al., 1987). During a crisis, groups matter all the more. Regardless of its form, social identity is not simply an individual's awareness of being a member of certain social groups, but also, above all, carries with it the values and emotional significance attached to this membership (Tajfel, 1972). We deem our in-groups as better, having more agency and a higher status.

Social identity enriches individuals, making them stronger and healthier, as it enables them to feel worthy (enhances their self-esteem), gives them meaning and purpose, and increases their sense of control and self-efficacy (e.g., Cruwys et al., 2014; Greenaway et al., 2015; Jetten et al., 2015). It is not only a source of social support (Haslam et al., 2012); being in a group is even said to be "healing", that is, group membership has a positive effect on an individual's health and wellbeing (Haslam et al., 2009; Jetten et al., 2012). These palliative properties of groups are further intensified during a crisis. What is of key importance here is the cognitive construal of group membership (how

DOI: 10.4324/9781003254133-4

50 *Individuals, Groups, and Society in Pandemics*

you think of yourself as a group member), rather than the identification itself (I am a woman). Tajfel (1972) emphasized that groups became important to us when they were positively differentiated or distinct from other groups. Therefore, social identity is shaped by the fundamental process of social comparison, whereby people continuously compare themselves to others in ways that grants them an advantage. During the COVID-19 pandemic, countries tended to compare themselves to others in terms of numbers of coronavirus tests, cases, and deaths. The resulting comparisons are important because they shape our beliefs about how we are faring and, thus, contribute to our choice of the most optimal strategy for handling the pandemic. Before the COVID-19 outbreak in Europe and the US, no country considered it reasonable to compare themselves to China, and, as a consequence, no preventive steps were taken sufficiently early. Even in countries where the disease was spreading at lightning speed, as in Italy, China's example was not followed. Countries seemed to wait for other European countries to respond, and, as a result, restrictions were introduced far too late.

Factors playing a crucial role in the process of identity construction include the individual's social history (defining yourself as a member of a group important to you in the past), social context (identifications created must be meaningful in the social context), and social influence (which makes you think of yourself the way others would like you to; Reicher et al., 2005; Haslam and Turner, 1992). What is also important is whether we perceive the group as supportive, successful, and collaborative, or rather focus on its failures and mistakes, and see it as inferior to others. Even if we belong to a low status group (for instance, an ethnic, religious, or sexual minority), we can engage in constructing a positive identity by enhancing the group's status (for instance, by recalling its achievements), thinking about intergroup boundaries as permeable (i.e., membership of another group is easily attained), and by perceiving the group's status relative to other groups as stable and legitimate (Tajfel and Turner, 1979; Ellemers, 1993; Haslam et al., 2009). Notably, the status of groups plays a role in coping with a crisis, and the more stratified the society, the more crucial this role becomes. In response to COVID-19, in many countries, high status groups, i.e., those that had much to lose (e.g., businesses and contacts), could be seen to press their governments to take steps that would allow them to maintain the status quo (such as lifting lockdowns, unfreezing the economy, and providing fiscal stimuli; Haslam et al., 2020).

All kinds of social divisions can prevent the fulfillment of a group's potential. People who perceive themselves to be members of an unattractive (stigmatized or underprivileged) group, when faced with difficulty, tend to choose individual strategies, since they know their group will not provide them with appropriate support. For this reason, they often turn away from their in-group, and fail to cooperate with its members. For example, women who experience various forms of sexism are unlikely to engage in joint efforts to improve women's status. Instead, they strive to find their place in a world ruled by men. This mindset of being a member of an inferior group – or one that is simply underprivileged in the current context – can be disastrous in times of crisis because it prevents people from seeing themselves as group members with a shared social identity, which makes it less likely they will work for the common good (Drury, 2012). These chosen strategies are not just individual ones but are also oriented toward acting in their own self-interest and pursuing their own individual goals, with no consideration for other people's needs. Notably, in times of crisis, the "nation" category frequently becomes a significant and inalienable entity, and possesses great motivational potential. However, if the nation is narrowly defined by those in power in such a way that many groups are excluded from it (atheists, leftists, the green left, the homonormative), or exclude themselves (underprivileged groups), it is hard to build community and make use of its potential by invoking this category in a crisis situation. According to Haslam and colleagues (2020), social identity may be used to influence society by making it more cohesive, activating collective action, and shaping positive intergroup relations.

It should be noted, however, that a sense of community has some negative aspects, too, especially when the community is threatened (by a disease or a financial crisis). We know that threats to the in-group tend to decrease outgroup tolerance (Haslam et al., 2020). During the COVID-19 pandemic, we were witness to violent attacks on Asians in Italy and the US. This type of risk can be expected to increase in the future, fuelled by politicians endeavouring to explain the negative effects of the pandemic, and hunting for scapegoats and excuses for their own inadequacies. One way of doing so is to point fingers at certain aliens (e.g., the Chinese as the culprit behind "the Wuhan virus"). In fact, a threat to the in-group leads to generalized biases against various groups, as well as institutions that were clearly unprepared for the pandemic (the European Union). The upshot of this is that we can anticipate increased xenophobic and anti-EU behaviour.

Still, the threat can be utilized for the common good, but this would require courageous, effective, and prudent leaders. By including others who are suffering (human beings, Europeans) in the "us" category, leaders can show how we can unite in the fight against the virus and how we can come to each other's aid instead of competing for resources. All this necessitates coordinated efforts of individuals, communities, and governments, carried out in a spirit of goodwill. Happily, joint efforts of this kind have already been undertaken. As laudable as such individual efforts are, it is clear that without cooperative, unity-building activities at the governmental level, the desired outcomes will not be produced at the scale needed.

In this context, it is also worth taking into consideration affective factors, such as moral emotions (Schnall et al., 2008) and the sense of existential threat (Becker, 1973). We know, for instance, that the fear of contracting a virus leads to disgust, which, in turn, is manifested as increased judgement of others (as being more ungenerous, insensitive, and lacking in empathy). We may, therefore, find messages concerned with offering assistance to others

52 *Individuals, Groups, and Society in Pandemics*

to be less effective than anticipated, especially when these "others" are the potential casualties of the pandemic. Conversely, if such moral emotions as compassion, or a set of feelings known as "moral elevation", are successfully evoked, prosocial behaviour may arise (Schnall and Roper, 2012). Moral role models (such as celebrities, artists, and other highly respected people) play an important role in inspiring others to mimic such behaviour; consider the example of the European footballer Robert Lewandowski and his wife Anna, who donated 1,000,000 EUR to the fight against the coronavirus.

A second affective factor is the experience of existential threat caused by exposure to information about COVID-19 deaths, which leads not only to clinical symptoms of anxiety disorders (US data) but also to collective efforts to protect the in-group (Wohl et al., 2012; Tabri et al., 2020). This goes some way to explaining why people stock up on supplies (so that their in-group members, their family, do not run out of food and other essentials). It is also the reason for persistent violations of lockdown rules by members of groups who dismiss this preventative measure as ineffective (for example, teenagers at parties). In a highly polarized society, it may also cause deeper divides and increased biases, discrimination, and exclusion, which may lead us to expect a higher level of social aggression. On the other hand, the sense of an existential threat can also be used for promoting collective prosocial efforts to protect broadly defined in-groups (Europeans, humans), and initiating such behaviours is where religious leaders, for instance, could play a significant role.

During a pandemic, it is not only outgroups who may threaten us. Our loved ones can also pose a threat, and coming from this subset of in-group members (i.e., people we are close to), these threats are highly dangerous as they damage solidarity, trust, and cooperation. Analyses of past pandemics show that when people become suspicious of their family and friends, social bonds are weakened and in-group identification decreases. This dis-identification can be understood as an inclination to psychologically distance oneself from the threatened in-group; this phenomenon is most clearly seen in those who were not previously closely related to the group (Greenaway et al., 2015; Sani, 2008).

Shared social identity decreases risk perception and increases risk taking. This was demonstrated by an analysis of people's behaviour during the HIV pandemic (Hammer et al., 1996). It turned out people were less careful when their sex partner was someone they trusted and felt close to. Similar behaviour can be observed nowadays, for instance, at mass gatherings, which, despite knowing they act as sources of infectious disease outbreaks, we show little wariness of attending when such events are organized by people we trust (i.e., members of our in-group; Pandey et al., 2013). This is due to the fact that we do not perceive our in-group as risk-related, but rather perceive it as a source of safety, comfort, and wellbeing (Cruwys et al., 2019; Novelli et al., 2010). In addition, the moral emotion of disgust is less likely to be evoked toward our in-group members.

2.2 COMPLIANCE, MIMICKING, AND FOLLOWING, OR HOW TO INFLUENCE GROUPS

In times of crisis, it is essential that people behave in accordance with directives from leaders, authority figures, or others in power (Cialdini and Goldstein, 2004; Uhl-Bien et al., 2014). Compliant behaviour of this kind is more likely to occur when people see society's problems as their own, see others adhering to the rules, and trust those in power. Conventionally, it was believed that people automatically obeyed those in authority (Milgram, 1974), the assumption being that, simply by dint of the overwhelming influence of authority, actions would be carried out unquestioningly, thoughtlessly, and instinctively. Recent studies have shown, however, that people will only follow instructions when they trust the authority, identify with others (the group), and consider the goal to be worth sacrificing their own self-interest for (Haslam et al., 2004; Dolinski and Grzyb, 2017; Haslam and Reicher, 2017). Hence, instead of merely issuing a directive, it is better to appeal to their group sensitivity by demonstrating to them that a specific behaviour is in the interest of a group they are committed to (Tyler and Blader, 2003). Research also shows that rule adherence is motivated by identification with the authority or the institution that the policy in question applies to (Bradford et al., 2015). It is also promoted by internalization of tax law rules (Hartner et al., 2010) and organization rules (Blader and Tyler, 2009). Similar effects will undoubtedly occur during a crisis such as a pandemic, as will be discussed in more detail in Chapter 3.

In order to reduce virus transmission during a pandemic, behaviours and habits must undergo change, and a key factor in making this change possible is adherence to social norms. Research has documented the effects of social norms on a variety of behaviours, such as donating money to charitable causes (van Teunenbroek and Bekkers, 2020), alcohol consumption (Bruckner et al., 2011), waste sorting (Cialdini et al., 1990), water conservation (Ferraro and Price, 2013), and risky driving (Simons-Morton et al., 2014), among others. We know social norms strongly influence human behaviour: People closely watch the activities of others, and what meets with approval (or not) becomes a major factor in individual choices (Cialdini et al., 1990; Thøgersen, 2008; Wenzel, 2004). This phenomenon, referred to as informational influence, emerges more powerfully under threat and uncertainty, and when the outcome of a behaviour is critical to the actor. Normative influence, in turn, occurs when people engage in certain behaviours to obtain social approval, and is related to higher conformity. In this context, any information about norm violations, especially by in-group members, is deleterious, as it suggests such behaviour not only readily occurs but also is fully accepted. Therefore, the promotion of positive health behaviours (such as hand washing or avoiding contact with others) will only be successful if a group has a well-established belief that these practices are effective. However, if a group (for example,

54   *Individuals, Groups, and Society in Pandemics*

elderly people) holds a widespread belief that these measures are ineffective, any such promotion will fail to make a difference. In a divided society, different groups hold to different norms which they consider important, and thus adhere and conform to, due to the fact that norms are closely related to social and political identities. Hence, different norm models should be developed for different groups (for the young, the elderly, office workers, drivers, etc.) while bearing in mind that political divides matter, too.

Research also shows that messages about norms that are supposed to develop over time (dynamic norms) are effective in promoting behaviour change (Sparkman and Walton, 2017). In other words, messages aiming to encourage specific behaviours should suggest that what is required today will become a norm in the near future. This is especially important during a pandemic, when we are asked to engage in behaviours that are completely new and not commonly accepted.

Psychology has a long tradition of seeing human beings as irrational, driven by emotions, impulsive, and, what is more, affected by cognitive limitations. For years, the metaphor of the cognitive miser, who always tries to minimize the amount of cognitive effort (Fiske and Taylor, 1984), was popular in the field. Later it was demonstrated that humans were rather motivated tacticians, able to shift between different modes of behaviour depending on their motivation (Kruglanski, 1989b; Gigerenzer, 2018). The first of these two perspectives has been recently adopted by behavioural economics, which argues that while human beings are irrational, their irrationality can be used to serve the common good (in accordance with the rules or the policy that is being implemented; Thaler and Sunstein, 2003). This approach suggests individuals should make choices, but their choices need to be guided, since people are incapable of making the right decisions on their own. Their behaviour can be successfully influenced by using subtle reinforcements, called nudges, that is, through an appropriate arrangement of cues and stimuli in the environment. These nudge techniques, proposed in the 1980s by Robert Cialdini (1984) in his book titled *Influence: The New Psychology of Modern Persuasion*, have been used to attempt to motivate people to sort their waste, to save money for retirement, or to consent to organ donation. Recently, Capraro and colleagues (2019) have demonstrated the effectiveness of such moral nudges. In their experiments, subjects were encouraged to engage in prosocial behaviour, but before making the actual choice, they were asked to think about what the morally right thing to do was. The authors also showed that the effects of moral nudges were not limited to an immediate increase in altruistic behaviour; the positive tendencies persisted over time and spilt across contexts. This is a notable finding because earlier studies had suggested that, even when people did a good deed for others, they were inclined to be selfish in their subsequent behaviour (or in future contexts) – and vice versa (Sachdeva et al., 2009; Blanken et al., 2015). The reason underlying this tendency is that prosocial behaviour is typically costly and its maintenance requires proper self-regulation, something which is missing or significantly impeded in real-life situations. However, the role of religious faith runs counter to this prevailing everyday force, since moral nudges, by definition, refer to morality. Thus, nudge techniques that shape behaviour can be particularly effective in a highly religious society (e.g., Poland).

During a pandemic, nudges can be implemented to motivate people to wash their hands frequently, maintain social distance, stay at home, avoid shaking hands, shun large gatherings, and self-isolate when they suspect they may be infected. But while these techniques work for straightforward behaviours (Thaler and Sunstein, 2009), their effectiveness has not been proven in dealing with complex problems because radical behaviour change requires identity-based norm internalization, and nudges do not allow this to happen (Mols et al., 2015). Thus, nudges can be used to elicit a specific behaviour, but they do not lead to profound, lasting change. The latter has to be based on people's engagement in collective efforts, organized around a shared meaning. Without norm internalization (as mentioned earlier), we will return to our old habits as soon as the choice architecture changes. For example, people will sanitize their hands as long as a dispenser is installed at the entrance of a premises, but will discontinue the habit in its absence. What is more, even if certain norms have been established, people may still fail to do what is expected of them.

Effective interventions should aim to reinforce the desired behaviours and engage people in new ones, based on what really matters to them. One main approach deployed to produce such changes in behaviour is through reference to relevant and valued group memberships, since it is only when people define themselves as group members and believe certain norms are vital to the group, and essential for its survival in the future, that they are motivated to work strenuously to change their behaviour (Cruwys et al., 2021). Advocates of this approach recommend leaders should not treat people as passive followers (which is consistent with the logic of nudging), but rather as autonomous individuals whose power becomes clearly visible when they join forces to achieve goals important not just to them as individuals, but also to the group as a whole (Steffens et al., 2018).

Leaders are of paramount importance in times of crisis since we seek guidance in situations of confusion and uncertainty (Turner, 1991) and pay attention to how society around us reacts. So, during a crisis, an effective leader creates a shared group identity and fosters the related feeling that "we are in it together". Fine examples of community building during the current pandemic have been notably provided by female leaders: Mette Frederiksen (Denmark), Sanny Martin (Finland), and Erny Solberg (Norway; Tu, 2020). The sense that the crisis is affecting everyone to the same extent is vital, as it encourages people to consider sacrificing their personal goals for the community. An instance of this is the directive to wear face masks, which is meant to protect others more than individuals themselves.

56 *Individuals, Groups, and Society in Pandemics*

A leader's influence is effective when:

- We deem the leader to be acting in the interests of the community rather than for the favoured few (Jacinda Ardern, New Zealand's Prime Minister, serves as a positive example here; Deutsche Welle DW news, 2020; *Guardian News*, 2020). Positioning oneself above society is perceived negatively, as illustrated several times during the pandemic, including when Jarosław Kaczyński, the leader of Poland's ruling party, paid his respects at his brother's (the late President Lech Kaczyński's) tomb in a cemetery closed to the general public (including those who lost their loved ones in the same presidential plane crash in 2010); when Catherine Calderwood, Scotland's Chief Medical Officer, was seen out walking after instructing her department's staff not to; and when David Clark, New Zealand's Health Minister, went mountain biking, breaking the rules of the country's lockdown (McKay, 2020).
- The leader's actions and efforts ensure we fully comprehend the meaning of what is happening around us (Jetten et al., 2020; Muldoon et al., 2019; Williams and Drury, 2009).
- The leader can be seen to be making key decisions, using expert knowledge, drawing conclusions from comparable situations in the past, and taking preventative steps for the future (Boin et al., 2013).
- The leader is known to take responsibility for his or her actions (Haslam et al., 2020).

A threat such as the COVID-19 pandemic has negative consequences, but if appropriately channeled and/or managed, it can also have positive effects. This requires social trust (in institutions and the government), which is low in many societies. Although restoring trust in the government among a significant number of people will in all probability be infeasible, exemplary leadership could facilitate this process. Happily, a relatively brief period is required to rebuild trust in various social groups (increased trust in physicians/scientists has already been noted) and toward certain institutions (such as emergency and rescue services).

2.3 COOPERATION: COMMUNAL AND INDIVIDUALISTIC ORIENTATIONS

Handling any crisis requires coordinated cooperation at multiple levels: individual, group, and societal. Cooperation is far from easy and is quite unlikely to occur spontaneously, as such behaviour requires people to bear some costs for the benefit of others (Nowak, 2006) and to put others' interests ahead of their own (Van Lange et al., 2018). Typical strategies employed to promote cooperation involve rewarding those who cooperate (Rand and Nowak, 2013) and punishing those who fail to do so (Yamagishi, 1986). Although these methods are expensive, time-consuming, and demand a great deal of focused attention, we naturally cooperate with our kin (a reasonable strategy from an evolutionary perspective) and members of groups we identify with. Cooperation is also engendered when we believe others act accordingly and we perceive mutual aid as a norm which determines our in-group's wellbeing or survival (Fischbacher et al., 2009; Kraft-Todd et al., 2015).

Confronted with the current pandemic-related threat, community plays a valuable role in helping people cope with uncertainty, both materially and symbolically. The material aspect involves supporting each other, in particular, financially. Research (Weber and Hsee, 2000) that compared high-risk behaviours in communities living in collectivist and individualistic cultures found that members of the former (the Chinese) were willing to take higher financial risks than members of the latter (Americans). To interpret these findings, Weber and Hsee (1999, 2000) proposed the cushion hypothesis, according to which, in collectivist cultures (compared to individualistic ones) individuals have wider and more reliable social networks (Hofstede, 2001; Hofstede et al., 2010), enabling them to rely on others' support in the event of a loss (see also Choi et al., 2008; Illiashenko, 2019). This idea has been supported by more recent studies (Schneider et al., 2017), which suggest that, even in a highly individualistic country such as the United States, differences in financial risk taking are related to differences in the strength of social networks. The stronger an individual's social network, the higher their willingness to accept risk. In their models of interpersonal relationships, both Clark and Mills (1993, 2012), and Fiske (1992, 2004) emphasize that people's willingness to engage in altruistic, selfless helping behaviour, without expecting any reward or reciprocity, and without calculating whether such reciprocal gestures (if any) will be comparable to the original behaviour, is a prototypical value of a community. It is worth remembering that communal support can also be symbolic. Communal orientation is inseparably linked to experiencing such emotions as elevation, love, or compassion – feelings that create and strengthen interpersonal bonds, and become a source of support when individuals are under threat (Fiske, 2019; Fraley, 2019; Mikulincer and Shaver, 2017; Fiske et al., 2017; Seibt et al., 2018).

These psychological characteristics of the communal orientation support the intuitive belief that it can play a critical role in coping with epidemic-related uncertainty. This applies to regulating both health protective behaviours and behaviours that reduce economic risks. Communal support seems particularly important during forced isolation or when individuals experience a sense of dread caused by the chronic fear of contracting the disease. In economic terms, the community may provide material or emotional support when people lose their jobs or have to suspend a business activity that represents their basic source of income.

Still, communal orientation is merely one of several different ways of shaping interpersonal relationships, i.e., one of many possible social orientations. Apart from the communal orientation, psychologists and anthropologists describe the exchange or market pricing orientation (Clark and Mills, 1993, 2012; Fiske, 1992, 2004; Fiske and Haslam, 2005; Rai and Fiske, 2011), which involves applying business thinking to non-business domains, such as marriage (Clark et al., 2010; Halawa and Olcon-Kubicka, 2018). An individual interprets the exchange processes as an investment, and focuses primarily on its rate of return ("Will the relationship be profitable for me?", "How much can I gain from this?"). According to Fiske (1992), a prototypical attribute of exchange (or market pricing) orientation is the proportionality of the expenditure–outcome relationship, regardless of how expenditures are measured (as money, time, effort, psychological support, etc.). While communal orientation emphasizes emotion and affection, exchange orientation values logic and rationality.

Research shows that both types of social orientation may be activated in response to changing external conditions (Gasiorowska and Zaleskiewicz, 2020; Zaleskiewicz, Gasiorowska et al., 2020; Zaleskiewicz et al., 2017; Lodder et al., 2019; Vohs, 2015). Interestingly, exchange relationship orientation increases when people experience uncertainty and a lack of control. For example, in a series of experiments by Gasiorowska and Zaleskiewicz (2020), when subjects were reminded, even subtly, that in some situations the course of events were beyond their control, their social preferences shifted toward being more exchange oriented. Other studies have found that the exchange orientation in interpersonal relationships has a negative effect on people's emotional functioning (Jiang et al., 2014; Ma-Kellams and Blascovich, 2013; Mead and Stuppy, 2014; Vohs, 2015). As demonstrated by Molinsky, Grant, and Margolis (2012), the activation of market pricing orientation in social relationships reduces compassionate behaviour, even leading people to perceive the expression of compassion in an organizational context as unprofessional.

We encounter a paradox here. On the one hand, we anticipate that the trauma related to the pandemic, and to any substantial economic risks, will be reduced by an enhanced communal orientation, characterized by the willingness to provide help and emotional support. Numerous studies bear this expectation out. Other experiments, however, indicate the opposite effect may occur: Uncertainty and a perceived lack of control, both natural consequences of an unpredictable epidemic-related situation, may increase the individualistic and unemotional exchange orientation, which is more associated with a tendency to calculate and pursue one's own self-interest. In a crisis, activation of either the communal orientation (focused on mutual help and cooperation) or the individualistic orientation (characterized by conflict and competitiveness) can emerge and it is the group's characteristics, norms, and shared values that will automatically influence which of the two prevails. Through appropriate management of the group process, however, every group's energy can be redirected toward the common good, and toward activating the group's full potential. Achieving this demands outstanding leadership and social trust, a subject we will return to in the next section.

2.4 WHEN GROUP COMMITMENT IS LOW

A lack of social identification may have the detrimental effect of cultivating conspiracy theories or beliefs that some powerful forces are vying to dominate the world. These beliefs hold explanatory power about the reasons for events, the beneficiaries, and the blame-worthy perpetrators (Weigmann, 2018). Conspiracy theories are surprisingly resistant to criticism since they postulate that conspirators act secretly and use disinformation to cover up their actions, so that even those who make efforts to debunk conspiracy theories may themselves be seen to form a part of the conspiracy (Douglas et al., 2017). Significantly, individuals prone to conspiratorial thinking feel weak and powerless (van Prooijen, 2017), have a lower sense of control (Bruder et al., 2013), and trust in people and institutions less (Goertzel, 1994). In general, they are less likely to identify with their own society, and more liable to be outsiders. Among the beliefs they espouse are that positive social norms and values have lost their regulatory quality, and that the world is now a treacherous place (Moulding et al., 2016). Haslam and colleagues (2020) have shown that conspiracy beliefs are associated with a lack of trust in governmental COVID-19 policies (in Australia, the UK, and the US), feelings of loneliness induced by isolation, and pandemic-related stress. What is abundantly clear is that, even though conspiracy thinking emerges in times of uncertainty, it comes about as a result of weak social identification and may lead to further alienation, lower social trust, and disruption of social bonds (Haslam et al., 2018), all of which are particularly harmful during a crisis. To make matters worse, conspiracy theories are also reinforced by such influences as propaganda, disinformation, and historical lies (van Prooijen, 2019).

Polarization is another barrier to coordinated action in any circumstances, but it is particularly damaging in a crisis, for a slew of reasons. First, uncertainty reinforces social differences and, consequently, the perception of these differences. In fact, polarization is regularly perceived as higher than it actually is, and these perceptions then impact people's behaviour (Enders and Armaly, 2019). Second, a polarized society is reluctant to engage in cooperative efforts, and lacks an understanding of the idea of the common good since it appears not to exist; instead, what seems to prevail are the interests of those supporting a particular political party. Third, polarization causes some people not to adhere to the restrictions imposed by their political opponents.

There are two dimensions to polarization. The first one involves attitudes toward issues that differentiate people with specific political views, and supporters of differing political parties. Incredibly, COVID-19 became a political issue in many countries (Pennycook et al., 2020), including Poland, where it featured in the recent presidential campaign. The second dimension concerns emotions (affective polarization) such as appeal, trust, and respect. This type of polarization means that anything consistent with the policy and opinions of the party we identify with feels better, more appropriate, and more exemplary, whereas things suggested by our political opponents feel objectionable (Kahan, 2017; Van Bavel and Pereira, 2018). Affective polarization decreases trust, including trust in information from a politically unsupported source, and, thus, contributes to the rejection of essential public health guidelines (Hetherington and Weiler, 2015). Kossowska, Szwed, and Czarnek (2020) have demonstrated in the Polish context that political beliefs and strong party

60 *Individuals, Groups, and Society in Pandemics*

identification lead to biased perceptions of reality, consistent with the official party narrative. A number of psychological mechanisms activated and reinforced by polarization have been described. The first one is the fit principle (Oakes et al., 1994), that is, interpreting the coronavirus threat in terms of an in-group–outgroup conflict ("us" versus "them"), or seeing the disease and everything that is related to it through the lens of party identification. Another mechanism is party identity protective cognition (Kahan, 2017), leading to perception biases (see Kossowska, Szwed, & Czarnek, 2020). For example, in the United States, Republicans are more concerned about their civil rights and liberties being violated than they are fearful of the virus, resulting in reduced adherence to COVID-19 restrictions (Allcott et al., 2020; Butchireddygari, 2020). Similarly, in Poland people with left-wing beliefs fear the coronavirus outbreak more and are thus more likely to comply with COVID-19 guidelines, as long as these guidelines are based on expert knowledge related to the spread of the virus (Kossowska et al., 2021). We should bear in mind that polarization also heats up public emotions, increases intergroup conflict and tension, erodes social trust and solidarity (Arvan, 2019; Enders and Armaly, 2019), and leads to a sense of anomie whereby people stop seeing themselves as members of a community (Liu and Hilton, 2005).

2.5 COLLECTIVE BEHAVIOUR: PROTESTS

Dissatisfaction with social and economic conditions may sometimes erupt into social unrest (protests, riots, demonstrations). According to Besta and colleagues (2019), social mobilization can only occur when people make appropriate social comparisons, notice their disadvantaged situation and the resulting deprivation, and perceive it as outrageously unfair. Protests are most likely to be initiated not by those who are truly struggling, but rather by those whose situation has become slightly worse, who have then noticed the negative change and consider it unjust. So, social unrest begins with relative deprivation among a small section of the population (Smith et al., 2012), but then the probability of people taking action rises when this feeling pertains to the entire group (not just individuals), and when the perception of unfair deprivation is accompanied by anger (Smith et al., 2012; van Zomeren et al., 2008). Unlike other negative emotions, such as sadness or fear, anger motivates behaviours that may change the undesirable situation. Counterintuitively perhaps, research shows that anger is likely to result in legitimate, normative behaviours, such as taking part in demonstrations or signing petitions, and not necessarily to actions that violate social norms (Tausch et al., 2011; Besta et al., 2019).

In addition, the more group members identify with their in-group, the stronger their sense of injustice related to the group's disadvantaged situation. This means that individuals who strongly identify with their group are not only more inclined to take action due to concern about their in-group, but also subjectively perceive the situation as more negative, which additionally boosts their motivation to change the status quo (Kawakami and Dion, 1995).

Compared to individuals with lower in-group identification, they also have a firmer belief that collective action can alter the situation. Finally, research has found that the relationship between social identity and engagement is bidirectional, that is, not only does group identification lead to higher engagement, but higher engagement in actions for one's group also promotes stronger group identification (Klandermans, 2002). This is relevant to our discussion of the pandemic and its effects since fear and uncertainty experienced during a crisis facilitate social mobilization. Nevertheless, it is worth knowing when mobilization culminates in real change, and when it merely brings about chaos and destruction in society.

Politicized identity is an especially strong predictor of collective action (van Zomeren et al., 2008). Politicization of identities occurs when group members start to realize they are involved in power relations within society and become aware that another group possesses more power and control. This comes with the recognition that the status quo can only be improved by transforming the power structure, and thus their motivation is sparked to engage in collective action to bring about such change (Radke et al., 2016; Simon and Klandermans, 2001; Sturmer and Simon, 2004). Researches describe two mechanisms by which politicized identities foster collective action. First, identifying with a specific social movement enhances our understanding of the political situation, which makes injustice more readily noticeable, enables us to identify actors responsible for it, and then devise possible remedies. Second, politicized identities strengthen the belief that protest and other actions of the sort have a chance at succeeding. The significance of politicized identities has also been demonstrated for collective action in solidarity with an outgroup (for example, a vulnerable or disadvantaged one). When politics permeates every aspect of people's lives – as in Poland or the United States – this type of identity becomes particularly salient, releasing group energy. We have seen this with demonstrations in Poland (entrepreneurs demanding to be treated more seriously by the government during the pandemic crisis) and in the United States (where there have been protests against the introduction of pandemic-related restrictions).

Studies on the collective identity of disadvantaged groups (Klandermans, 2000; Simon and Klandermans, 2001; Vollhardt, 2015) confirm that when members of various underprivileged groups notice similarities between themselves, they are more liable to solidarize and act in another group's interest (Subašić et al., 2011). For example, becoming aware of racism experienced by one's own group leads to increased openness, and feelings of closeness and sharing a common fate with other groups suffering ethnic discrimination (Craig and Richeson, 2012). Disadvantaged groups may be joined by privileged ones, when the latter become cognizant of the injustice experienced by members of the former. This can only happen, though, if they come to recognize the faults of the system they inhabit, a realization which is quite unlikely to occur as members of privileged groups customarily fail to notice their own privilege (Kraus et al., 2017).

Collective action in support of outgroups can also result from identification with all human beings, referred to as global identity (McFarland et al.,

62   *Individuals, Groups, and Society in Pandemics*

2019). In this case, the reference group is all humankind, without differentiating between ethnic or national groups. The development of this type of identity is determined by both personality and environmental factors. Global human identification is promoted by openness to experience, empathy, and universalism (Hamer et al., 2019). Other contributing factors include intercultural contact (Sparkman and Eidelman, 2018), norms accepted in one's everyday environment, and global awareness (Reysen and Katzarska-Miller, 2013). People's engagement and commitment to a particular cause is also determined by their social circles and networks (Besta et al., 2019).

Protests are not always organized but rather break out spontaneously. Living in a state of continuous threat leads to the probability of social turmoil becoming higher. Riots are likely to be provoked in response to specific actions taken by the government or law enforcement agencies: use of force, flouting norms, or blatantly unfair treatment of certain persons. In a crowd, people will commit acts they would never do on their own. Historically, Le Bon (1985) believed one's individual self was lost in a crowd, which in turn results in the loss of the standards of evaluation responsible for making people's behaviour rational and norm compliant. Today, we know this is not true (McPhail, 2017; Reicher, 2001). What happens in a crowd of people does not result from random events. Naturally, violence and conflict may flare up, but they are the exception rather than the rule (Barrows, 1981). In fact, even the most violent of crowds behaves in an orderly, patterned way, and their behaviour can be seen to be socially meaningful (Davis, 1973).

It seems, however, that contrary to Le Bon's argument, people do not act devoid of standards or limitations but in accordance with collective standards, and shared identity and morality. Reicher (1984, 1987) posits that our identity is not "lost in the crowd", but rather there is a shift from an individual to a social identity. Thus, the standards regulating our behaviour do not drop dramatically. Instead, other norms, values, and beliefs become salient in a crowd – those specific to a group. It represents a cognitive shift: People start thinking in terms of the group, perceiving themselves as group members that are motivated by a shared understanding of law. There is also a relational shift: People feel closer to each other, initiate conversation, and share their stories and resources. The sharing and social support provided by the group are vital in a crisis. Finally, there is an affective shift – the feelings of closeness, support, and agency are rewarding, and they serve to reduce the negative feelings so common during a crisis. This explains why people may experience negative emotions related to their actual circumstances and, at the same time, positive feelings arising from a sense of community (Hopkins et al., 2019).

Conflict and social divides become activated in a crowd, which is why crowds are likely to turn against another group, such as the police or other demonstrators. However, violence and conflict are not inherent attributes of a crowd, but may become such depending on the crowd's values or beliefs. While the annihilation of the opposing group is a value for certain groups (for example, football hooligans versus the police), it is not necessarily a universal feature. In fact, there is always some kind of interaction between the parties (Neville and Reicher, 2018). Still, clear social divides promote violence, as illustrated by the police's violent behaviour during the protests by entrepreneurs in Warsaw (in May 2020) against ineffective state support during the pandemic (Siałkowski and Krawczyk, 2020).

2.6 PERCEPTION OF SOCIAL INEQUALITIES

History tells us that the poor are hardest hit by pandemics (Hays, 2005; Jetten and Peters, 2019), and the COVID-19 pandemic follows this pattern. The poor are at a higher risk of contracting and dying from the disease, and they experience more pandemic-related stress (Faheem et al., 2020). To compound matters, they are also more likely to fall prey to misinformation and, as a result, to ignore health recommendations (Pirisi, 2000). Finally, they are less able to comply with restrictions designed to protect citizens' health, such as performing remote work or social distancing (Bedford et al., 2020). Therefore, it is essential that limited resources, aid, and support reach the poorest in society.

Social inequalities and rising poverty are highly probable long-term effects of the current pandemic. It has already been estimated that for any one percentage point decline in the global economy, more than 10 million people worldwide fall into poverty (International Food Policy Research Institute, 2020). We know economic inequalities have a negative effect on wellbeing (Helliwell and Huang, 2008; Lillard et al., 2015; Oishi et al., 2011) and damage intergroup relations, thus hindering the maintenance and development of harmonious social relationships. This is due to the fact that inequality increases perceived intergroup differences in wealth, status, power, and influence (Wilkinson and Pickett, 2010; Jaśko and Kossowska, 2013). With growing inequality, wealth becomes the basis for social evaluations, which results in frequent intergroup comparisons and leads to a clear in-group–outgroup categorization ("us" versus "them"; Cheung and Lucas, 2016). This contributes to lower cooperation and increased competitiveness among individuals and groups, a decline in intergroup trust, and higher levels of violence and social unrest (Nishi et al., 2015; Elgar, 2010; Dorling and Lee, 2014). What is more, perceived inequality makes people less likely to see themselves and their group as an integral part of a society that is going through a crisis and overcoming it together (Uslaner and Brown, 2005). Society then splits into subgroups with dissimilar, often conflicting goals, making it difficult to implement a coordinated policy and provide support for every group.

Researchers note that inequalities influence not only the way we perceive social reality (for example, as a zero-sum game – one person's wealth is always linked with another's poverty), but also the value we place on the wealth itself (its desirability stems from its determination of the value of individuals and groups). As a result, individual and group strivings focus on the collection and possession of material goods; even more importantly, ownership becomes an important determinant of the particular value of individuals and groups.

For example, in a study conducted in 27 countries by Durante and colleagues (2017), higher perceived inequality made people see individuals with a higher socioeconomic status (SES) as less warm, and those with a lower SES as less competent. Moreover, excessive stereotyping of groups, higher in countries with objectively greater inequalities, promotes the legitimization of negative attitudes and behaviour toward the poor. Under such circumstances, there is little room for solidarity, assistance, and support for those in need.

In this context, a key aspect of societal inequalities is the perceived fairness of any existing differences. A sense of injustice and unfair treatment is a major motivation to strive for change in the social order (Besta et al., 2019). We know from existing research that inequality is perceived as unfair when (a) boundaries between groups differing in income and wealth are impermeable (so, no matter how hard you try, it is hard to improve your social position and economic status); (b) the social system is unstable; and (c) wealth differences result from illegitimate actions (Jetten et al., 2017). As an example, Davidai and Gilovich (2015) have demonstrated that Americans believe that it is more probable that people advance and become wealthier than that their lives come to be downgraded, and they suffer a loss of their wealth or status. Such perceptions of group mobility may contribute to an underestimation of the level of inequality (Norton and Ariely, 2011) and, thus, to justifications for inequalities (Chambers et al., 2015; Day and Fiske, 2016), which, in turn, leads to their acceptance (Shariff et al., 2016). Research suggests that when inequality is longstanding – that is, the social system is more stable (for example, the caste system in India) – existing inequalities are felt to be more legitimate (Blanchar and Eidelman, 2013). When people perceive that wealth has been gained in legitimate ways, inequalities are seen as justified and fair. However, if they believe inequality has resulted from illicit behaviour (corruption, fraud, exploitation, nepotism, chance, or pure luck), they are more likely to regard it as a social problem (Tyler, 2011). Note that different wealth groups vary in their responses to inequality. For those at the bottom of the wealth hierarchy, a larger gap between the rich and the poor increases a sense of relative deprivation, which in turn fuels resentment and dissatisfaction (Smith et al., 2012). Richer groups are more focused on maintaining and protecting their status and wealth, and one status-protection strategy is to hold a belief in their own superiority, to despise poorer groups and to treat them unequally (Hays and Blader, 2017).

Experiencing uncertainty, which is inherent in any crisis, including a pandemic, leads to increased perceptions of intergroup differences in wealth. Richer groups are perceived as those who have easier access to healthcare, medicines, and scarce goods, and so intergroup differences are seen as threatening, unjustified, and unfair. This leads to increased competition, lower trust, and more negativity in intergroup relations (Jetten et al., 2015). We have already discussed how groups with a strong sense of community fare better in times of disaster. Perceived inequalities lead to each group being left to cope on its own, and so those having more resources (or readier access to resources) do better (Muldoon et al., 2019).

3 SOCIETAL LEVEL

Małgorzata Kossowska, Natalia Letki,
Tomasz Zaleskiewicz, and Szymon Wichary

3.1 INSTITUTIONAL TRUST

Each social relationship progresses more smoothly and effectively when it is based on trust. Trust-based relationships require less expenditure to ensure their effectiveness (enforcement costs; Tyler, 2021). Both theoretical work and empirical research show that trust is a multidimensional phenomenon; it may refer to trust in various institutions and social groups, as well as trust in people in general (Uslaner, 2018; Bauer and Freitag, 2018; Newton et al., 2018). Indicators of institutional trust used interchangeably in empirical studies include trust in various institutions, support for the government and other political institutions, and evaluations of their quality and competence. Even though trust has been mentioned earlier in the book, so far, we have mainly discussed the mechanisms of its development. In this section, we will focus on institutional trust – in the state and its institutions.

Trust in institutions can be defined as the confidence that institutions will act in the best interests of citizens (Levi and Sacks, 2009), based on beliefs about their quality and competence (Keele, 2005). These legitimizing beliefs give legitimacy to the actions of the state, particularly a democratic state (Levi and Sacks, 2009). Legitimacy is essential for citizens to be willing to comply with laws and restrictions (Grimes, 2006; Letki, 2006; Marien and Hooghe, 2011), and to support and assist the state in performing its responsibilities (Yang and Holzer, 2006). It is obvious, then, that in the context of attempts to prevent the spread of SARS-CoV-2 and reduce the number of COVID-19 infections and deaths, decision makers' actions can only be effective if the decision makers themselves enjoy trust-based legitimacy. During a pandemic, the situation on the ground is invariably dynamic and unpredictable, characterized by incomplete information about the disease and its consequences. In times of uncertainty, factors that would normally justify the authorities' actions must be substituted by trust in institutions and the state.

Often it is necessary to introduce far-reaching regulations affecting citizens' behaviour, even in their private and professional lives. When personal freedom has to be substantially limited (for example, by imposing restrictions on free movement or a ban on pursuing important life goals such as working,

DOI: 10.4324/9781003254133-5

66   *Individuals, Groups, and Society in Pandemics*

getting married, or attending a loved one's funeral), and if the legitimacy of the state and its institutions is at a low level, this may increase the necessity of the use of coercive measures. This is illustrated by what happened in South Africa in 2007, when protests against poor conditions in forced isolation facilities for tuberculosis patients led to an eruption of violence, and the use of firearms by the police (Baleta, 2007). Research on police legitimacy and the acceptance of the use of force by police shows that legitimacy is a key factor leading to public support for such actions, but only at a reasonable level and in acceptable circumstances (Gerber and Jackson, 2017; Bradford et al., 2017). Still, it is not easy to predict what circumstances will be regarded as "acceptable" by the public, so the use of coercive measures (for example, financial penalties for violating stay-at-home restrictions) should be kept to a minimum. In the short run, coercion can be effective, but when used over a longer period, it will diminish trust in the state and its institutions and, consequently, reduce their legitimacy. In the context of the pandemic, one example of the negative effects of excessive use of force and punishment was the way citizens circumvented the ban on going outside by borrowing other people's dogs for walking, or by organizing gatherings on the pretext of shopping. In such circumstances, people tend to focus on maneuvering their way around restrictions, rather than complying with them. When restrictions are perceived as right and appropriate, then they are not ridiculed and subverted in this way.

Although institutional trust is conceptualized as forming the basis of legitimacy, empirical studies often use it as a measure of legitimacy of the state and its institutions. Other commonly used measures include the levels of compliance and political protest. Both types of behaviour are seen as direct consequences of low legitimacy, so legitimacy constitutes a link between institutional trust and citizens' attitudes toward the state and its institutions. Therefore, on the one hand, the level of compliance with pandemic-related guidelines and restrictions arises from the level of legitimacy of the state and its institutions; on the other, it can be regarded as a useful measure of legitimacy. In hindsight, in the comparison to be made of how the coronavirus pandemic unfolded in various countries, we will be able to analyze the legitimacy of their governments, as gauged by their citizens' compliance with pandemic-related restrictions. That said, the need for controversial regulations may arise at various stages of a pandemic and the concomitant crisis, so it is critical that decision makers' actions do not cause a loss of legitimacy as a result of their implementation.

3.1.1 SOURCES OF INSTITUTIONAL TRUST

Trust in institutions is based on a positive perception of these entities, and this has two dimensions: rational (or calculative) trust, which results from inferring future behaviour from that observed in the past; and relational trust, which is based on the similarity of values and identities (Earle, 2010). The first, rational trust, may reflect commonly available information and/ or direct experience, whereas the second, relational trust, is a source of preconceptions about institutions, and influences their evaluation, which, in effect, is the basis of rational trust. Thus, the level of trust is the sum of evaluation-based trust and identity-based trust (Citrin and Stoker, 2018). In other words, trust in institutions is only partly determined by how well they respond to pandemic- and crisis-related challenges; trust (or the lack of it) is also a reflection of preexisting support (or lack of support) for these institutions. Supporters of a government facing a pandemic will trust it more, on average, than people who voted for opposition parties in the election. Still, even those in support of the government may cease trusting it as a result of their evaluations of the government's policies in response to a crisis.

3.1.2 EVALUATION-BASED TRUST

Evaluation may concern the outcomes of actions (performance) or the quality of procedures and the extent to which they are complied with (procedure). In both cases, citizens' expectations play an important role as a reference point for evaluation. Furthermore, evaluation can be based on direct experience and subjective perceptions of one's own situation, or on second-hand knowledge (for example, from the media). Finally, because of differences in accessibility and perceived responsibilities of institutions at various levels (central or local), in the process of generating trust, there is a disparity between assessments of political institutions compared to those of street-level bureaucracy. With regard to the current pandemic, evaluations of performance will primarily concern the effectiveness of steps taken to reduce the spread of SARS-CoV-2, whereas evaluations of procedure will focus on decision makers' adherence to the rule of law and maintenance of equal handling of citizens (for example, equal access to treatment), as well as the transparency and reliability of information surrounding their actions.

3.1.3 TRUST IN POLITICAL INSTITUTIONS

State institutions (such as the government, parliament, the prime minister, the president, and political parties) are generally perceived in terms of subjective evaluations of national-level politics and its influence on citizens' lives, with media reports being the main source of information about government policies. In other words, citizens have little direct contact with state institutions, so they cannot form their own personal, first-hand views about them, instead having to rely on information supplied by the media. Evaluations of the effectiveness of the government's actions and their influence on people's lives reflect the calculative aspect of trust, but are strongly determined by political or party affiliation (partisan-based evaluation/satisfaction), which in turn corresponds to relational trust. It follows that the same information concerning the positive or negative outcomes of actions taken by the government or its agencies – for example, reports about various restrictions imposed during the pandemic – will be interpreted by people

68   *Individuals, Groups, and Society in Pandemics*

differently, depending on their attitudes toward the government and particular political parties. What makes understanding the sources of the evaluations of institutional effectiveness even more problematic is the fact that individuals make such evaluations considering their own circumstances (for example, having to provide care for their children who are staying home to have online classes) or the situation of the society (the effects of the spread of the coronavirus, or the consequences of a financial crisis expected to be caused by the pandemic). Perceptions of the latter are based on media reports, which are processed by individuals in line with their preexisting attitudes toward the government and its institutions.

Research on forming judgements about policy quality and effectiveness has focused on evaluations of one's own financial situation and the economic situation of the country (Alford and Hibbing, 2004; Rudolph, 2003a, 2003b). Citizens with more positive perceptions of the country's macroeconomic performance place more trust in institutions, especially in the government (Chanley et al., 2000; Ellinas and Lamprianou, 2014; Wroe, 2016), and this effect is stronger in times when economic issues are seen as particularly relevant (Hetherington and Rudolph, 2008). Moreover, the negative effect of poor perceived economic performance is much stronger than the positive effect of good performance (Hetherington and Rudolph, 2015). We can safely assume that the same mechanism of judgement formation will operate during the COVID-19 crisis: People's attention will focus on the government's responses to the pandemic, and, in turn, their subjective perceptions of the effectiveness of these responses will have a particularly strong effect on the level of institutional trust. Additionally, negative evaluations will play a more important part in this process than positive ones. Still, once people become accustomed to the pandemic, trust in institutions will come to be less dependent on evaluations of their performance vis-à-vis the crisis.

Comparisons of personal (egotropic) economic perceptions and perceptions of the state of the country's economy (sociotropic) show that the latter have a slightly stronger effect on the perception of institutions, which is also powerfully influenced by political preferences (Evans and Andersen, 2006; Hansford and Gomez, 2015). The relationship between political preferences and the interpretation of facts also holds true for other policies (for example, immigration, international, military, health, and education; Gaines et al., 2007). Furthermore, if citizens are forced to analyze and interpret complex or ambiguous information, their support (or lack of support) for the government causes their evaluations to be more polarized. When information is unambiguous, supporters and opponents of the government tend to have more closely aligned opinions (Parker-Stephen, 2013). This means the social benefits or costs (for example, protecting certain groups from the virus or a lack of such protections) should have a stronger effect on institutional trust than a person's individual situation. Given the complexity of the reporting on COVID-19, evaluations of the government's responses can be expected to be sharply politically polarized.

Research on how people seek out information needed to make a decision or form a judgement suggests that, in general, information seeking serves to confirm their preexisting opinions rather than check to see if they are valid (Valentino et al., 2009). A literature review on processing and interpreting information about health policy issues in the United States shows that both media messages and their interpretations by the audience are highly politicized, especially when medical information is incomplete or contradictory (Gollust et al., 2020). In experiments on people's satisfaction with institutional responses to a natural disaster such as Hurricane Katrina, the respondents blamed politicians of the opposite party for inadequate preparation for the hurricane. This effect was even more marked when the politicians' party affiliation was known (i.e., politicians of the opposite party were judged more negatively, while those of the supported party were evaluated more positively). Additional information concerning the politician's position and duties reduced the effect of partisan preferences on his or her evaluation, and made it more objective (Malhorta and Kuo, 2008). In the context of COVID-19, where even experts cannot claim to have comprehensive or thorough knowledge of the workings of the disease and the many viral variants, it is no wonder that citizens will be especially prone to processing and interpreting information through the lens of their political or partisan preferences. Those supporting the government will seek media reports confirming that its responses are effective and right, whereas those opposing the government will search for information attesting to the weaknesses and ineffectiveness of current government policies. Research shows that selective information processing, biased in favour of one's preferred candidate or party, is also prevalent in social media (Shin and Thorson, 2017). In other words, through their highly politicized reports about the government's decisions and their effects, the media, often the main source of information about current events, reinforces preexisting stances toward the government and other political institutions, rather than contributing to more objective evaluations of their actions.

While political preferences may serve as a substitute for the evaluation of the caliber of the government and its performance in the context of such complex issues as immigration or health policies, it is actually media coverage of political standards that has a strong, immediate, and far-reaching effect on trust in politicians, and in the system as a whole. Reports of immoral or dishonest behaviour, both in the public sphere (corruption, nepotism) and in private life (sex scandals) have a powerful negative effect on trust in politicians themselves and in the institutions they represent (Bowler and Karp, 2004; Maier, 2011). Therefore, media reports on politicians profiting from pandemic-related decisions (such as the purchase of medical equipment or tests) or violating restrictions they themselves have introduced (for example, breaching the lockdown rules or the requirement to wear masks) may have a particularly dramatic and negative effect on trust in institutions and their representatives (Soroka, 2006). An understanding of how media coverage

70   *Individuals, Groups, and Society in Pandemics*

of political scandals and unethical behaviour influences institutional trust is employed by the media, which uses sensational news around these topics to mobilize or demobilize support for government or opposition-related institutions by appealing to the political preferences of the citizenry.

3.1.4 TRUST IN PUBLIC INSTITUTIONS

Public institutions that citizens have direct contact with are evaluated based on their efficiency, performance, contact quality, and ability to deliver the expected service (Orr and West, 2007), and their perceptions are dependent neither on political or partisan preferences, nor on the election cycle (Jilke, 2018). This explains why local public institutions (street-level bureaucracy) are usually more trusted than central institutions (Rothstein and Stolle, 2003; Wallace and Latcheva, 2006; Jilke, 2018). An individual may have a negative opinion about the functioning of the healthcare system, as an indicator of the government's quality, but, at the same time, have a positive view of the general practitioner or local hospital they have had first-hand experience with. Positive evaluations and trust in local institutions delivering healthcare and public services depend primarily on their availability, efficiency, and quality of service. It is also critical for the authorities to consult with citizens about their decisions, which has a positive effect on their perceived legitimacy and increases people's willingness to comply with the authorities' decisions (Grimes, 2006). It is unclear to what extent evaluations of local institutions influence evaluations of central government, and vice versa (Van de Walle and Bouckaert, 2003).

In the context of a pandemic, decentralization and public consultation in decision making may not be feasible, since so much depends on central co-ordination and effective implementation of measures designed to prevent the spread of the disease. Still, it is institutions at the local level that are responsible for delivering public services related to healthcare and institutional support, as well as for enforcing centrally imposed restrictions and regulations. Any inefficiencies among frontline services, such as the sanitary service, hospitals, or the police, will not only have a negative impact on their perceived quality and citizens' trust in them, but also may be interpreted as reflecting a general weakness of the state.

3.1.5 PROCEDURAL FAIRNESS

A distinct branch of research on the sources of positive evaluations of both political and public institutions focuses on the quality of processes. This means that procedures, and the extent to which they are followed, with a special emphasis on fairness and impartiality, are seen as crucial for the development of institutional trust (Tyler, 2021; Tyler and Huo, 2002; Sunshine and Tyler, 2003). The assumption is that citizens perceive their relationship with the state and its representatives as a psychological contract. Positive

Societal Level 71

perceptions of institutions are influenced more by expending efforts to fulfill the duties arising from this contract than the actual outcome itself (Feld and Frey, 2007). Moreover, studies of citizens' attitudes and behaviour in the context of compliance with the law point to procedural fairness as the main determinant of an institution's legitimacy and, thus, of people's willingness to comply with its regulations. We know that high levels of legitimacy are more effective in motivating citizens to cooperate with the state and its institutions than deterrence. This can be clearly seen in studies on people's willingness to accept a court sentence, comply with police decisions (Esaisson, 2010; White et al., 2016; Mazerolle, Antrobus et al., 2013, Mazerolle, Bennett et al., 2013; Hough et al., 2010), and to cooperate with local authorities (Grimes, 2006). Furthermore, studies consistently show that the fear of sanctions has less of an impact on people's willingness to cooperate than the perceived level of procedural fairness, and at the same time, the latter increases the effect of punishment or legal sanction (Augustyn and Ward, 2015; Verboon and van Dijke, 2011).

Surveys have been used to explore the direct effect of procedural quality on trust in a number of institutions: the police (Nix et al., 2015), government officials (Van Ryzin, 2011), local authorities (Grimes, 2006), and courts (Grootelaar and van den Bos, 2018). Using respondents' subjective evaluations as a measure of procedural quality, these studies have shown that perceptions of procedural standards have a much stronger effect on institutional trust than the actual outcome of the process. Indeed, both experimental studies (Murphy et al., 2014) and those measuring procedural efficacy with objective ecological indicators of institutional quality (such as the World Bank's Worldwide Governance Indicators or the Transparency International Corruption Perceptions Index) support these conclusions (van Ryzin, 2011; van der Meer and Hakhverdian, 2017).

The studies discussed above appear to be of particular relevance to forming positive evaluations and, hence, developing institutional trust in the context of a pandemic. The dynamic and unpredictable situation related to a virus such as SARS-CoV-2, and the resulting necessity to mobilize a variety of the state's and citizens' resources, do not necessarily lead to optimal policy outcomes. If it turns out that certain measures are insufficient or that some key resources have been exhausted, this will inevitably diminish an institution's efficiency and performance. That said, we must bear in mind that one of the key determinants of citizens' evaluations of institutional performance and, consequently, their trust in institutions, is the belief that specific actions were taken in good faith, with due diligence, and in accordance with the law.

When it comes to political institutions and central administrative institutions, the most commonly used indicator of high procedural standards is the level of corruption, that is, the abuse of public resources or offices for personal gain (Kurer, 2005; Hetherington and Rudolph, 2008; Hibbing and Theiss-Morse, 2002). A belief that institutions are corrupt significantly decreases institutional trust, as demonstrated by correlational, comparative, and

72   *Individuals, Groups, and Society in Pandemics*

experimental studies (Villoria et al., 2013; Chang and Chu, 2006; Erlingsson et al., 2016; van der Meer and Hakhverdian, 2017; Wallace and Latcheva, 2006; Ares and Hernández, 2017). It follows, then, that allegations in the media that some individuals or groups have privileged access to COVID-19-related services (such as free tests), or that people with political connections have profited from decisions related to the purchase of medical equipment, may substantially undermine trust in the government and its institutions.

3.1.6 INSTITUTIONAL TRUST UNDER CRISIS

RISK PERCEPTION

Research on the relationship between institutional trust and perceptions of and responses to risk finds that trust in institutions is a significant factor that can account for citizens' attitudes and behaviours, while recognizing the importance of both calculative and relational trust (van der Does et al., 2019). These studies explore different types of risks, for example, natural (floods, hurricanes, and earthquakes), technology, and terrorist risks. Not all of the studies focus on all dimensions of risk, but their findings, in general, demonstrate a negative effect of trust on risk perception. That is, individuals with high levels of trust in institutions responsible for handling risks are less afraid of being directly affected by the risks (Basolo et al., 2009; DeYoung and Peters, 2016; Han et al., 2017). In these studies, while institutional trust did not have an obvious effect on taking preparedness measures, two studies on how institutional trust influences flood risk perception (in the Netherlands and China) demonstrated that high levels of trust in institutions responsible for flood risk management actually decreased citizens' willingness to take individual protective measures and to prepare for the crisis. Their reluctance can be explained by the reduction in the perceived probability of the hazard, and the increase in people's reliance on government support should the crisis occur (Terpstra, 2011; Su et al., 2017). This effect was found for both calculative trust (the evaluation of the quality and capacity of institutions) and relational trust (trust in government). Trust in institutions (measured by a belief that they are competent) has a direct positive effect on people's willingness to prepare for future hazards by purchasing insurance, but, at the same time, decreases it indirectly by having a negative influence on the perceived risks (Peng et al., 2019).

This effect, found for natural hazards, can be also expected to occur during a pandemic: Individuals with higher levels of trust in government and its institutions, and with feelings of confidence about their competence and efficiency, will regard the threat of the virus as less serious and, as a result, may tend to engage in less preparation and preventive behaviour. This may also hold true for any expected government support during the economic crisis, one of the main consequences of the pandemic. Simply put, people will feel less threatened by the crisis if they place great trust in the government's policies for economic assistance.

Societal Level 73

MILITARY OR TERRORIST CRISIS

The literature shows that military or terrorist threats boost trust in political institutions. This phenomenon, known as the rally-round-the-flag effect, is manifested as the massive surge of support for the government and other institutions that occurs as a result of any mobilization in response to dramatic events at the national or international level (Hetherington and Nelson, 2003). This effect was observed in the United States after the September 11, 2001 attacks, when there was a dramatic increase in public approval for President George W. Bush (Hetherington and Nelson, 2003) and trust in government (Chanley, 2002). A quasi-experiment focusing on the 2015 terrorist attacks in France also demonstrated an uptick in trust in government (Coupe, 2017). Further evidence comes from a study on institutional trust in the context of the 2004 attacks in Madrid. This showed that there was a substantial rise in trust levels not only in political institutions, such as the government, the parliament, or political parties, but also in the police, courts, the army, and the media. While the upsurge in trust in political institutions persisted for up to 7 months after the attack, trust in the media grew immediately after the attack (for up to 7 days) but then declined. Increased trust in the army lasted the longest (up to 19 months after the attack; Dinesen and Jaeger, 2013).

What can explain this higher trust in government following terrorist attacks? Research findings indicate that it comes as a result of the increased importance of issues associated with defense and foreign policy, which causes people to perceive the government in terms of these two aspects; however, it has no effect on the perception of other government policies (Hetherington and Husser, 2012). Still, this increase in trust is very important, as it has direct bearing on public approval of higher government expenditure on measures to prevent and combat terrorism (Chanley, 2002). Given the sudden and volatile nature of a pandemic, which can cause a sense of threat analogous to a military attack, its onset is marked by a rise in trust in the government and its institutions, as well as public support for their crisis management policies (Bol et al. 2021; see also section 9.4.5). Indeed, a very recent study, based on panel data from Sweden, shows that the COVID-19 pandemic can be linked to enhanced institutional trust (Esaiasson et al., 2020). Another study, using Dutch data, demonstrates a rallying effect as a result of a national health crisis whereby the severity of the COVID-19 epidemic comes to the fore as the dominant determinant of political trust (Schraff, 2020).

ECONOMIC CRISIS

Research shows that an economic crisis has a clearly negative impact on institutional trust. This is true for both political and public institutions (Ervasti et al., 2019; O'Sullivan et al., 2014), as well as transnational institutions such as the European Parliament (Dotti Sani and Magistro, 2016). Studies of the relationship between trust in EU institutions and in national political institutions have found that support for the EU is largely a reflection of support for and trust in the national government (Armingeon and Ceka, 2014). A decrease in both types of trust as a result of an economic crisis has proved to be the most dramatic in the countries hit hardest by the crisis, especially among the most economically disadvantaged citizens (Dotti Sani and Magistro, 2016; Armingeon and Ceka, 2014; Foster and Frieden, 2017). Finally, a comparison of the effects of evaluations of healthcare and educational institutions, and perceptions of macroeconomic performance, on trust in political institutions during the economic crisis in Greece demonstrated that, while the crisis did not increase the effects of evaluations of macroeconomic performance, it substantially enhanced the impact of evaluations of social welfare institutions on trust (Ellinas and Lamprianou, 2014).

These research findings are critically important in efforts to anticipate how trust and support for the government will be influenced by the economic crisis caused by the pandemic. Although initially a pandemic-related sense of threat led to increased institutional trust, the resulting economic crisis can be expected to decrease it substantially, especially when the direct epidemic risk has subsided and macro- and microeconomic issues become more of a priority for the majority of citizens.

NATURAL CRISIS

A study on institutional trust in the context of Hurricane Katrina demonstrated that levels of trust were contingent on whether the respondent had direct, first-hand experience of the evacuation or was merely an observer exposed to media coverage of the event. This effect varied depending on which institutional level was involved, be it central, federal, or local. Individuals with personal experiences of the evacuation (survivors) showed a higher level of trust in central institutions than those who had viewed it from afar (observers). Of significance is the fact that attention to media coverage increased trust in local institutions and decreased trust in central institutions in both groups, but the effect was stronger for survivors of the hurricane (Reinhardt, 2015). By comparison, when it comes to COVID-19, there are also people directly affected by the epidemic and observers who receive information from media sources. However, a pandemic differs from a natural disaster in that there are no clear procedures and action plans with specific institutional actors responsible for their implementation at the national, regional, or local level. Regulations are frequently created on an *ad hoc* basis in response to the rapidly shifting conditions. Therefore, it is no easy task to determine whether and to what extent conclusions from studies on the dynamics of institutional trust during a natural disaster can be extended to an understanding of the circumstances of the pandemic.

Societal Level 75

PANDEMIC

Past pandemics, such as avian influenza (bird flu) or influenza A (H1N1), provide an insight into the dynamics of institutional trust in a context practically identical in many ways to the COVID-19 crisis. In 2009, a series of telephone surveys were conducted in the Netherlands concerning respondents' perceptions of the country's health situation, sense of health safety, and trust in government. The findings show that trust in government, which was initially high, decreased dramatically over time (after about 3 months) and then remained at a stable, but still relatively high, level (Van der Weerd et al., 2011). The study also found that trust in government had a positive effect on people's willingness to vaccinate, but had no impact on their willingness to engage in additional protective measures, such as adopting special hygiene procedures. This willingness depended primarily on perceived risk, and, as we know, trust in government decreases risk perceptions (as is the case with natural disasters). Still, we should be mindful of the fact that the scale of past pandemics was much more modest, and the attendant social, political, and economic challenges, as well as health risks, were not commensurate to the COVID-19 pandemic. Direct evidence comes from an analysis of survey data from 15 countries of Western Europe, which indicates that trust in government and support for the ruling party (or the prime minister) are strongly negatively related to the number of COVID-19 deaths. Conversely, the introduction of epidemic-related restrictions significantly increases both trust in government and support for the prime minister and the ruling party (Bol et al., 2021).

Research by Albertson and Gadarian (2015) summarizes the relationships discussed in this section. It shows that internal risks (those associated with the government's actions) have a different effect on institutional trust than external risks (such as a pandemic or terrorism). The latter lead to a substantial increase in trust, at least in the short run, whereas the former reduce it, since they are more clearly linked to weak, inefficient, or incoherent government policies.

3.1.7 INSTITUTIONAL TRUST AND COMPLIANCE

Research on the willingness of citizens to obey the law, and adhere to guidelines and regulations imposed by institutions, has focused on the effects of legitimacy and institutional trust as factors that motivate citizens to cooperate, even when the outcomes of cooperation are not entirely beneficial to them. The positive effects of trust and legitimacy offer a constructive alternative to punishment and surveillance. As a consequence, compliance reduces the costs incurred by enforcing citizens' cooperation with the state while ensuring a higher level of such cooperation than would otherwise arise from their sense of moral obligation, or fear of punishment. Scholz and Lubell describe trust in institutions as a heuristic that is necessary for the development of conditional

76 *Individuals, Groups, and Society in Pandemics*

cooperation between citizens and the state, whereby the readiness of citizens to cooperate is contingent on their trust in government institutions and their perceived legitimacy. This model is applied to explain payment of taxes (Scholz and Lubell, 1989; Frey and Torgler, 2007), cooperation with local institutions (Grimes, 2006), support for compliance with the law (Letki, 2006; Marien and Hooghe, 2011), and a willingness to accept institutional decisions, even if they are perceived as unfair or unfavourable (Esaiasson, 2010).

In-depth interviews investigating the effects of Hurricane Katrina revealed that low trust in local and federal institutions was the main cause for non-compliance with the mandatory evacuation order and the rejection of the advice concerning evacuation among residents. Their distrust reflected their lack of confidence in the competency of government officials and their intention to act in citizens' best interests (Cordasco et al., 2007). Comparable conclusions arise from survey research: Institutional trust is the main determinant of people's behaviour under threat (Kim and Oh, 2015). With regard to pandemics, research shows that trust in institutions directly responsible for healthcare (e.g., the ministry of health – Prati et al., 2011; the healthcare system – Rudisill, 2013) has a strong positive effect on their readiness to adhere to restrictions and guidelines. Studies on emergency situations have found that in such circumstances risk perceptions are as important as, if not more important than, institutional trust.

3.2 SOCIAL CAPITAL

There are two basic dimensions of social capital: cognitive (trust and reciprocity norms) and behavioural (networks of interconnections and relationships). Social capital complements the categories of human, economic, and physical capital, and public infrastructure. This means it can be utilized to achieve a variety of individual and collective goals. A related concept, social trust (also known as generalized trust), is trust in people in general, including unfamiliar others. Both theoretically and empirically, trust in others is related to the norm of generalized reciprocity, which moves us to offer assistance without any expectation of direct reciprocation (Putnam, 2000). The sources of social capital are not fully understood: Some see it as a product of socialization (Uslaner, 2002); others as a result of interactions with different people and in different contexts (Glanville and Paxton, 2007); and still others emphasize that whom we trust depends on the culture we grew up in (Delhey et al., 2011). The behavioural dimension – formal and informal social networks – develops spontaneously as a by-product of the social activity of individuals, and the contexts in which they operate (Cattell, 2001; Gesthuizen et al., 2009). Across cultures, these social networks vary in size and structure due to cultural differences in everyday interactions.

With regard to the object of trust and the structure of social networks, social capital is divided into two main categories: bonding and bridging social capital. The former refers to connections within a group, and the latter refers to ties between groups. Both types serve important social functions, but most people prefer interactions with members of their own group (homophily), even though in many circumstances it would be optimal to extend one's social interactions and cooperate with members of other groups (McPherson et al., 2001). Networks are typically seen as two-dimensional, and include formal networks (for example membership in organizations and associations) and informal ones (relationships with friends and family). To understand the status of networks, one should consider the extensiveness and intensiveness of these social networks, that is, what resources they include and what resources they provide access to (Reeskens and van Oorschot, 2014; Letki and Mierina, 2015). All these dimensions with respect to the development and functioning of social networks are significant in that they define the utility of social capital for individuals and groups. Research into the mechanisms of social capital development and the ways it is utilized stresses the relevance of social inequalities, which, on the one hand, determine what resources are present in existing networks and, on the other, what resources are reproduced by social capital (Lin, 2000; Stanton-Salazar and Dornbusch, 1995; Cleaver, 2005).

3.2.1 SOCIAL CAPITAL AS A DETERMINANT OF COMPLIANCE

Trust in others is a key determinant of cooperation in the context of public goods (Fischbacher et al., 2001; Frey and Meier, 2004; Gächter et al., 2004). Of course, a vital public good during a pandemic is public health, which can only be sustained by reducing the spread of the virus. Small groups have mechanisms necessary to effectively monitor and enhance cooperation and adherence to norms and rules in situations where no-one can be excluded from the utilization of certain goods (as discussed earlier). Knowledge concerning the behaviour of other group members, and the ability to influence their behaviour, enables each group member to estimate the probability that the public good in question – in this case, public health – will be created, and, consequently, to assess how reasonable it is to make their own contribution, for example, by complying with the requirement to wear face masks.

This contrasts with situations with very large groups (e.g., society as a whole), in which people remain largely anonymous. Due to the large group size and the lack of direct interactions with most group members, they are deprived of knowledge concerning the behaviour of others, and are unable to monitor or correct others' behaviour. In these circumstances (a large-N situation), since the decision about whether to make an individual contribution to a public good cannot be based on direct observation, trust becomes paramount. In society at large, trust takes over both the informative function (informing us about others' behaviour and the resulting probability that the public good in question will be produced) and the normative function, since beliefs about other people's trustworthy behaviour become the basis for an individual's decisions on what behaviour is appropriate and desirable. Research

78 *Individuals, Groups, and Society in Pandemics*

shows that people's aversion to being perceived as a "leech" is stronger than their aversion to being "played for a sucker" or taken advantage of (Hibbing and Alford, 2004). This tendency, combined with the previously mentioned reciprocity norm, increases the willingness of subjects to behave fairly, that is, to comply with the norms accepted by the majority. When applied to co-operation for a public good, this means that trust, or a belief that others are making their rightful contributions, motivates people to cooperate. Hence, social trust can increase cooperation with state institutions, as long as it in-volves trust in others in the context of adhering to the rules and restrictions imposed by those institutions.

Apart from laboratory and natural experiments (e.g., Fischbacher et al., 2001; Frey and Meier, 2004; Gächter et al., 2004), the positive effect of so-cial trust on individuals' contributions to public goods in large-N situations has been demonstrated in the context of payment of taxes. According to the conditional cooperation model, confidence that other citizens are honest tax-payers is a key element (along with trust in government) of the trust heuristic that makes people significantly more willing to pay taxes (Scholz and Lubell, 1989). Similar conclusions come from studies on pro-environmental behav-iour, which is also strongly determined by social trust (Sønderskov, 2009; 2011; Macias, 2015).

Transposing these observations into the context of the COVID-19 pan-demic is fairly straightforward: Confidence that other members of a com-munity are adhering to pandemic-related guidelines and restrictions is a key factor motivating each individual in the community to comply with these guidelines and restrictions. It should be emphasized, however, that during a pandemic the intended outcome of cooperation may not be achieved, that is, the public good in question may not be successfully created, even if the level of free riding is relatively low. This is due to the specific nature of pandemics, where even relatively few people violating pandemic-related rules may lead to the spread of the disease. Such imbalances do not exist for tax fraud or anti-environmental behaviours.

So, on the one hand, social trust should have a positive effect on compli-ance, as it serves as a heuristic which reinforces behaviours consistent with the public interest; but on the other hand, its effect can be negative since it fosters the illusion that the effectiveness of collective behaviour is unreal-istically high, in this case, for example, that it will lead to the achievement of herd immunity. By doing so, trust in others can decrease perceived risk, leading to opportunistic behaviour ("I don't have to adhere to COVID-19 recommendations, other people's behaviour will protect me"). During a cri-sis, a feeling of being strongly networked can also have a negative impact by instilling a belief that the network of support and mutual help will effec-tively reduce the negative effects of the crisis. As a result, individuals who see themselves as surrounded by strong support networks perceive the crisis as less threatening, and thus may expend less effort in preparing for it or taking measures to prevent it. In fact, this effect has been observed for comparable natural disasters, such as fires or floods (Bihari and Ryan, 2012; Babcicky and Seebauer, 2017).

3.2.2 SOCIAL CAPITAL AS A SOURCE OF SUPPORT AND RESOURCES

According to classical sociological theory, social capital is conceptualized as a resource that can be derived from an individual's social networks (Granovetter, 1983, 2018; Paldam, 2000; Portes, 1998). This means that if we suffer a shortage of resources, we can compensate for this by relying on those of others in our network. These resources include emotional and organizational support, and also information and financial capital. Of course, our social network connections can be weak or strong. It is worth noting that weak ties, due to their heterogeneity (connections with those in distant parts of the social network), are a better source of stratified resources, such as financial capital or information (for example, about employment opportunities), whereas strong ties (e.g., connections with friends and family) provide emergency and emotional support but do not have the potential to facilitate an individuals' social mobility or to help them radically change their life circumstances (Narayan, 1999; Woolcock, 2001). Naturally, access to resources depends on being connected to other people whose resources may be obtained through the network (Burt, 2000; Portes, 1998). For this reason, the size of one's social network is not the sole or even the most crucial criterion for assessing social capital; the actual resources existing among those in the network are of equal importance.

There is no doubt that during a crisis, for example a pandemic-related one, social capital becomes a critical resource for many, since the availability of traditional institutional mechanisms of support may be limited, or may prove inefficient. An instance of this is when school closures during the COVID-19 pandemic meant that distance learning was introduced. At this juncture, access to education became strongly dependent on the resources of a student's family and on its cultural capital. For children living in low-income and poorly educated families, a factor of major importance for their development and education was whether their parents' social connections were capable of ensuring access to such resources as the equipment required to participate in online classes or the skills necessary to provide educational support.

3.2.3 SOCIAL CAPITAL AND WELLBEING

Happiness, life satisfaction, and psychological wellbeing are largely dependent on social capital, both individual and collective (i.e., the social capital of the local community, or another reference group an individual operates within). Due to the strong relationship between psychological wellbeing and

80   *Individuals, Groups, and Society in Pandemics*

physical health, it is difficult to clearly separate the mechanisms that link individual and collective social capital with wellbeing and health, hence studies on both types of wellbeing are discussed together in this section.

Strong ties are a source of social support, that is, emotional, informational, and instrumental support (practical assistance with everyday problems; Szreter and Woolcock, 2004; Umberson and Montez, 2010; Umberson et al., 2010). All three functions become particularly important during a crisis, when the customary ways of obtaining resources are limited or unavailable. That is what happened to families affected by domestic violence, whose members were previously able to use institutional support but lost access to it as a result of lockdown. Although there is no detailed data available on this issue across countries affected by COVID-19, the number of calls to helpline services soared. In addition, in some countries (like France and Spain), special code messages were introduced to be used at grocery stores or pharmacies as signals of domestic violence. The increased use of these coded communications suggest the problem has substantially risen. Social capital (especially strong ties) is of key importance in such circumstances as it can provide psychological and material support, serving, at least partly, as a substitute for standard institutional support.

Social interactions, especially informal ones, can also protect an individual's wellbeing (the various domains of life satisfaction) in unfavourable economic conditions (Colombo et al., 2018; Lahad et al., 2018). Although social trust and informal networks tend to have a positive effect on job satisfaction, this effect was not found in countries most severely affected by the recent economic crisis, such as Greece, Spain, Cyprus, or Ireland (Lange, 2015). This finding is consistent with conclusions reached by another study demonstrating that, under extreme economic stress, the buffering effect of social trust against mental health issues such as depression disappeared (Economou et al., 2014).

In the UK, trust in other people, though made significantly lower as a result of the economic crisis, remained an important factor that improved wellbeing, whereas formal networks had no such effect (Lindström and Giordano, 2016). Similar conclusions were drawn from data collected in new democracies: Even though the effects of social trust on various dimensions of wellbeing were attenuated by the experience of an economic crisis, after the crisis they were still positive and of high statistical significance (Habibov and Afandi, 2015). Also, the social capital of an entire community (studied using measures aggregated at the level of a town or city) substantially contributes to happiness and wellbeing. Formal networking decreases the negative impact of higher unemployment resulting from a crisis (Helliwell et al., 2014).

3.2.4 SOCIAL CAPITAL AND HEALTH

Communities with higher levels of social capital have better indicators of health (Ehsan et al., 2019). This is true for both subjective indicators, for example self-rated health (Kawachi et al., 1999; Mohnen et al., 2011), and objective indicators, such as vaccination coverage and mortality rate (Nagaoka et al., 2012; Rönnerstrand, 2014; Hernandez et al., 2019), based on studies measuring the behavioural, networking aspect of social capital. Research also shows that, although the relationship between social capital and health is positive and occurs regardless of the level of social inequality, it is weaker in neighbourhoods with higher levels of social capital (Islam et al., 2006). This is consistent with research pointing to social capital as providing resources which are particularly important where other types of resources are limited or unequally distributed (Letki and Mierina, 2015).

Research on mechanisms linking social capital with health emphasizes the role of social support provided by strong ties, especially within the family, which significantly reduces mortality by providing direct care and assistance, and also by helping to obtain professional medical care (Shor et al., 2013; Kawachi et al., 1999). Similarly, qualitative studies using in-depth interviews suggest that social networks play an important role in reducing the negative impact of social exclusion on wellbeing and health, but highlight the limited amount and efficiency of social capital in low-status groups. This is in accordance with quantitative research highlighting intergroup inequalities in terms of the richness of their social networks (Cattell, 2001).

Another important factor is the information effect of social capital, although this is a feature of mainly higher-status networks. Research shows that individuals with higher (college) education have more college-educated people in their networks, which has a positive effect on their likelihood of being vaccinated against A/H1N1. The mechanisms accounting for this point to the information effect (network members as sources of high-quality information) and the influence of social ties on attitudes toward vaccination (college-educated individuals, who have more positive attitudes toward vaccination, formed the subjects' social networks), which reinforced the positive effect of the respondents' own educational attainment (Hernandez et al., 2019). The neighbourhood-based social capital of parents, and the resulting health communication strategies, are also important factors reinforcing the effect of knowledge about the A/H1N1 virus, as well as parents' willingness to vaccinate their children (Jung et al., 2013). Other studies have noted the positive effect of social trust (at the ecological level) on immunization uptake, without any empirical verification of the mechanisms linking the two variables (Rönnerstrand, 2014). The influence of networking on health-protective behaviours during an influenza pandemic, such as vaccine uptake, mask wearing, and hand washing, is also positive, but only for informal social networks, that is, networks of local connections with family and friends, measured by the availability of social support. In contrast, formal networks (membership in organizations) have no effect on behaviour in a pandemic (Chuang et al., 2015).

Thus, the relationship between social capital and public health is multidimensional: Not only do strong ties provide psychological support, care, and access to professional services, but they are also a source of happiness and wellbeing associated with a sense of belonging and feeling cared for by our

82   *Individuals, Groups, and Society in Pandemics*

loved ones. In this sense, the effect of social capital is universal. Still, as far as the quality of information in an individual's social network is concerned, it reflects the social status of those in the network. Being apprised of quality information is of key importance for risk perceptions and the person's willingness to comply with pandemic-related measures.

3.2.5 INEQUALITIES IN SOCIAL CAPITAL USE

As mentioned earlier, literature on the use of social capital as a pool of resources emphasizes that the composition of social networks is highly dependent on social position (Lai et al., 1998), and thus their utility is stratified. Lower-status groups rely primarily on strong ties, which are homogeneous, and therefore poor in instrumental resources, such as knowledge, information, or financial capital (Pichler and Wallace, 2009; Letki and Mierina, 2015). This state of affairs is particularly relevant in a crisis, since when there is intense competition for resources, it is social networks, not institutions, that serve as the main means of resource distribution. This has been demonstrated by studies on job hunting or bankruptcy prevention strategies in countries going through a political transformation or an economic crisis (Clarke, 2000; Gerber and Mayorova, 2010; Johnson and Mitton, 2003; Aidis et al., 2008). These studies indicate that members of high-status groups use social capital to maintain or improve their status, whereas resources available in social networks within low-status groups are so modest that they can only go as far as helping people to merely survive. These inequalities in resources within social networks are significant in the context of crisis preparedness, but there is no research showing how critical they could be during a crisis, or in coping with its consequences.

Comparative studies also show that resources obtained from social networks provide cushioning from poverty, especially when welfare state functions become limited. Informal networks (family and friends) may prevent the necessity of lowering one's standard of living or taking out loans during an economic crisis (Reeskens and van Oorschot, 2014). Households varying in social status utilize their networks with different outcomes (Wetterberg, 2007). For those in the lower social classes, strong ties are the main source of social resources, which makes it more difficult for them to access instrumental resources, such as financial capital or information about employment opportunities (Letki and Mierina, 2015). One should remember, however, that owing to its low cost and egalitarian nature, social support available through strong ties becomes particularly important during a crisis.

Given the stratification of social network types, the effect of networking on the spread of viruses deserves special attention. Research on social contacts shows that interactions within strong ties are usually physical, frequent, and of long duration (Mossong et al., 2008; Leung et al., 2017), and as such carry a greater risk of virus transmission. This suggests that the risk of infection during an epidemic of a respiratory tract disease (such as COVID-19) may be greater in lower-status groups.

3.2.6 CRISIS AND SOCIAL CAPITAL

While social capital – trust and networks – is a major resource attenuating the negative impact of a pandemic (and the resulting economic crisis) on people's lives, the level of social capital, especially trust, is significantly decreased by unfavourable economic conditions. Drawing on data from the 2006–2012 European Social Survey, Iglič and colleagues (2020) demonstrate that different dimensions of social capital showed wide-ranging responses to Europe's economic crisis: There was a decline in social trust, but it was not as affected by the crisis as social networks were, both formal and informal. According to the authors, the decreases in social trust and formal networking are best explained by political factors, and the decline in informal networks by economic variables. However, longitudinal studies conducted in the UK show that the economic crisis significantly decreased social trust but not formal networks (membership in organizations and associations; Lindstrom and Giordano, 2016). In a different context, Indonesia, an economic crisis there in the 1990s did, in fact, lead to a decline in formal social capital, whereas informal social capital increased, with informal networks serving as a substitute for institutional support, especially for poor families (Wetterberg, 2007).

A positive picture emerges from research on social capital and pro-social behaviours in the context of natural disasters: Experiments show that in tsunami-hit villages the level of social trust was significantly higher there than in those that did not go through the same experience. When support from family and friends was included in the model, the effect of the natural disaster on trust was not statistically significant, which suggests that help and support obtained when struggling with the disaster led to increased trust (Cassar et al., 2017).

During a pandemic, while there is increased demand for social capital, special challenges arise related to sustaining this social capital, particularly within formal and informal networks. Apart from the negative social and economic consequences (unemployment, impoverishment, exclusion, higher inequality), people may experience the directly damaging effects of quarantine and restricted social contact, namely, social networks become weakened or even broken. However, the most recent study, based on panel data from Sweden, shows that the COVID-19 pandemic has (slightly) increased social trust (Esaiasson et al., 2020).

One should also mention here research suggesting that in times of natural disasters, when personal, real-life interactions were not possible, people eagerly used the internet to sustain and create social capital. Though developed virtually, without personal contact, it transpired that it was capable of performing all the functions attributed to traditional social capital, that is,

84 *Individuals, Groups, and Society in Pandemics*

expressive (supportive) functions and instrumental-informational ones (Procopio and Procopio, 2007).

3.2.7 SOCIAL CAPITAL AND COMMUNITY RESILIENCE

The significance of social capital for cooperation in large-N situations, and its role as a source of social support, information, and financial resources, make it an important factor promoting post-crisis community recovery. The literature highlights the crucial role of trust and existing networks in coordinating efforts, exchanging information, and developing norms that promote social support, as well as providing assistance within these networks. Studies on the effects of crises and disasters make use of the concept of community resilience, referring to the collective ability of a community (a neighbourhood or a geographical area) to deal with stress and efficiently resume the rhythms of daily life through cooperation following a disorganizing event (Aldrich and Meyer, 2015). Social capital in the form of trust and reciprocity norms, along with formal and informal networks, is an important component of community resilience, primarily due to its positive effect on wellbeing and health (Norris et al., 2008; Cutter et al., 2010). Various research approaches, applied in different cultural and geographical contexts, lead to the same conclusion: Social capital is a key factor enabling social, economic, and infrastructural community recovery following earthquakes, hurricanes, and floods, with significant indicators of social capital including membership in formal organizations, social support, and being a member of a religious and ethnically homogeneous community (Aldrich and Meyer, 2015; Sherrieb et al., 2010).

Research on particular cases shows that bonding social capital alone is often insufficient to ensure successful recovery following a crisis or a disaster; what is also needed is bridging social capital (Elliott et al., 2010; Hawkins and Maurer, 2010). Moreover, the use of social capital for reconstructing a community affected by a crisis and its consequences is associated with evident inequalities: Communities with a lower socioeconomic status are significantly less able to mobilize social capital than more advantaged groups (Elliott et al., 2010; Poortinga, 2012). Thus, the COVID-19 pandemic can be expected to increase both individual and group-level social inequalities. Returning to normal – or creating a "new normal" – will be a much greater challenge in countries and communities with low levels of social capital.

4 COMMUNICATION IN TIMES OF PANDEMIC

Małgorzata Kossowska, Natalia Letki,
Tomasz Zaleskiewicz, and Szymon Wichary

4.1 MEDIA AND MENTAL HEALTH DURING PANDEMIC[1]

During a pandemic people want to know what is going on, so they intensely seek information, mainly through the media (Nielsen et al., 2020). Research shows social media sites, such as Facebook, Twitter, Reddit, and YouTube, have become the main source of health information for people around the world, and a global platform for communication about health, illness, and health risks. The reasons for this are that by making it possible to follow the course of the pandemic, these media outlets satisfy the need for knowledge, understanding, and control; and by offering an opportunity to take part in thematic groups, they meet the need for belonging. As a result, people feel well-informed, in control of the situation, and a sense of togetherness.

Having said all this, research does show that social media also fuels fears and concerns. For many, intensive consumption of information online during a pandemic leads to increased distress and anxiety, lowered mood, impaired functioning, and increased attention to anything negative, unpleasant, and threatening (Thompson et al., 2020). Then, in a vicious cycle that is difficult to break, the more anxious we are, the more we focus on negative information, which further increases anxiety. Needless to say, the consequences for our mental and physical health can be severe.

The media itself is also a source of unsubstantiated claims, phony knowledge, and misinformed opinions – all types of disinformation that are particularly harmful during an epidemic crisis (Wang et al., 2019). Since the outbreak of COVID-19, erroneous information has spread as rapidly and widely as the virus itself (OECD, 2020). "We're not just fighting an epidemic; we're fighting an infodemic," said Tedros Adhanom Ghebreyesus, Director-General of the World Health Organization, at a conference on security in Munich, Germany, in February 2020.

4.1.1 DISINFORMATION DURING THE COVID-19 PANDEMIC

Analyses carried out during past pandemics show that about 20–30% of YouTube videos about infectious diseases contain false, inaccurate, or misleading

DOI: 10.4324/9781003254133-6

information (Tang et al., 2018). More detailed analyses performed during the Zika pandemic found that 24% of YouTube videos contained misleading information (Bora et al., 2018), and that Facebook posts conveying false data about the disease were more popular than those providing accurate and reliable information (Sharma et al., 2017). Finally, an analysis of Reddit posts during the 2014 Ebola epidemic in West Africa showed that news shared on Reddit was more sensational than traditional media coverage and did more to amplify fear and uncertainty than news outlets informed by expert knowledge (Kilgo et al., 2019).

The damaging effects of disinformation concerning COVID-19 cannot be overestimated. According to the OECD report (2020) on COVID-19 disinformation, data from Argentina, Germany, South Korea, Spain, the United Kingdom, and the United States show that about one in three persons has been exposed to false or misleading COVID-19 information on social media, taken it seriously, and subsequently used it to inform their decisions. Studies cited in this report suggest disinformation is disseminated significantly more widely than information about the disease from reliable sources like the World Health Organization (WHO), the United States Centers for Disease Control and Prevention (CDC), or the European Centre for Disease Prevention and Control (ECDPC). According to the CDC report, one third of adult American respondents, misled by false information about antiviral effects of bleach or other household cleaning products, have ingested them at least once, in the belief that they could prevent COVID-19. False information encouraged people to defy COVID-19 recommendations, such as social distancing, quarantine, and mask wearing, thus contributing to the spread of the disease.

The harmful effects of disinformation go beyond public health issues. According to the previously mentioned OECD report (2020), in the United Kingdom, the false claim that radio waves emitted by 5G towers make people more vulnerable to COVID-19 has led to more than 30 arson attacks and other acts of vandalism against telecom equipment and facilities, and about 80 incidents of harassment against telecom employees, while in the Netherlands, 15 such arson attacks have been recorded. Meanwhile, in Australia, the European Union, and the United States, disinformation pointing to minorities as the cause of the pandemic has fueled animosity against ethnic groups, contributing to a rise in discrimination and violence. A new term has even been coined to describe this phenomenon: "coronaracism." Comparable patterns of behaviour have been observed during past pandemics. During the SARS epidemic, when fake news spread about a local SARS outbreak in New York City's Chinatown, the district was quickly identified as a site of contagion, despite the fact that, in reality, there was not a single case of SARS in Chinatown (Taylor, 2019). Similarly, when a hoax website posted fake news claiming that Hong Kong would be sealed off as an infected region during the 2003 SARS epidemic, panic-stricken crowds stormed grocery stores to stock up on food to create long-term personal supplies for themselves (Cheng and Cheung, 2005).

No single reason for spreading false information exists – they are myriad. Some people use online platforms to disseminate conspiracy theories, for example that COVID-19 is a biological weapon, a product of 5G technology, or part of a greater plan to redesign the population. Others spread rumours about allegedly effective COVID-19 treatments, such as the intake of diluted bleach, the consumption of bananas, or switching off all electronic devices. Still others attempt to exploit the pandemic to turn a profit, by selling fake testing kits, masks, and treatments, informing people that their products will prevent or cure the disease. This type of information is disseminated deliberately, to mislead people and make money, or simply for the purposes of social destabilization.

4.1.2 WHY DOES FAKE NEWS SPREAD SO FAST?

False news spreads faster and reaches more people than true stories (Vosoughi et al., 2018). Researchers found that whereas true information rarely spread to more than 1,000 people, the top 1% of false news typically reached between 1,000 and 100,000 people. Moreover, it took the truth six times longer than false information to travel to 1,500 people. Although these effects were found for all categories of information, they were particularly strong for political news. Given the fact that the COVID-19 pandemic (and the surrounding strategies to address it) has been politicized in many countries, the information circulating is in some ways tantamount to political news. This means than political preferences serve as a filter for the selection of pandemic-related information.

Beyond these factors, it is also simply the case that sharing false information appeals to people enormously, and those engaging in online debates are particularly likely to share inaccurate or exaggerated content (Chadwick et al., 2018). False news encourages people to pass it on since it provokes strong emotions: fear, disgust, moral outrage, and surprise. Conversely, research indicates that factually accurate information is not so willingly shared, although can still inspire emotions, albeit different ones: anticipation, sadness, and joy (Brady et al., 2019; Vosoughi et al., 2018). What appears to matter, then, is not the specific, consistent emotions involved, but rather the level of arousal stirred up by the news; and it so happens that false information generates higher levels of arousal than the truth. It follows that the probable reason to share such provocative information is a strategy to reduce the emotional tension it has produced on encountering it.

False but novel information is also something we are willing to share, and once repeated many times, this false news comes to be perceived as true. This is because the very act of repetition makes information easier to process (an experience referred to as processing fluency), which in turn leads to positive perceptions of false information (Dechêne et al., 2010), thereby increasing its subjective credibility (Pennycook et al., 2018; Effron and Raj, 2019). Moreover, research has found that the illusory truth effect for false news occurs despite its low general credibility, and even when such information is explicitly marked as having been questioned by fact-checkers or is inconsistent with the subject's beliefs (Pennycook et al., 2020). Naturally, this effect does not occur for completely incredible or outlandish information, which is promptly rejected out of hand. According to Fragale and Heath (2016), people are more likely to share information consistent with their beliefs. In this scenario, the mechanism of disinformation would go as follows: false information is encountered and matches an individual's beliefs; because people assume that their beliefs are true, and that true beliefs come from credible sources, they thus deem the false information credible – otherwise their beliefs would turn out to be false, a notion people cannot afford to accept.

Believing and disseminating false information has little to do with low intelligence or limited knowledge about the subject in question. In general, people have the ability to distinguish true from fake news, but, nevertheless, are more likely to share the latter (Pennycook and Rand, 2019). One might expect that people who receive false information would be more likely to engage in discussions, or to attempt to check or verify the news. This is not the case, however. Shin and Thorson (2017) demonstrated that sharing false information did not have a corrective function. People tend not to discuss, analyze, or verify such information; they either accept it or reject it, which gives rise to the formation of closed groups of people holding certain opinions (Pariser, 2011; Sunstein, 2018). These and other studies suggest that even when people recognize information as false, they are still inclined to pass it on.

Tracking the path of disinformation spread about COVID-19, it has been found to move top-down, from politicians, celebrities, and other prominent figures, to ordinary internet users, as well as horizontally, between users. However, the impact of these two sources of disinformation differs dramatically. Studies cited by the OECD report (2020) show that top-down disinformation constitutes only 20% of all misleading claims about COVID-19 but has a huge impact by generating 69% of total social media engagement. Conversely, while the majority of COVID-19 disinformation on social media is created from the bottom-up, by ordinary users, most of these posts seem to make a significantly weaker impression. Therefore, it should be concluded that influential public figures bear a great deal of responsibility for the problem of disinformation and unfounded rumours about COVID-19.

People are increasingly likely to access news and other content through news aggregator websites, social media platforms, and file sharing sites. Unlike traditional media, such as TV news or newspapers, online platforms deliver automated and personalized content, using data about a user's past online activity, their social network connections, location, etc. In effect, content personalization algorithms lead to a user's repeated exposure to the same (or similar) content and ads. Moreover, some platforms display news next to other types of content, such as ads or content from other users, which makes it considerably more difficult to distinguish truth from falsehood.

4.1.3 COMBATTING COVID-19 DISINFORMATION

A variety of measures have been taken to reduce the spread of false and misleading information about COVID-19. For example, some online platforms automatically refer their users to official sources whenever they search for information about the pandemic. These platforms ban ads for medical face masks and ventilators and make efforts to detect and remove false, misleading, and potentially harmful content related to COVID-19, for instance by closing online stores or removing offers that contain false or misrepresentative claims about products said to prevent or treat the disease. Moreover, Facebook, Google, LinkedIn, Reddit, Twitter, and YouTube published a joint statement declaring their willingness to cooperate with government public health agencies in combatting fraud and misinformation about COVID-19.

The OECD report (2020) on combatting pandemic-related disinformation describes the following initiatives to tackle disinformation:

1. **Highlighting, displaying, and prioritizing content from authoritative sources**. The report notes that platforms such as Facebook, Instagram, TikTok, and Pinterest are now automatically redirecting users searching for COVID-19 content to information from the WHO. Similarly, Google launched a dedicated COVID-19 microsite and an "SOS Alert," which directs people searching for "coronavirus" to news and other content from the WHO. YouTube features awareness-raising and advertising videos from public health agencies on its homepage and highlights content from authoritative sources in response to searches for information on COVID-19. Twitter points its users to the latest information from trusted sources and Snapchat has also partnered with the WHO to create filters and stickers that provide guidance on how to prevent the spread of the virus.

2. **Cooperation with fact-checkers and public health authorities to report and remove disinformation**. The report notes that Facebook cooperates with fact-checkers to debunk false rumors about COVID-19, label that content as false, and notify people attempting to share such content that it has been confirmed as false. Facebook has partnered with the International Fact-Checking Network (IFCN, http://www.poynter. org/ifcn), an organization that supports similar initiatives around the world to develop and promote best practices in preventing disinformation. The goal of this cooperation is to launch a $1M grant programme to increase Facebook's activity in this area, for example by removing content flagged as false by public health authorities. The report adds that Google donated $6.5M to fact-checkers focusing on coronavirus. In turn, Twitter broadened the definition of harm on its platform to address content conflicting with guidance from authoritative sources.

3. **Offering free advertising to authorities**. According to the report, Facebook, Twitter, and Google have granted free advertising credits to

90   *Individuals, Groups, and Society in Pandemics*

the WHO and national health authorities to assist them with disseminating critical information about COVID-19.

These initiatives are important as they facilitate access to accurate, reliable information about COVID-19. Still, they have limited impact and the fight with disinformation remains a daunting challenge. The OECD's report identifies the reasons why the COVID-19 disinformation crisis is not easy to resolve. First, its authors believe that as a result of the pandemic, online platforms like Facebook, Google, and Twitter have faced a shortage of staff capable of moderating online activity by flagging and removing undesirable content. Consequently, they have increased their reliance on algorithms – automated monitoring technologies. We know, however, that these technologies cannot detect every instance of disinformation. Furthermore, in order to prevent legal problems, they are programmed to err on the side of caution, which increases the risk of false positives. For example, YouTube has noted an increase in video removals as a result of the platform's greater reliance on automated moderation systems and, inadvertently, there have been multiple incidents of automated monitoring systems flagging COVID-19 content from reliable sources as spam. Therefore, there is a risk that moderating content without adequate human supervision, to suppress COVID-19 disinformation, may limit the availability of reliable information about the disease. In addition, the report notes that without appropriate transparency regarding the content monitoring process, algorithms may violate people's freedom of expression.

Facebook and Instagram have banned ads claiming that a product is an effective cure or that it prevents the contraction of COVID-19, as well as ads for masks, hand sanitizers, surface disinfecting wipes, and COVID-19 testing kits. Twitter has implemented comparable measures under its Inappropriate Content Policy. Similarly, Google and YouTube prohibit any content, including ads, that seeks to profit from the pandemic, and on this basis have banned ads for personal protective equipment. These measures deter scammers trying to sell fake COVID-19-related products and help to protect consumers against price gouging. Unfortunately, the report notes they may also make it more difficult for people to find and buy hygiene products online. Some commentators argue disinformation is hard to eliminate without infringing not only on users' freedom of expression but also their right to privacy and self-determination.

It should be noted here that not all online platforms have chosen not to profit from false or misleading content. Examples of such harmful practices are identified by initiatives like the Tech Transparency Project (https://tech-transparencyproject.org), EUvsDiSiNFO (https://euvsdisinfo.eu), or EU DisinfoLab (https://www.disinfo.eu). The last of these three concluded that "the moderation process of [...] debunked conspiratorial content has been slow and inconsistent across platforms [...]."

In order to find an effective long-term solution to the flood of disinformation, we need systematic research. Regular transparency reviews of the procedures used by online platforms to detect and deal with COVID-19 disinformation would help researchers, policymakers, and the platforms themselves to identify best practices in this area. The European Commission has recently called on platforms to voluntarily issue such transparency reports on a monthly basis. If that became a requirement and, particularly, if it were expanded to include other pieces of legislation, then international, multi-stakeholder cooperation (involving governments, health organizations, tech companies, and citizens) on common action standards could help to significantly increase the efficiency of existing measures as well as reduce their cost.

4.1.4 IMMUNITY TO FAKE NEWS

Online platforms cannot stand alone in their efforts to combat disinformation. Governments, public health organizations, international organizations, media associations, tech companies, and, finally, citizens themselves must join forces in this fight. All the parties need to work together to improve people's media and digital literacy skills. If users are able to identify the source of what they read, who wrote it, and who sponsored it, and if they know why this information (as opposed to any other) is shown to them, they will be less likely to be influenced by false data (Guess et al., 2020). They should also know it is relatively easy to verify information using websites such as factcheck.org (https://www.factcheck.org) or Snopes (https://www.snopes. com). There are also semi or fully automated algorithms for detecting disinformation in online content, for example FakerFact (http://www.fakerfact. org, now retired), a browser extension that reviews a site and suggests what type of content it provides. We can also use other sophisticated tools to detect whether the source of information is a bot or a human user (e.g., Botometer; Davis et al., 2016).

Numerous studies show disinformation is tough to fight against; disclaiming, debunking, or simply withdrawing false information are all of little use (van der Linden, 2017; Nadarevic and Aßfalg, 2017; Walter and Murphy, 2018). Roozenbeek and Linden (2019a suggest people should be inoculated against fake news; just as vaccination protects us from a range of diseases, special "vaccines" could help us build an immunity to false information. To test their assumptions, Roozenbeek and Linden (2019), in a large-scale study with 15,000 participants, developed an online game in which players produced fake news using common misinformation techniques, such as polarization, invoking emotions, floating conspiracy theories, trolling people online, deflecting blame, and impersonating fake accounts. The game is based on an assumption that exposing people to misinformation strategies, warning them about how they are used, and simply familiarizing them with these techniques helps to build a cognitive immunity to protect them from real misinformation. The results suggest that people's improved ability to detect misinformation, and understand how it works and how they can protect themselves, makes them less susceptible to fake news, regardless of their education, age, or political orientation.

Other studies have demonstrated that prompting people to engage in fact checking (Brashier et al., 2020) or to think about accuracy (Pennycook and Rand, 2019) markedly improves their immunity to false information and makes them less willing to share it. According to Pennycook and colleagues (2020), people believe in fake news about COVID-19 as they tend to respond intuitively. Prompting them to adopt the right attitude ("Be accurate and correct, check facts before sharing") makes them engage in reflective, critical thinking, which helps them to discern falsehood from facts.

4.2 RISK COMMUNICATION

It is somewhat paradoxical to expect people to show appropriate and rational responses (e.g., behaviour consistent with safety rules) while being menaced by a global pandemic, despite lacking any expertise about the threat they are dealing with, or its potential short- and long-term consequences. Therefore, what becomes particularly crucial in this context is effective communication about the threat and its related level of risk. Risk communication refers to an interactive process by which information is exchanged between various actors, for example, researchers as senders (or communicators) of a message and the general public as the receiver, with the purpose of improving the audience's understanding of the nature of the risk, its magnitude (for instance, the probability of negative consequences), and what protective actions should be taken (Bostrom et al., 2018; Lundgren and McMakin, 2018). With regard to a pandemic, key information to be communicated includes the nature of the epidemic risk, its dynamics (in what ways and how fast the virus spreads), how easy it is to get infected, whether people differ in their immunity to the virus, what the infection fatality ratio is, and what can be done to reduce the probability of infection.

4.2.1 SIMPLE AND CLEAR MESSAGES

A major problem related to the communication of information about a pandemic and health recommendations is the complexity of messages. Messages that are complex and change over time are quite unlikely to be retained in people's memory. Simple messages containing one to three elements can be recalled, giving them the potential to change behaviour. A theory that might be of some help here is the dual coding principle (Clark and Paivio, 1991), which posits that messages are better called to mind if they convey their content via two sensory modalities: visual and auditory. Thus, a simple message should be presented as an image with a verbal commentary (or some other type of audio background) that makes reference to the message content.

Research suggests that some ways of presenting information make it significantly easier to understand complex problems and draw the right conclusions.

One such thinking tool, helpful in the context of health behaviours and risk taking, is the use of natural frequencies to represent information about disease-related risk. Natural frequencies represent probability information in terms of actual cases rather than percentages. Let us say that instead of writing that the case fatality rate of a disease is 4%, you cite the figures in this manner: Out of 29,788 people diagnosed with the disease, 1,256 died. If the message is conveyed in this fashion, a crucial part of the information, the base rate, gives the recipient a general idea of the magnitude of the problem. Gigerenzer and colleagues (Hoffrage and Gigerenzer, 1998; Gigerenzer, 2011) have demonstrated that the use of natural frequencies significantly improved diagnostic inferences for a variety of diseases and medical tests, even among doctors who, by definition, ought not to make diagnostic errors (see also section 1.6 on risk perception).

When it comes to the affective and motivational aspects of messages on health behaviours, numerous studies indicate that manipulating risk appraisals can increase risk avoidance at the level of self-reported intentions as well as actual behaviour (Sheeran et al., 2014). This effect is moderated by self-efficacy: If a message emphasizes the risks linked with a hazard, that is, presents a clear picture of its potential detrimental consequences and the associated negative emotions, then such a message will be particularly effective; however, this works only if the recipient's self-efficacy is enhanced, in other words, if they believe they are capable of coping with the hazard.

Relatively simple colour manipulations may also contribute to the effectiveness of health messages. Research on the effects of the colour red suggests it has a singular influence on perception and attention, attracting attention more than any other colour (Kuniecki et al., 2015). This has significant implications in many domains (Elliot and Maier, 2012; Meier et al., 2012); for example, the use of red in persuasive messages makes them more effective (Gerend and Sias, 2009), most probably as it helps to focus people's attention on the message presented.

4.2.2 APPROPRIATE MESSAGE FRAMING

One of the mechanisms that leads to an increased sense of threat is not the direct experience of risk but learning of risks vicariously (for example, learning about a pandemic through reading, watching, and conversing about it), which results in higher levels of anxiety. Therefore, appropriate messaging with the public on the subject of risk plays a central role in reducing the harmful effects of a pandemic. One way of doing this is by ensuring that messages are properly framed so that the focus is not solely on risk but promotes the right mindset, which is crucial as it affects wellbeing, behaviour, and physiology. Research shows that certain mindsets about the nature of ageing (for example, ageing as inevitable decline) may contribute to a decrease in preventive behaviours, a higher incidence of cardiovascular diseases, and shorter life expectancy. Similarly, mindsets about stress (seen as a debilitating factor) bring about impaired physiological responses and increased maladaptive behaviour (Crum et al., 2013; Zion et al., 2019). Thus, during the COVID-19 pandemic, people's mindsets about their ability to cope with the pandemic risk are of paramount importance.

A question arises as to which mindset vis-à-vis the COVID-19 pandemic will be more successful in promoting positive health behaviours. Should it be framed as a disaster that requires sacrifice to be handled? Or should the message conveyed be that the pandemic is a challenging situation that creates new possibilities? Currently, people are exposed to hopelessly contradictory messages ("COVID-19 is like the flu; we can cope with the flu, so we don't need any special precautions" or "COVID-19 is a disaster that will kill thousands of people"), which contribute to inconsistent behaviours (for example, people focus on complying with hygiene and isolation rules but at the same time do their shopping in crowded supermarkets). Consistent information about COVID-19 would seem to be more effective: that it is a disease which can be managed; that a healthy human body can handle and withstand it, if basic hygiene rules are observed (hand washing, self-isolation, or quarantine); and that positive change is possible.

The framing of these messages should be tailored for specific target groups, seeing as different groups have different beliefs about the pandemic, its causes, ways of dealing with it, etc. When messages about the pandemic are shared in social media discussion groups, people's beliefs grow in strength, so these shared beliefs must be taken into account. Research on the effects of using the word "panic" (such as panic buying) in times of disaster, like the current pandemic, deserves special attention in this context. Panic suggests people are behaving irrationally and competing for scarce resources, driven by a desire to increase their own and their loved ones' chances of survival. To frame messages more positively, cooperation with the media (including social media) would seem necessary to maximize the certainty of better outcomes.

4.2.3 RISK COMMUNICATION MODEL

Bruine de Bruin and Bostrom (2013) proposed a four-step model for the design of risk communication. The four steps of the process include: (1) identifying what people should know to engage in appropriate behaviours when facing a risk (conducting research, meta-analyses, and literature reviews; carrying out exchanges of knowledge among experts – holding expert panels etc.); (2) identifying what people think (and how they feel) about the risk and how they make decisions (large-sample surveys and opinion polls, qualitative studies, interviews); (3) designing communication content (detecting gaps between expert knowledge and lay beliefs, matching the information format to recipients' knowledge and cognitive skills, testing communications); (4) testing the effectiveness of communication content (randomized control trials).

A large proportion of the problems with communicating risk arise in phase two, i.e., misidentifying people's beliefs and opinions about the subject in question (Bruine de Bruin and Bostrom, 2013; Willis et al., 2011; Zaleskiewicz et al., 2002). For example, message senders may fail to recognize that recipients' beliefs about risk are strongly associated with emotions (Engdahl and Lidskog, 2012; Finucane, 2008). Thus, when experts intend to communicate risk (as is the case during a pandemic), the first thing to explore is people's lay or naïve theories about the subject (Furnham, 1988; Levy et al., 1999; Plaks et al., 2009). We know that, for instance, when it comes to economic risks (e.g., higher unemployment, reduced demand for some services, lower prices for certain products), existing evidence suggests that lay understanding of even basic economic phenomena can be far from the reality (Boyer and Petersen, 2018; Leiser and Shemesh, 2018). It seems we have not evolved to automatically understand the rules of economics, in contrast to our evolutionarily adaptive ability to spontaneously interpret natural phenomena in the domain of biology (Ziv and Leiser, 2013). For example, people demand increased government spending on programmes they consider important, failing to understand that more funding in one area requires cutbacks in others (Faricy and Ellis, 2014). In their book, Leiser and Shemesh (2018) offer a case in point that illustrates our lack of intuitive understanding of how economics works. When people are asked how to attract artists to the downtown area, they suggest offering subsidies so that artists can afford high rents. However, principles of economics would indicate that this will increase demand for housing while the supply remains unchanged, which, in turn, will cause price rises on the real estate market and the establishment of a new market equilibrium. In other words, the social outcomes achieved will be precisely the opposite of the ones intended. A final concrete illustration also concerns people's generally naïve knowledge of economic risk. As demonstrated by research on economic literacy (discussed in more detail in section 1.6), a large proportion of people cannot see that diversification is essential for risk control and that by diversifying their investment portfolio they can reduce its overall risk (Lusardi and Mitchell, 2014); this misapprehension of economic fundamentals attests to a significant inconsistency between our intuition and the mechanisms responsible for risk levels.

According to researchers studying the psychological aspects of judgement and decision making (e.g., Finucane et al., 2000; Slovic et al., 2004; Slovic and Peters, 2006), these biases in understanding phenomena involving some kind of risk (not just in economics, but also in the social, health, or environmental domains), may be related to people's use of the affect heuristic. This is a mental shortcut whereby information producing the same affective response (positive or negative) is assigned to the same conceptual category. As a result, people are unable to intuitively grasp that higher gains (having a positive affective value) are achieved by taking higher risks (characterized by a negative affective value). For instance, entrepreneurs can prosper if they accept higher business risks (Zaleskiewicz, Bernady, and Traczyk, 2020). The use of the affect heuristic has been shown for perceptions of environmental risks (Finucane et al., 2000), and in the context of financial risk (Kaustia et al., 2009; Statman et al., 2008; Shefrin, 2014). Although there is actually a positive correlation between risk and the profitability of financial instruments, people perceive this correlation as negative (that is, they believe you can grow rich without taking any risks, and they wrongly perceive investments that yield little in the way of profits to be highly risky). We can assume, therefore, that naïve theories of risk that people, for their own purposes, use to interpret the nature and magnitude of specific hazards in various sets of circumstances are based on affective factors, resulting in biased perceptions of the relationship between the level of risk and any expected benefits (defining this relationship as negative, whereas it is actually positive). If these properties of risk perception are not accounted for in the process of designing risk messages, communication will not be effective; it will mislead the recipients instead of promoting good decision making (for example, messages focusing solely on potential benefits are conducive to the perception of low risk).

Another problem occurring at the border between step 1 and step 2 of the previously discussed risk communication model (i.e., between expert knowledge and people's naïve beliefs) is related to the fact that lay people may not only have different perceptions of risk mechanisms but also question the very existence of the risk itself. Research on communicating climate change risks shows us the importance of people's lay beliefs about the existence and potential effects of the hazard. Studies of American adults show that the vast majority do not associate the increasing phenomenon of global warming with any negative health impacts (Leiserowitz, 2005). Respondents said the overall number of deaths and illnesses due to global warming each year was a few hundred, and believed it would be several thousand in 50 years, which represents a vast underestimation. What is more, very few Americans associated global warming with severe weather phenomena such as hurricanes and droughts. A similar problem has been found by studies testing people's beliefs about the existence of the pandemic, its risks, and its potential causes. In a YouGov poll conducted for *The Economist* on a representative sample of 1,500 US adult citizens on March 8–10, 2020, 13% of respondents said the statement "Coronavirus is a hoax" was definitely true or probably true. Among those who acknowledged the existence of the virus, 49% considered the statement "The coronavirus is a man-made epidemic" to be definitely true or probably true. This sort of response reflects a belief in some kind of conspiracy theory and is entirely inconsistent with current scientific knowledge (Andersen et al., 2020). These findings suggest that those designing messages about the current epidemic risk should take into account the discrepancy between expert knowledge and lay beliefs among the receivers of messages in the communication process.

Note

1 Dr. Gabriela Czarnek has contributed to this chapter.

5 SUMMARY

Małgorzata Kossowska, Natalia Letki,
Tomasz Zaleskiewicz, and Szymon Wichary

In this section we would like to briefly summarize each chapter, listing the barriers that prevent, or may potentially prevent, people from engaging in positive health behaviours.

5.1 EMOTIONS REGULATE HEALTH-RELATED DECISION MAKING

1. **Emotions perform multiple important functions.** Experiencing certain emotions is a signal that the individual has encountered a challenge in the environment, which produces a specific motivational response. For example, we would expect the feeling of anxiety induced by an awareness of the epidemic risk to motivate people to engage in protective behaviours, and as such, to have a mobilizing function. However, if anxiety is too low or not present at all, the motivation to take protective measures (such as wearing a face mask or using hand sanitizer) will also be low, leading to an increased risk of infection, or even death.

   Feelings also have functions that play a role in social interactions. One example of an emotion serving an important communicative function is anger, which is responsible for supporting the process of goal pursuit. Individuals who strictly follow hygiene rules may respond with anger against those who ignore or violate them (for example, refuse to wear masks, do not disinfect their hands when entering a store, or violate the rules of isolation). In other words, expressing anger is an effective way of making others comply with safety measures. Although experiencing anger facilitates goal attainment, it may also lead to uncontrolled aggressive outbursts. Another emotion, fear, mobilizes the body and activates defensive behaviour, but it may also lead to widespread panic when affective responses are transferred from person to person – an effect known as emotional contagion. One more important emotion experienced during a pandemic is disgust, which amplifies moral judgements. Under the influence of disgust (related to toxin or pathogen threats) people are more likely to categorize other people's behaviour as violating moral norms, and to condemn such behaviour.

DOI: 10.4324/9781003254133-7

2. **Emotions affect cognitive functioning.** Threat-related affective states characterized by high arousal (such as the aforementioned anxiety, fear, or disgust) reduce our cognitive capacity, thus increasing the tendency for selective information processing. As a result of this, we attend more to information which is congruent with our current emotional state, and are more able to encode and recall such information. When experiencing anxiety, people use simplified rules for decision making: In anxiety-provoking situations, not all the choice alternatives are considered; instead, just a few highly relevant cues are utilized. One's time perspective is also shortened: decisions are made in a way that focuses in on a shorter time horizon. In addition, threat-related emotional states lead to preference potentiation. That is, in high arousal situations, decision makers are more determined to choose their preferred options and devote less attention to considering alternative choices. When increased anxiety is felt, people are less likely to take risks compared to when they are anxiety-free. Affective states also influence trust and cooperation: Positive emotions promote cooperation, while stress and negative emotions tend to reduce it.

3. **Health anxiety.** This type of anxiety refers to the "tendency to be alarmed by illness-related stimuli, including but not limited to, illness related to infectious diseases" (Taylor, 2019, p. 49). When individuals face an epidemic risk, their experience of high levels of health anxiety may result in maladaptive responses. Indeed, people with extremely high health anxiety can show unreasonably strong reactions to any information about the possibility of getting infected. This may take the form of excess healthcare utilization or cyberchondria, characterized by excessive online searches for medical information. Conversely, individuals with low levels of health anxiety may ignore preventive recommendations as they simply do not feel the need to protect themselves.

   The following factors have been linked to health anxiety:

   - misinterpretation of health-related stimuli;
   - specific beliefs about health and disease – selective retrieval of memories about previous illnesses and biased interpretations of these;
   - hypervigilance to any physiological symptoms that may signal illness; and
   - maladaptive coping – a tendency to engage in or avoid behaviours that seem to prevent or facilitate infection (for example, compulsive handwashing and sanitizing).

5.2 PERCEPTION OF RISK

One of the most important questions to answer in the context of pandemic risk is how good people are at estimating risk. If they perceive the pandemic as highly risky, it can be assumed that people will be more likely to engage in protective behaviours and observe safety rules (such as hand sanitizing, mask wearing, or self-isolation).

During a pandemic, people take diverse risks, including:

- Functional risks: Will the new measures work and turn out to be equally effective?
- Physical risks: Will I get hurt by the new solution?
- Financial risks: Will the new measures be more expensive?
- Social risks: Will I lose my reputation or bear costs related to social change?
- Time risks: Will the new measures be more time-consuming and, if yes, will the time investment pay off?

Understanding the emotional and cognitive mechanisms underlying the perceptions of the different types of risks will help to predict whether individuals will or will not engage in specific behaviours.

1. **How do people estimate risk?** Objectively, the level of risk is related to two parameters: the severity and probability of negative consequences. In the context of a pandemic, this would include indicators such as the probability of being infected by the disease, the odds of dying if one becomes infected, the number of people exposed, etc. Research in cognitive psychology suggests people are not particularly good at processing these values, and intuitive risk estimates are weakly correlated with objective measures of riskiness. People are more driven by their emotional and intuitive perceptions of risk than by quantitative assessments. A key problem in this context is people's misunderstanding of what probabilities are and what they mean. Intuitively, it might by quite tricky to process information such as: "The probability of dying if you develop COVID-19 is 2%." Research suggests probabilistic information can be conveyed more effectively using natural frequencies, for example: "Out of 100 people who will develop COVID-19, two will die." One should also remember that sensitivity to changes in probability is decreased when people experience strong anxiety.

2. **The feeling of risk.** Psychometric studies within the psychometric paradigm show that risk perception is related to two dimensions, referred to as "unknown risk" and "dread risk." The former is of a cognitive nature, and the latter connected to emotional factors. Thus, we may call it a dual-process model of risk perception. When it comes to the cognitive dimension of risk perception, things perceived as hazardous are those that are novel, poorly understood (both by laypersons and by scientists), or rare. As regards the emotional dimension, perceived risk is higher when people do not feel in control, when they think they are exposed to risk involuntarily, and when they believe that any potential losses will be catastrophic. The coronavirus risk may appear high since it is poorly

100   *Individuals, Groups, and Society in Pandemics*

understood and difficult to manage, and, of course, may have unknown consequences for the future. However, when perceived control of that risk increases (which reduces anxiety) or more resources describing the phenomenon become available (leading to higher perceived knowledge about the pandemic), people's assessments of risk may plummet.

3. **Perceived risk and preventive behaviours.** Research on risk perception explores not only how people spontaneously assess risks, but also how these perceptions are related to their preventive behaviours. Findings from meta-analytical studies show that:

   - Individuals who perceive the risk of infection to be higher are more likely to get vaccinated.
   - Individuals who see themselves as more susceptible to a disease are more likely to be vaccinated.
   - Those who perceive the potential consequences of a disease as more severe are more likely to take vaccines.

   Studies have also found that providing knowledge about risks and enhancing self-efficacy both increase people's motivation to take preventive actions and adhere to safety rules.

4. **Individual differences in risk perception.** There are significant individual differences in risk taking, depending on age, sex, and personality, as well as motivational and affective factors. Sex has been found to moderate the effect of stress on risk taking – in men, risk taking is increased by stress, while in women, it is decreased. In addition, men are also more inclined to take risks than women. As for age differences, elderly people are more likely to use simple decision-making heuristics than younger people, and risk taking also decreases with age. Moreover, age moderates the effect of stress on risk taking: Stress decreases risk taking even further in elderly people, but increases it among the young. Finally, risk taking is positively related to such personality traits as impulsivity, sensation seeking, extraversion, and openness to experience, whereas it is negatively related to neuroticism and agreeableness.

5.3 DECISION MAKING IN A PANDEMIC

We have mentioned the important function of habits. It is worth noting here that habits are hard to change and, for many of us, such change is neither pleasant nor straightforward. Moreover, people may experience conflicting goals (health versus comfort), and their decisions often require making tough trade-offs.

1. **Trade-offs.** Decision makers sometimes have to make comparisons and trade-offs between different values, which may lead to conflict in decision making. The problem is not emotionally arduous when such comparisons are made within the same value category – for example, when a consumer chooses between a cheaper product in larger packaging and a more

expensive product in smaller packaging. It is when people have to weigh values that are hard to compare, such as money and the feeling of uncertainty, that psychological complications occur. Moreover, it can become a particularly thorny problem to decide between values that seem completely incommensurate, such as health and finance. Unfortunately, during a pandemic, people are repeatedly faced with such appalling dilemmas. For example, should we close businesses (to ensure isolation) at the cost of higher unemployment and pay cuts?

2. **Barriers to trade-offs.** The most extreme cases of people's reluctance to make trade-offs are those where a decision maker believes that some values (such as life, health, or freedom) cannot be compared to or traded for anything else. These are referred to as sacred values. During the COVID-19 pandemic, strong emotions, taking the form of moral outrage, were triggered by media reports that in some countries politicians decided not to introduce strict lockdowns (thus increasing the probability of infection and death among the most vulnerable, such as the elderly) in order to protect certain economic values (for example, to avoid a dramatic rise in unemployment).

3. **Unwanted choices.** It is also interesting to consider the behavioural consequences of putting people in a situation where they have to make unwanted or (as they see it) unacceptable trade-offs (such as the ones that must be made under threat). Both earlier and more recent studies demonstrate that in such circumstances people are likely to show decision aversion and do what they can to avoid making their own decisions (for example, they procrastinate or attempt to shift the responsibility for the decision onto someone else). They can also engage in different kinds of rationalizations, for example, by making efforts to denigrate one of the choices.

4. **Tokenism and habituation.** We have also noted how people are prone to tokenism, that is, to expending merely symbolic efforts to solve an issue, which do not really contribute to alleviating the problem (for example, "I wash my hands and I don't have to do anything else"), while being fully convinced of their active commitment. Finally, we are at risk of growing accustomed to the pandemic, regarding it as the normal state of affairs and seeing the coronavirus as a part of the landscape. We believe acknowledging these various barriers will help to not only understand people's behaviour (or the lack of it) but also take any appropriate measures.

5.4 BELIEFS, IDEOLOGY, AND VALUES

1. **Community as a value.** When under threat, faced with pandemic-related risks, we are repeatedly reminded of the role of community as a value that allows people to cope with uncertainty, both materially and symbolically. The material aspect involves providing support to each other, in particular that of a financial nature. Communal support can also

be purely symbolic or emotional. Communal orientation is inseparably linked to experiencing such emotions as elevation, love, or compassion – feelings that create and strengthen interpersonal bonds, and become a source of support under threat.

2. **Communal versus exchange orientation.** Communal orientation is one of several different ways of shaping interpersonal relationships, in other words, one of many possible social orientations. Apart from communal orientation, psychologists and anthropologists describe exchange (or market pricing) orientation, which involves applying business thinking to non-business domains, such as marriage. In this mode, an individual interprets social exchange processes as an investment and focuses primarily on its rate of return ("Will the relationship be profitable for me?", "How much can I gain?"). A prototypical attribute of exchange orientation is the proportionality of the expenditure–outcome relationship, regardless of how expenditures are measured (as money, time, effort, psychological support, etc.). Where communal orientation emphasizes emotion and affection, exchange orientation values logic and rationality.

3. **What contributes to the two types of orientation – communal and exchange?** Exchange orientation increases when people experience uncertainty and a lack of control. Other studies have found that exchange orientation in interpersonal relationships impairs people's emotional functioning. It has been demonstrated that the activation of market pricing orientation in social relationships reduces compassionate behaviour and causes people to perceive any expression of compassion in the organizational context as unprofessional. Here we are confronted with a paradox. On the one hand, we expect that the trauma related to the pandemic and to substantial economic risks will be reduced by an enhanced communal orientation, which is characterized by a willingness to provide help and emotional support. On the other hand, experiments suggest the opposite may also be true: Uncertainty and a perceived lack of control, which come as a natural consequence of an unpredictable situation such as an epidemic, may be conducive to the development of an individualistic and unemotional exchange orientation, which is associated with a tendency to calculate and pursue one's own self-interest.

4. **Social comparisons.** We have devoted much attention to group and intergroup relationships. In this context, significant barriers arise from comparisons to others, which are facilitated by:

    - certain social norms (for example, non-compliance as a norm, or beliefs such as "My house, my rules"); and
    - perceived inequalities (if dilemmas arise concerning the distribution of resources that involve any sort of inequalities, actual or perceived, people's willingness to cooperate decreases).

5. **Ideology.** Other factors that make people less likely to follow expert advice can be categorized as related to beliefs and ideologies. These include:

- their worldview – beliefs that the coronavirus is not a real problem but rather part of some political game (for example, the virus seen as a hostile ideology);
- the tendency to sustain and defend the status quo;
- conspiracy beliefs and theories; and
- polarization.

5.5 SEEKING INFORMATION

1. **Ignorance** or a lack of knowledge about the existence and scale of the problem, about its causes, and about ways to manage it, as well as conflicting or inconsistent media messages, constitute a major barrier to engaging in positive health behaviours. People may fail to seek information because they disregard the problem. This is usually the case when certain members of society suffer no losses related to the problem, or are unaware of any losses being incurred, or when they are uncertain about whether the problem really exists and how serious it is. People may underestimate the significance of the problem (for example, because of its location – a belief that it does not affect "their own" area; or because of time – a belief that the effects of the pandemic are not immediate and will only emerge in the future). Additionally, they may be overly optimistic and believe the problem will solve itself somehow. Finally, certain individuals may also have low perceived control of their predicament, and consequently fail to take action, as they hold the belief that anything they do will be ineffective or meaningless.
2. **Experts.** When making decisions, people turn to external sources of information in two cases: (1) when there is an excess of information that they cannot process; (2) when there is a scarcity of information, or the information they already have is barely understandable. Of the two, the latter seems to be the one that holds true during the pandemic. To deal with the shortage of information, one source used by decision makers to obtain information about risks related to SARS-CoV-2 is experts, such as epidemiologists and physicians, whereas for information about the economic consequences of the pandemic, one may turn to economists and financial analysts. However, individuals without an adequate educational background may encounter a serious challenge: How can they find out who really is an expert and who is not? Unfortunately, people are prone to cognitive and motivational biases in evaluating the quality and credibility of experts.
3. **When we do not trust experts – denial, reactance, and confirmation bias.** When trust is low, even the widest and most generous assistance programmes are seen as insufficient and unsuccessful. Trust-related barriers involve the denial or minimization of the problem, as well as reactance (those who do not believe the information provided

by the government or scientists react strongly against guidance and orders, treating them as restrictions on their personal freedom). One of the biases in evaluating expert authority is associated with people's desire to confirm their existing beliefs and opinions, which leads to confirmation bias or to egocentric advice discounting, i.e., filtering information through one's personal beliefs. Generally, these biases can be described as motivated reasoning and selective processing of information to make it consistent with one's goals.

4. **When experts are reliable.** Research suggests people are likely to attribute more reliability to experts who confirm their preexisting beliefs, which, of course, can lead to strong biases in decision making. If someone believes the epidemic risk is extremely high and will have serious social consequences, they will be more likely to trust experts who express similar opinions and, at the same time, will discount advice from those claiming that the risk of contracting the disease is low. On the other hand, when an individual believes the risk is not very real, they will reject expert opinions of the sort that say the risk of infection is high, and so will be unlikely to follow hygiene guidelines. This effect is caused by factors related to protecting one's self-esteem, by people's belief that they possess objective knowledge on a subject, and that those who disagree are prone to error. In addition, it is caused by the fact that information consistent with one's beliefs is simply easier to process. Hence, it appears that in order to correctly predict whether people will respond positively to experts' recommendations during a pandemic, we have to learn and understand what people think about them. In other words, what matters is not only the clarity and power of experts' messages, but also their consistency (or inconsistency) with citizens' opinions.

5.6 TRUST IN INSTITUTIONS

1. **Trust in institutions is the fundamental indicator of their legitimacy.** Citizens' willingness to comply with orders and regulations related to a crisis situation depends on how much they trust the government and its agencies. The question of sources of trust is a complex one, since on the one hand, citizens' attitudes toward the state and its institutions are determined by emotional factors and associated with identity (for example, political identities), and on the other, they are based on how people evaluate the quality of actions taken by the state and its institutions, with these evaluations themselves being determined by identity-related factors (the same government measures can be evaluated differently depending on whether the government has been formed by a political party we support or one we oppose). Perceptions of the response of state institutions are largely based on media coverage and second-hand information, whereas "frontline" or local institutions are evaluated based on contact quality. Research shows that effectiveness measured in terms

of outcomes (for example, financial results) is less significant for creating trust in institutions than their perceived fairness or adherence to the adopted procedures (procedural fairness). Most studies point to procedural fairness as the main determinant of citizens' compliance with the law – even if it is perceived as unfavourable.

2. **What contributes to institutional trust?** External risks (such as military threats and, perhaps, a pandemic) give rise to a sudden mobilization and high levels of trust in institutions (a phenomenon known as the rally-round-the-flag effect), but this increase is short lived. Risk perceptions are another factor influencing people's willingness to comply with orders and regulations in a crisis situation. Importantly, high institutional trust decreases perceived risk, so individuals with high levels of trust in the government and its agencies are less likely to engage in preparation and preventive behaviours.

3. **The role of local institutions.** When it comes to COVID-19, citizens will interpret the effectiveness of government policies through the lens of their political preferences and the perceived fairness or impartiality of pandemic-related actions. "Frontline" institutions (street-level bureaucracy) have a significant role to play: It is their quality that should be particularly important in encouraging cooperation with the government, as it will become the main source of information about the levels of procedural fairness that exist.

5.7 SOCIAL CAPITAL

1. **Social capital helps to cope with difficulties.** Individual social capital involves resources that can be reached through family, friends, and acquaintances (for example, having highly educated people with good access to information in one's social networks has a positive effect on the person's position in terms of understanding actual risks and available strategies). Social capital as individual resources (social networks) is of key importance in crisis: It ensures emotional support and everyday instrumental support (via strong ties, i.e., family and friends), as well as access to resources beyond those in our possession (via weak ties, i.e., acquaintances and their acquaintances). Strong ties are essential for an individual's psychological wellbeing (all the more so in a crisis) and are directly related to health (both subjectively rated and assessed using objective measures). Apart from that, social capital has an indirect effect on health by protecting people from poverty and exclusion. Importantly, the structure of ties or connections that make up social capital reflects social inequalities: Low-status individuals rely primarily on strong ties, with their social networks being homogenous and comprised of other low-status individuals. So, in a crisis, strong ties will help poor and uneducated people to survive but will not allow them to bounce back and improve their socioeconomic position or prospects.

2. **Social capital has a collective aspect, too**, because it defines the prevailing means of interaction, and thus influences group effectiveness and its costs. The cognitive dimension of social capital involves generalized trust and reciprocity norms. These are of key importance during a pandemic because of their significance for people's contributions to public goods (in this case, health) in large-N contexts. Trust in others, in terms of their fair compliance with the law, determines our own willingness to comply, because in large-N situations only confidence in other people's fair behaviour grants meaning to our own contributions to a public good. In a large-N situation, when the group is too large to influence individual behaviour through informal sanctions, a high level of social capital is necessary to reduce free-riding, and during a pandemic, even low rates of free-riding (for example, a relatively small number of people refusing to wear face masks) may undermine collective efforts. Social trust on its own, without the norm of reciprocity, may lead to opportunistic behaviour such as free-riding. Research shows, however, that while high levels of social trust and reciprocity norms are associated with feeling responsible for the community and the common good, they also lead to increased perceptions of opportunistic behaviours as exploitative; seeing yourself as exploiting others is more psychologically costly than being aware that you have been taken advantage of.

3. **Community resilience.** The social capital of a group is the main component of what we refer to as community resilience, or the collective ability to recover from a disaster or crisis. Support for victims, information about available help, and the collective memory of the community structure and relationships among its members are some positive consequences of social capital, which help the community to recover more rapidly.

4. **Social capital in a crisis.** Unfortunately, crisis situations may erode social capital, though data on this subject is inconclusive. While social ties still maintain their fundamental functions of psychological and organizational support, when dramatic events occur, a decrease in the levels of formal social capital and generalized trust follows. On the other hand, in communities that have experienced dramatic events (such as natural disasters), the support provided by neighbours and family members leads to much higher levels of trust in others. Moreover, the internet seems to play a positive role in the fundamental function of providing support, and online contact may successfully fulfill all the basic tasks of social capital.

5.8 RISK COMMUNICATION

1. **What is risk communication?** By risk communication we mean an interactive process by which information is exchanged between various actors (for example, researchers as senders or communicators of a message and the general public as the receiver), with the purpose of improving

the audience's understanding of the nature of a risk, its magnitude (for example, the probability of negative consequences), and what protective actions should be taken. With regard to a pandemic, the key information to be communicated includes the nature of the epidemic risk, its dynamics (in what ways and how fast the virus is spreading), how easy it is to catch the disease, whether people differ in their immunity to the virus, what the infection fatality ratio is, and what can be done to reduce the probability of infection.

2. **The steps of the risk communication process.** The four steps of the process include:

   - identifying what people should know to engage in appropriate behaviours when facing a risk;
   - identifying what people already think (and how they feel) about the risk and how they make decisions;
   - designing communication content; and
   - testing the effectiveness of communication.

   A large proportion of problems with communicating risk arise at step two, i.e., from misidentifying people's beliefs and opinions about the subject in question. For example, message senders may fail to recognize that recipients' beliefs about risk are strongly associated with emotions, which means that messages focused solely on conveying knowledge will be ineffective and unlikely to produce the desired effects, such as compliance with hygiene rules.

3. **What is communicated during a pandemic?** During a pandemic, it is important to communicate not only health risks but also economic risks. Research suggests that people have very limited knowledge about economic phenomena and display low financial literacy (defined as a set of practical skills in personal financial management). Moreover, perceptions of economic risk are influenced by the affect heuristic, which can be described, in essence, as a tendency to perceive things that are profitable as low in terms of risk, and to see things that produce very little profit as highly risky, even though in real markets the opposite is the case. In other words, there is a positive correlation between risk and profit, but in people's minds this correlation seems to be negative.

4. **Message complexity.** A major problem related to the communication of information about a pandemic and health recommendations is the complexity of messages. Messages that are complex and change over time are quite unlikely to remain in people's memory. Simple messages containing one to three elements can be recalled, which opens up the possibility that these types of communication will actually change behaviour. The dual coding principle says messages are more effectively brought to mind if they convey their content via two sensory modalities: visual and auditory. Thus, a simple message should be presented as an image with a verbal commentary (or some other type of audio content relevant to

the message). Certain formats of presentation make it significantly more straightforward to understand complex problems and draw the right conclusions. One illustration of this is natural frequencies, which represent probability information in terms of actual cases rather than percentages. By using natural frequencies, people are assisted in drawing correct conclusions about diseases and medical tests.

5. **Manipulating risk appraisal in messages** increases risk avoidance. This effect is moderated by self-efficacy: If a message emphasizes the risk related to a hazard, that is, presents a clear picture of its potential adverse consequences and the related negative emotions, then such a message will be particularly effective if the recipient's self-efficacy is enhanced, that is, if they believe they are able to cope with the hazard.

6. **Colour manipulations in messages.** Research on the effects of the colour red suggests it has a special influence on perception and attention. The use of red in persuasive messages makes them more effective.

7. **Communicating things people do not believe.** Communicating risks can also be challenging because people may simply deny their existence. It is not rare for people to believe that the coronavirus is a fabrication of sorts, so they therefore take the view that there is no need to take any preventive measures.

References

Ahorsu, D. K., Lin, C. Y., Imani, V., Saffari, M., Griffiths, M. D., & Pakpour, A. H. (2020). The fear of COVID-19 scale: Development and initial validation. *International Journal of Mental Health and Addiction*, 1–9. https://doi.org/10.1007/s11469-020-00270-8

Aidis, R., Estrin, S., & Mickiewicz, T. (2008). Institutions and entrepreneurship development in Russia: A comparative perspective. *Journal of Business Venturing*, 23(6), 656–672.

Albertson, B., & Gadarian, S. K. (2015). *Anxious Politics: Democratic Citizenship in a Threatening World*. Cambridge, UK: Cambridge University Press.

Aldrich, D. P., & Meyer, M. A. (2015). Social capital and community resilience. *American Behavioral Scientist*, 59(2), 254–269.

Alford, J., & Hibbing, J. (2004). The origin of politics: An evolutionary theory of political behavior. *Perspectives on Politics*, 2(4), 707–723. doi:10.1017/S1537592704040460

Allcott, H., Boxell, L., Conway, J., Gentzkow, M., Thaler, M., & Yang, D. Y. (2020). *Polarization and Public Health: Partisan Differences in Social Distancing During the Coronavirus Pandemic*. NBER Working Paper No. w26946. https://ssrn.com/abstract=3574415

Alter, A. L., & Oppenheimer, D. M. (2009). Uniting the tribes of fluency to form metacognitive cation. *Personality and Social Psychology Review*, 13, 219–235.

Andersen, K. G., Rambaut, A., Lipkin, W. I., Holmes, E. C., & Garry, R. F. (2020). The proximal origin of SARS-CoV-2. *Nature Medicine*, 26, 450–452.

Arendt, H. (2006). *Eichmann in Jerusalem: A Report on the Banality of Evil*. New York: Penguin Classics.

Ares, M., & Hernández, E. (2017). The corrosive effect of corruption on trust in politicians: Evidence from a natural experiment. *Research & Politics*, 4(2). https://doi.org/10.1177/2053168017714185

Armingeon, K., & Ceka, B. (2014). The loss of trust in the European Union during the great recession since 2007: The role of heuristics from the national political system. *European Union Politics*, 15(1), 82–107.

Armitage, R., & Nellums, L. B. (2020). COVID-19 and the consequences of isolating the elderly. *Lancet Public Health*. https://doi.org/10.1016/S2468-2667(20)30061-X

Arndt, J., Cox, C. R., Goldenberg, J. L., Vess, M., Routledge, C., Cooper, D. P., & Cohen, F. (2009). Blowing in the (social) wind: Implications of extrinsic esteem contingencies for terror management and health. *Journal of Personality and Social Psychology*, 96(6), 1191–1205. https://doi.org/10.1037/a0015182

Arndt, J., Routledge, C., & Goldenberg, J. (2006). Predicting proximal health responses to reminders of death: The influence of coping style and health optimism. *Psychology & Health*, 21(5), 593–614. https://doi.org/10.1080/14768320500537662

Arndt, J., Schimel, J., & Goldenberg, J. L. (2003). Death can be good for your health: Fitness intentions as a proximal and distal defense against mortality salience. *Journal of Applied Social Psychology*, 33, 1726–1746.

Arndt, J., Vail, K. E. III, Cox, C. R., Goldenberg, J. L., Piasecki, T. M., & Gibbons, F. X. (2013). The interactive effect of mortality reminders and tobacco craving on smoking topography. *Health Psychology*, 32(5), 525–532. https://doi.org/10.1037/a0029201

Arnsten, A. F. (2009). Stress signalling pathways that impair prefrontal cortex structure and function. *Nature Reviews Neuroscience*, 10(6), 410–422.

Arvan, M. (2019). The dark side of morality: Group polarization and moral epistemology. *The Philosophical Forum*, 50, 87–115.

Ashby, F. G., & Isen, A. M. (1999). A neuropsychological theory of positive affect and its influence on cognition. *Psychological Review*, 106(3), 529.

Attwell, K., & Freeman, M. (2015). I Immunise: An evaluation of a values-based campaign to change attitudes and beliefs. *Vaccine*, 33(46), 6235–6240.

Augustyn, M. B., & Ward, J. T. (2015). Exploring the sanction–crime relationship through a lens of procedural justice. *Journal of Criminal Justice*, 43(6), 470–479.

Babalola, S. (2011). Maternal reasons for non-immunization and partial immunization in northern Nigeria. *Journal of Paediatrics and Child Health*, 47, 276–281.

Babcicky, P., & Seebauer, S. (2017). The two faces of social capital in private flood mitigation: Opposing effects on risk perception, self-efficacy and coping capacity. *Journal of Risk Research*, 20(8), 1017–1037.

Baleta, A. (2007). Forced isolation of tuberculosis patients in South Africa. *The Lancet Infectious Diseases*, 7(12), 771.

Baron, J. (2006). *Thinking and Deciding*. Cambridge University Press.

Barrett, L. F. (2013). Psychological construction: A Darwinian approach to the science of emotion. *Emotion Review*, 5, 379–389.

Barrows, S. (1981). *Distorting Mirrors*. Yale University Press.

Basolo, V., Steinberg, L. J., Burby, R. J., Levine, J., Cruz, A. M., & Huang, C. (2009). The effects of confidence in government and information on perceived and actual preparedness for disasters. *Environment and Behavior*, 41(3), 338–364.

Bauer, P. C., & Freitag, M. (2018). Measuring trust. *The Oxford Handbook of Social and Political Trust*. Oxford University Press.

Baumeister, R. F. (1989). The Optimal margin of illusion. *Journal of Social and Clinical Psychology*, 8, 176–189.

BBC. (2020). Worldwide coronavirus deaths pass 600,000. (July 10). https://www.bbc.com/news/live/world-53462322

Beattie, J., & Barlas, S. (2001). Predicting perceived differences in tradeoff difficulty. In E. U. Weber, J. Baron, & G. Loomes (Eds.), *Conflict and Tradeoffs in Decision Making* (pp. 25–64). Cambridge University Press.

Beattie, J., Baron, J., Hershey, J. C., & Spranca, M. D. (1994). Psychological determinants of decision attitude. *Journal of Behavioral Decision Making*, 7(2), 129–144.

Bechara, A., & Damasio, A. R. (2005). The somatic marker hypothesis: A neural theory of economic decision. *Games and Economic Behavior*, 52(2), 336–372.

Bechara, A., Damasio, H., Tranel, D., & Damasio, A. R. (2005). The Iowa Gambling Task and the somatic marker hypothesis: Some questions and answers. *Trends in Cognitive Sciences*, 9(4), 159–164. https://doi.org/10.1016/j.tics.2005.02.002

References 111

Becker, E. (1973). *The Denial of Death*. New York, NY: Free Press.

Becker, M. W., & Leinenger, M. (2011). Attentional selection is biased toward mood-congruent stimuli. *Emotion*, 11(5), 1248.

Bedford, J., Enria, D., Giesecke, J., et al. (2020). COVID-19: Towards controlling of a pandemic. *The Lancet*. https://doi.org/10.1016/S0140-6736(20)30673-5

Benin, A., Wisler-Scher, D., Colson, E., Shapiro, E., & Holmboe, E. (2006). Qualitative analysis of mothers' decision-making about vaccines for infants: The importance of trust. *Pediatrics*, 117, 1532–1541.

Benjamin, D. J. (2019). Errors in probabilistic reasoning and judgment biases. In B. D. Bernheim, S. DellaVigna, & D. Laibson (Eds.), *Handbook of Behavioral Economics: Foundations and Applications 2* (pp. 69–186). North-Holland: Elsevier. https://doi.org/10.1016/bs.hesbe.2018.11.002

Besta, T., Jaśko, K., Grzymała-Moszczyńska, J., & Górska, P. (2019). *Walcz, Protestuj, Zmieniaj Świat*. Sopot: Smak Słowa.

Bihari, M., & Ryan, R. (2012) Influence of social capital on community preparedness for wildfires. *Landscape and Urban Planning*, 106, 253–261.

Biliński, J. (2020). Epidemia obnażyła zapaść, w jakiej jest polski system ochrony zdrowia. https://pulsmedycyny.pl/epidemia-obnazyla-zapasc-w-jakiej-jest-polski-system-ochrony-zdrowia-opinia-987179

Blackwell, S. E., Rius-Ottenheim, N., Schulte-van Maaren, Y. W., Carlier, I. V., Middelkoop, V. D., Zitman, F. G., Spinhoven, P., Holmes, E. A., & Giltay, E. J. (2013). Optimism and mental imagery: A possible cognitive marker to promote well-being? *Psychiatry Research*, 206, 56–61.

Blader, S. L., & Tyler, T. R. (2009). Testing and extending the group engagement model: Linkages between social identity, procedural justice, economic outcomes, and extrarole behavior. *Journal of Applied Psychology*, 94(2), 445–464. https://doi.org/10.1037/a0013935

Blanchar, J., & Eidelman, S. (2013). Perceived system longevity increases system justification and the legitimacy of inequality. *European Journal of Social Psychology*, 43, 238–245.

Blanken, I., van de Ven, N., & Zeelenberg, M. (2015). A meta-analytic review of moral licensing. *Personality and Social Psychology Bulletin*, 41(4), 540–558. https://doi.org/10.1177/0146167215572134

Bobevski, I., Clarke, D. M., & Meadows, G. (2016). Health anxiety and its relationship to disability and service use: Findings from a large epidemiological survey. *Psychosomatic Medicine*, 78, 13–25.

Boin, A., Kuipers, S., & Overdijk, W. (2013) Leadership in times of crisis: A framework for assessment. *International Review of Public Administration*, 18(1), 79–91. https://doi.org/10.1080/12294659.2013.10805241

Bol, D., Giani, M., Blais, A., & Loewen, P. J. (2021). The effect of COVID-19 lockdowns on political support: Some good news for democracy? *European Journal of Political Research*, 60(2), 497–505.

Bonaccio, S., & Dalal, R. S. (2006). Advice taking and decision-making: An integrative literature review, and implications for the organizational sciences. *Organizational Behavior and Human Decision Processes*, 101(2), 127–151.

Bora, K., Das, D., Barman, B., & Borah, P. (2018). Are internet videos useful sources of information during global public health emergencies? A case study of YouTube videos during the 2015–16 Zika virus pandemic. *Pathogens and Global Health*, 112(6), 320–328. https://doi.org/10.1080/20477724.2018.1507784

112 *Individuals, Groups, and Society in Pandemics*

Bostrom, A., Böhm, G., & O'Connor, R. E. (2018). Communicating risks: Principles and challenges. In M. Raue, E. Lermer, & B. Streicher (Eds.), *Psychological Perspectives on Risk and Risk Analysis* (pp. 251–277). New York: Springer.

Bowler, S., & Karp, J. A. (2004). Politicians, scandals, and trust in government. *Political Behavior*, 26(3), 271–287.

Boyer, P., & Petersen, M. B. (2018). Folk-economic beliefs: An evolutionary cognitive model. *Behavioral and Brain Sciences*, 41, 1–51.

Brackett, M. A., Rivers, S. E., Bertoli, M. C., & Salovey, P. (2016). Emotional intelligence. In L. Feldman Barrett, M. Lewis, & J. M. Haviland-Jones (Eds.), *Handbook of Emotions* (pp. 513–531). New York: The Guilford Press.

Bradford, B., Hohl, K., Jackson, J., & MacQueen, S. (2015). Obeying the rules of the road: Procedural justice, social identity, and normative compliance. *Journal of Contemporary Criminal Justice*, 31, 171–191.

Bradford, B., Milani, J., & Jackson, J. (2017). Identity, legitimacy and "making sense" of police use of force. *Policing: An International Journal*, 15, 731–742.

Brady, W. J., Wills, J. A., Burkart, D., Jost, J. T., & Van Bavel, J. J. (2019). An ideological asymmetry in the diffusion of moralized content on social media among political leaders. *Journal of Experimental Psychology: General*, 148(10), 1802–1813. https://doi.org/10.1037/xge0000532

Brashier, N. M., Eliseev, E. D., & Marsh, E. J. (2020). An initial accuracy focus prevents illusory truth. *Cognition*, 194, 104054. https://doi.org/10.1016/j.cognition.2019. 104054

Brewer, M. B., Hong, Y. Y., & Li, Q. (2004). Dynamic entitativity: Perceiving groups as actors. In V. Yzerbyt, C. M. Judd, & O. Corneille (Eds.), *The Psychology of Group Perception* (pp. 19–30). New York: Psychology Press.

Brewer, N. T., Chapman, G. B., Gibbons, F. X., Gerrard, M., McCaul, K. D., & Weinstein, N. D. (2007). Meta-analysis of the relationship between risk perception and health behavior: The example of vaccination. *Health Psychology*, 26(2), 136.

Brook, A. T. (2005). *Effects of contingencies of self-worth on self-regulation of behavior.* Unpublished doctoral dissertation. Ann Arbor: University of Michigan.

Brown, K., Fraser, G., Ramsay, M., et al. (2011). Attitudinal and demographic predictors of measles-mumps-rubella vaccine [MMR] uptake during the UK catch-up campaign 2008–09: Cross-sectional survey. *PLoS ONE*, e19381.

Bruckner, T., Scheffler, R. M., Shen, G., et al. (2011). The mental health workforce gap in low- and middle-income countries: A needs-based approach. *Bulletin of the World Health Organization*, 89(3), 184–194.

Bruder, M., Haffke, P., Neave, N., Nouripanah, N., & Imhoff, R. (2013). Measuring individual differences in generic beliefs in conspiracy theories across cultures: The Conspiracy Mentality Questionnaire (CMQ). *Frontiers in Psychology*, 4, Article 225, 1–15.

Bruine de Bruin, W., & Bostrom, A. (2013). Assessing what to address in science communication. *Proceedings of the National Academy of Sciences*, 110, 14062–14068.

Burt, R. S. (2000). The network structure of social capital. *Research in Organizational Behavior*, 22, 345–423.

Butchireddygari, L. (2020). How concerned are Americans about coronavirus so far? *Five Thirty Eight* (March 13). https://fivethirtyeight.com/features/how-concerned-are-americans-about-coronavirus-so-far/

References 113

Byer, B., & Myers, L. B. (2000). Psychological correlates of adherence to medication in asthma. *Psychology, Health & Medicine*, 5(4), 389–393.

Byrnes, J. P., Miller, D. C., & Schafer, W. D. (1999). Gender differences in risk taking: A meta-analysis. *Psychological Bulletin*, 125(3), 367.

Capraro, V., Jagfeld, G., Klein, R., Mul, M., & van de Pol, I. (2019). Increasing altruistic and cooperative behaviour with simple moral nudges. *Scientific Report*, 9, 11880. https://doi.org/10.1038/s41598-019-48094-4

Carver, C. S., & Scheier, M. F. (2014). Dispositional optimism. *Trends in Cognitive Sciences*, 18, 293–299.

Carver, C. S., Scheier, M. F., & Segerstrom, S. C. (2010). Optimism. *Clinical Psychology Review*, 30, 879–889.

Cassar, A., Healy, A., & Von Kessler, C. (2017). Trust, risk, and time preferences after a natural disaster: Experimental evidence from Thailand. *World Development*, 94, 90–105.

Cattell, V. (2001). Poor people, poor places, and poor health: The mediating role of social networks and social capital. *Social Science & Medicine*, 52(10), 1501–1516.

Cavallo, J. V., Fitzsimons, G. M., & Holmes, J. G. (2009). Taking chances in the face of threat: Romantic risk regulation and approach motivation. *Personality and Social Psychology Bulletin*, 35(6), 737–751. https://doi.org/10.1177/0146167209332742

Centers for Disease Control and Prevention (CDC). (2018). *Influenza vaccination recommendations*, 2017–2018.

Chadwick, A., Vaccari, C., & O'Loughlin, B. (2018). Do tabloids poison the well of social media? Explaining democratically dysfunctional news sharing. *New Media & Society*, 20(11), 4255–4274. https://doi.org/10.1177/1461444818769689

Chambers, J., Swan, L., & Heesacker, M. (2015). Perceptions of US social mobility are divided (and distorted) along ideological lines. *Psychological Science*, 26, 413–423.

Chang, E. C. C, & Chu, Y. (2006). Corruption and trust: Exceptionalism in Asian democracies? *The Journal of Politics*, 68(2), 259–271.

Chanley, V. A. (2002). Trust in government in the aftermath of 9/11: Determinants and consequences. *Political Psychology*, 23(3), 469–483.

Chanley, V. A., Rudolph, T. J., & Rahn, W. M. (2000). The origins and consequences of public trust in government: A time series analysis. *Public Opinion Quarterly*, 64(3), 239–256.

Cheng, C. (2004). To be paranoid is the standard? Panic responses to SARS outbreak in the Hong Kong Special Administrative Region. *Asian Perspective*, 28, 67–98.

Cheng, C., & Cheung. M. W. (2005). Psychological responses to outbreak of severe acute respiratory syndrome: A prospective, multiple time-point study. *Journal of Personality*, 73, 261–285.

Cheung, F., & Lucas, R. (2016). Income inequality is associated with stronger social comparison effects: The effect of relative income on life satisfaction. *Journal of Personality Social Psychology*, 110, 332–341.

Chiou, L., & Tucker, C. (2018). *Fake news and advertising on social media: A study of the anti-vaccination movement* (No. w25223). National Bureau of Economic Research.

Choi, I., Choi, J. A., & Norenzayan, A. (2008). Culture and decisions. In D. J. Koehler, & N. Harvey (Eds.), *Blackwell Handbook of Judgment and Decision Making* (pp. 504–524). Oxford: Blackwell.

114 Individuals, Groups, and Society in Pandemics

Chorus, C. G., Pudāne, B., Mouter, N., & Campbell, D. (2018). Taboo trade-off aversion: A discrete choice model and empirical analysis. *Journal of Choice Modelling*, 27, 37–49.

Chuang, Y. C., Huang, Y. L., Tseng, K. C., Yen, C. H., & Yang, L. H. (2015). Social capital and health-protective behavior intentions in an influenza pandemic. *PloS ONE*, 10(4), e0122970.

Cialdini, R. B. (1984). *Influence: The New Psychology of Modern Persuasion*. New York: Quill.

Cialdini, R. B. (2009). *Wywieranie wpływu na ludzi - teoria i praktyka*. Gdańskie Wydawnictwo Psychologiczne.

Cialdini, R., & Goldstein, N. (2004). Social influence: Compliance and conformity, 55, 591–621.

Cialdini, R. B., Reno, R. R., & Kallgren, C. A. (1990). A focus theory of normative conduct: Recycling the concept of norms to reduce littering in public places. *Journal of Personality and Social Psychology*, 58(6), 1015–1026. https://doi.org/10.1037/0022-3514.58.6.1015

Citrin, J., & Stoker, L. (2018). Political trust in a cynical age. *Annual Review of Political Science*, 21, 49–70.

Clark, J. M., & Paivio, A. (1991). Dual coding theory and education. *Educational Psychology Review*, 3(3), 149–210.

Clark, M. S., & Mills, J. R. (1993). The difference between communal and exchange relationships: What it is and is not. *Personality and Social Psychology Bulletin*, 19(6), 684–691. https://doi.org/10.1177/0146167293196003

Clark, M. S., & Mills, J. R. (2012). A theory of communal (and exchange) relationships. In P. A. M. Van Lange, A. W. Kruglanski, & E. T. Higgins (Eds.), *Handbook of Theories of Social Psychology* (pp. 232–250). Thousand Oaks, CA: Sage Publications.

Clark, M. S., Lemay, E. P., Graham, S. M., Pataki, S. P., & Finkel, E. J. (2010). Ways of giving benefits in marriage: Norm use, relationship satisfaction, and attachment-related variability. *Psychological Science*, 21(7), 944–951.

Clarke, S. (2000). The closure of the Russian labour market. *European Societies*, 2(4), 483–504.

Clay, R. (2017). The behavioral immune system and attitudes about vaccines: Contamination aversion predicts more negative vaccine attitudes. *Social Psychological and Personality Science,* 8, 162–172. https://doi.org/10.1177/1948550616664957

Cleaver, F. (2005). The inequality of social capital and the reproduction of chronic poverty. *World development*, 33(6), 893–906.

Clifford, S., & Wendell, D. G. (2016). How disgust influences health purity attitudes. *Political Behavior*, 38, 155–178. https://doi.org/10.1007/s11109-015-9310-z

Coelho, M. P. (2010). Unrealistic optimism: Still a neglected trait. *Journal of Business and Psychology*, 25, 397–408.

Cokely, E. T., Galesic, M., Schulz, E., Ghazal, S., & Garcia-Retamero, R. (2012). Measuring risk literacy: The Berlin Numeracy Test. *Judgment and Decision Making*, 7(1), 25–47.

Collishaw, S. (2015). Annual research review: Secular trends in child and adolescent mental health. *Journal of Child Psychology and Psychiatry*, 56, 370–393.

Colombo, E., Rotondi, V., & Stanca, L. (2018). Macroeconomic conditions and well-being: Do social interactions matter? *Applied Economics*, 50(28), 3029–3038.

References 115

Confas, N., Carl, N., & Woodley of Menie, M. A. (2018). Does activism in social science explain conservatives' distrust of scientists? *The American Sociologist*, 49, 135–148. https://doi.org/10.1007/s12108-017-9362-0

Cooper, D. P., Goldenberg, J. L., & Arndt, J. (2010). Examining the terror management health model: The interactive effect of conscious death thought and health-coping variables on decisions in potentially fatal health domains. *Personality and Social Psychology Bulletin*, 36(7), 937–946. https://doi.org/10.1177/0146167210370694

Cooper, K., Gregory, J. D., Walker, I., Lambe, S., & Salkovskis, P. M. (2017). Cognitive behaviour therapy for health anxiety: A systematic review and meta-analysis – Corrigendum. *Behavioural and Cognitive Psychotherapy*, 45(6), 673.

Cordasco, K. M., Eisenman, D. P., Glik, D. C., Golden, J. F., & Asch, S. M. (2007). "They blew the levee": Distrust of authorities among hurricane Katrina evacuees. *Journal of Health Care for the Poor and Underserved*, 18(2), 277–282.

Corum, J., Grady, D., Wee, S., & Zimmer, C. (2020). Coronavirus Vaccine Tracker. (September 13). *The New York Times*. https://www.nytimes.com/interactive/2020/science/coronavirus-vaccine-tracker.html

Coupe, T. (2017). The impact of terrorism on expectations, trust and happiness – the case of the November 13 attacks in Paris, France. *Applied Economics Letters*, 24(15), 1084–1087.

Craig, M. A., & Richeson, J. A. (2012). Coalition or derogation? How perceived discrimination influences intraminority intergroup relations. *Journal of Personality and Social Psychology*, 102(4), 759–777. https://doi.org/10.1037/a0026481

Crum, A. J., Salovey, P., & Achor, S. (2013). Rethinking stress: The role of mindsets in determining the stress response. *Journal of Personality and Social Psychology*, 104(4), 716–733. https://doi.org/10.1037/a0031201

Cruwys, T., Greenaway, K., Ferris, L. J., Rathbone, J. A., Saeri, A. K., Williams, E., Parker, S. L., Chang, M. X-L., Croft, N., Bingley, W., & Grace, L. (2021). When trust goes wrong: A social identity model of risk taking. *Journal of Personality and Social Psychology*, 120(1), 57–83.

Cruwys, T., Haslam, S. A., Dingle, G. A., Haslam, C., & Jetten, J. (2014). Depression and social identity: An integrative review. *Personality and Social Psychology Review*, 18(3), 215–238. https://doi.org/10.1177/1088868314523839

Cruwys, T., Saeri, A. K., Radke, H. R. M., Walter, Z. C., Crimston, D., & Ferris, L. J. (2019). Risk and protective factors for mental health at a youth mass gathering. *European Child and Adolescent Psychiatry*, 28, 211–222.

Cutter, S. L., Burton, C., & Emrich, C. (2010). Disaster resilience indicators for benchmarking baseline conditions. *Journal of Homeland Security and Emergency Management*, 7, 1–22.

Czarnek, G., Kossowska, M., & Richter, M. (2019). Aging, effort, and stereotyping: The evidence for the moderating role of self-involvement. *International Journal of Psychophysiology*, 138, 1–10. https://doi.org/10.1016/j.ijpsycho.2019.01.009

Czarnek, G., Kossowska, M., & Richter, M. (2020). Stereotyping and effort mobilization in older age: The role of self-involvement. In G. Sedek, T. M. Hess, & D. R. Touron (Eds.), *Multiple Pathways of Cognitive Aging: Motivational and Contextual Influences*. Oxford University Press.

Czarnek, G., Kossowska, M., & Szwed, P. (2020). Political ideology and attitudes towards vaccines: Study Reports. https://doi.org/10.31234/osf.io/uwehk

Daley, M. F., Narwaney, K. J., Shoup, J. A., Wagner, N. M., & Glanz, J. M. (2018). Addressing parents' vaccine concerns: A randomized trial of a social media intervention. *American Journal of Preventive Medicine*, 55(1), 44–54.

Damasio, A. R. (2011). *Błąd Kartezjusza. Emocje, rozum i ludzki mózg.* Pozna: Rebis.

Danis, K., Georgakopoulou, T., Stavrou, T., Laggas, D., & Panagiotopoulos,T. (2010). Socio- economic factors play a more important role in childhood vaccination coverage than parental perceptions: A cross-sectional study in Greece. *Vaccine*, 28, 1861–1869.

Davidai, S., & Gilovich, T. (2015). Building a more mobile America – one income quintile at a time. *Perspectives on Psychological Science*, 10, 60–71.

Davis, C. A., Varol, O., Ferrara, E., Flammini, A., & Menczer, F. (2016). Bot or not: A system to evaluate social bots. *Proceedings of the 25th International Conference Companion on World Wide Web - WWW '16 Companion*, 273–274. https://doi.org/10.1145/2872518.2889302

Davis, N. Z. (1973). The rites of violence: Religious riot in sixteenth-century France. *Past & Present*, 59, 51–91.

Daw, T. M., Coulthard, S., Cheung, W. W., et al. (2015). Evaluating taboo trade-offs in ecosystems services and human wellbeing. *PNAS*, 112(22), 6949–6954.

Day, M., & Fiske, S. (2016). Movin' on up? How perceptions of social mobility affect our willingness to defend the system. *Social Psychological and Personality Science*, 8(3), 267–274. https://doi.org/10.1177/1948550616678454

Dechêne, A., Stahl, C., Hansen, J., & Wänke, M. (2010). The truth about the truth: A meta-analytic review of the truth effect. *Personality and Social Psychology Review*, 14(2), 238–257. https://doi.org/10.1177/1088868309352251

de Figueiredo, A., Johnston, I. G., Smith, D. M. D., Agarwal, S., Larson, H. J., & Jones, N. S. (2016). Forecasted trends in vaccination coverage and correlations with socioeconomic factors: A global time-series analysis over 30 years. *The Lancet Global Health*, 4(10), e726–e735. https://doi.org/10.1016/S2214-109X(16)30167-X

Delhey, J., Newton, K., & Welzel, C. (2011). How general is trust in "most people"? Solving the radius of trust problem. *American Sociological Review*, 76(5), 786–807.

Desclaux, A., Diop, M., & Doyon, S. (2017). Fear and containment: Contact follow-up and social effects in Senegal and Guinea. In M. Hofman & S. Au (Eds.), *The Politics of Fear: Medecins sans Frontieres and the West African Ebola Epidemic* (pp. 210–234). New York: Oxford University Press.

DeSteno, D., Bartlett, M. Y., Baumann, J., Williams, L. A., & Dickens, L. (2010). Gratitude as moral sentiment: Emotion-guided cooperation in economic exchange. *Emotion*, 10(2), 289–293. https://doi.org/10.1037/a0017883

Deutsche Welle DW news. (2020). Coronavirus: 5 things New Zealand got right. https://www.dw.com/en/jacinda-ardern-leadership-in-coronavirus-response/a-53733397

DeYoung, S. E., & Peters, M. (2016). My community, my preparedness: The role of sense of place, community, and confidence in government in disaster readiness. *International Journal of Mass Emergencies & Disasters*, 34(2), 250–282.

Dillard, A. J., McCaul, K. D., & Klein, W. M. P. (2006). Unrealistic optimism in smokers: Implications for smoking myth endorsement and self-protective motivation. *Journal of Health Communication*, 11, 93–102.

Dillard, A. J., Midboe, A. M., & Klein, W. M. P. (2009). The dark side of optimism: Unrealistic optimism about problems with alcohol predicts subsequent negative event experiences. *Personality and Social Psychology Bulletin*, 35, 1540–1550.

References 117

Dinesen, P. T., & Jager, M. M. (2013). The effect of terror on institutional trust: New evidence from the 3/11 Madrid terrorist attack. *Political Psychology*, 34(6), 917–926.

Ditto, P. H., & Lopez, D. L. (1992). Motivated skepticism: Use of differential decision criteria for preferred and nonpreferred conclusions. *Journal of Personality and Social Psychology*, 63, 568–584. https://doi.org/10.1037/0022-3514.63.4.568

Dolinski, D., & Grzyb, T. (2017). *Posłuszny do bólu*. Sopot: Smak Słowa.

Dolinski, D., Dolinska, B., Zmaczynska-Witek, B., Banach, M., & Kulesza, W. (2020). Unrealistic optimism in the time of coronavirus pandemic: May it help to kill, if so – whom: Disease or the Person?. *Journal of Clinical Medicine*, 9(5), 1464. https://doi.org/10.3390/jcm9051464

Dorling, D., & Lee, C. (2014). Inequality constitutes a particular place. In Pakes, F., & Pritchard, D. (Eds.), *Riot, Unrest and Protest on the Global Stage* (pp. 115–131). Basingstoke, UK: Palgrave Macmillan.

Dotti Sani, G. M., & Magistro, B. (2016). Increasingly unequal? The economic crisis, social inequalities and trust in the European Parliament in 20 European countries. *European Journal of Political Research*, 55(2), 246–264.

Douglas, K. M., Sutton, R. M., & Cichocka, A. (2017). The psychology of conspiracy theories. *Current Directions in Psychological Science*, 26, 538–542. https://doi.org/10.1177/0963721417718261

Drury, J. (2012). Collective resilience in mass emergencies and disasters. In J. Jetten, C. Haslam, & S. A. Haslam (Eds.), *The Social Cure: Identity, Health and Well-being* (pp. 195–215). London: Psychology Press.

Duan, L., & Zhu, G. (2020). Psychological interventions for people affected by the COVID-19 epidemic. *Lancet Psychiatry*, 7, 300–302.

Durante, F., Tablante, C., & Fiske, S. (2017). Poor but warm, rich but cold (and competent): Social classes in the stereotype content model. *Journal of Social Issues*, 73, 138–157.

Duszyński, J., Pyrć, K., Afelt, A., Ochab-Marcinek, A., Rosińska, M., Rychard, A., & Smiatacz, T. (2020). *Zrozumieć COVID – 19*. Warszawa: Wydawnictwo PAN.

Earle, T. (2010). Trust in risk management: A model-based review of empirical research. *Risk Analysis: An International Journal*, 30(4), 541–574.

Economou, M., Madianos, M., Peppou, L. E., Souliotis, K., Patelakis, A., & Stefanis, C. (2014). Cognitive social capital and mental illness during economic crisis: A nationwide population-based study in Greece. *Social Science & Medicine*, 100, 141–147.

Edmondson, D., Park, C. L., Chaudoir, S. R., & Wortmann, J. H. (2008). Death without God: Religious struggle, death concerns, and depression in the terminally ill. *Psychological Science*, 19(8), 754–758. https://doi.org/10.1111/j.1467-9280.2008.02152.x

Effron, D. A., & Raj, M. (2019). Misinformation and morality: Encountering fake-news headlines makes them seem less unethical to publish and share. *Psychological Science*, 31(1). https://doi.org/10.1177/0956797619887896

Ehsan, A., Klaas, H. S., Bastianen, A., & Spini, D. (2019). Social capital and health: A systematic review of systematic reviews. *SSM-Population Health*, 8, 100425.

Elgar, F. (2010). Income inequality, trust, and population health in 33 countries. *American Journal of Public Health*, 100, 2311–2315.

Ellemers, N. (1993). The influence of socio-structural variables on identity management strategies. *European Review of Social Psychology*, 4(1), 27–57. https://doi.org/10.1080/14792779343000013

Ellinas, A. A., & Lamprianou, I. (2014). Political trust in extremis. *Comparative Politics*, 46(2), 231–250.

118 *Individuals, Groups, and Society in Pandemics*

Elliot, A. J., & Maier, M. A. (2012). Color-in-context theory. *Advances in Experimental Social Psychology*, 45, 61–125.

Elliott, J. R., Haney, T. J., & Sams-Abiodun, P. (2010). Limits to social capital: Comparing network assistance in two New Orleans neighborhoods devastated by Hurricane Katrina. *The Sociological Quarterly*, 51(4), 624–648.

Enders, A. M., & Armaly, M. T. (2019). The differential effects of actual and perceived polarization. *Political Behavior*, 41, 815–839. https://doi.org/10.1007/s11109-018-9476-2

Engdahl, E., & Lidskog, R. (2012). Risk, communication and trust: Towards an emotional understanding of trust. *Public Understanding of Science*, 19, 703–717.

Erlingsson, G. Ó., Linde, J., & Öhrvall, R. (2016). Distrust in utopia? Public perceptions of corruption and political support in Iceland before and after the financial crisis of 2008. *Government and Opposition*, 51(4), 553–579.

Ervasti, H., Kouvo, A., & Venetoklis, T. (2019). Social and institutional trust in times of crisis: Greece, 2002–2011. *Social Indicators Research*, 141(3), 1207–1231.

Esaiasson, P. (2010). Will citizens take no for an answer? What government officials can do to enhance decision acceptance. *European Political Science Review*, 2(3), 351–371.

Esaiasson, P., Sohlberg, J., Ghersetti, M., & Johansson, B. (2020) How the coronavirus crisis affects citizen trust in institutions and in unknown others – Evidence from "the Swedish experiment." *European Journal of Political Research*, online first.

Evans, G., & Andersen, R. (2006). The political conditioning of economic perceptions. *The Journal of Politics*, 68(1), 194–207.

Faheem, A., Ahmed, N., Pissarides, C., & Stiglitz, J. (2020). Why inequality could spread COVID-19. *The Lancet Public Health*, 5, e240.

Faricy, C., & Ellis, C. (2014). Public attitudes toward social spending in the United States: The differences between direct spending and tax expenditures. *Political Behavior*, 36, 53–76.

Feinstein, J. S., Adolphs, R., Damasio, A., & Tranel, D. (2011). The human amygdala and the induction and experience of fear. *Current Biology*, 21(1), 34–38. https://doi.org/10.1016/j.cub.2010.11.042

Feld, L. P., & Frey, B. S. (2007). Tax compliance as the result of a psychological tax contract: The role of incentives and responsive regulation. *Law & Policy*, 29(1), 102–120.

Ferraro, P. J., & Price, M. K. (2013). Using non-pecuniary strategies to influence behavior: Evidence from a large scale field experiment. *Review of Economics and Statistics*, 95, 64–73.

Ferrer, R., & Klein, W. M. (2015). Risk perceptions and health behavior. *Current Opinion in Psychology*, 5, 85–89. https://doi.org/10.1016/j.copsyc.2015.03.012

Ferrer, R. A., Klein, W. M. P., Avishai, A., Jones, K., Villegas, M., & Sheeran, P. (2018). When does risk perception predict protection motivation for health threats? A person-by-situation analysis. *PLoS ONE*, 13(3), Article e0191994.

Finucane M. L. (2008). Emotion, affect, and risk communication with older adults: Challenges and opportunities. *Journal of Risk Research*, 11(8), 983–997. https://doi.org/10.1080/13669870802261595

Finucane, M. L., Alhakami, A., Slovic, P., & Johnson, S. M. (2000). The affect heuristic in judgments of risks and benefits. *Journal of Behavioral Decision Making*, 13(1), 1–17.

References 119

Fischbacher, U., Fong, C. M., & Fehr, E. (2009). Fairness, errors and the power of competition. *Journal of Economic Behavior & Organization*, 72(1), 527–545. https://doi.org/10.1016/j.jebo.2009.05.021

Fischbacher, U., Gaechter, S., & Fehr, E. (2001). Are people conditionally cooperative? Evidence from a public goods experiment. *Economics Letters*, 71(3), 397–404.

Fischer, A. H., & Manstead, A. S. R. (2016). Social functions of emotion and emotion regulation. In L. Feldman Barrett, M. Lewis, & J. M. Haviland-Jones (Eds.), *Handbook of Emotions* (pp. 424–439). New York: The Guilford Press.

Fischhoff, B., Slovic, P., Lichtenstein, S., Read, S., & Combs, B. (1978). How safe is safe enough? A psychometric study of attitudes towards technological risks and benefits. *Policy Sciences*, 9, 127–152.

Fiske, A. P. (1992). The four elementary forms of sociality: Framework for a unified theory of social relations. *Psychological Review*, 99, 689–723. https://doi.org/10.1037/0033-295X.99.4.689

Fiske, A. P. (2004). Four modes of constituting relationships: Consubstantial assimilation; space, magnitude, time and force; concrete procedures; abstract symbolism. In N. Haslam (Ed.), *Relational Models Theory: A Contemporary Overview* (pp. 61–146). Mahwah, NJ: Erlbaum.

Fiske, A. P. (2019). *Kama Muta: Discovering the Connecting Emotion*. London: Routledge.

Fiske, A. P., & Haslam, N. (2005). The four basic social bonds: Structures for coordinating interaction. In M. W. Baldwin (Ed.), *Interpersonal Cognition* (pp. 267–298). New York: Guilford Press.

Fiske, A. P., & Tetlock, P. E. (1997). Taboo trade-offs: Reactions to transactions that transgress the spheres of justice. *Political Psychology*, 18, 255–297.

Fiske, A. P., Seibt, B., & Schubert, T. (2017). The sudden devotion emotion: Kama Muta and the cultural practices whose function is to evoke it. *Emotion Review*, 11, 74–86.

Fiske, S. T., & Taylor, S. E. (1984). *Social Cognition*. New York: Random House.

Florian, V., & Mikulincer, M. (1998). Symbolic immortality and the management of the terror of death: The moderating role of attachment style. *Journal of Personality and Social Psychology*, 74(3), 725–734. https://doi.org/10.1037/0022-3514.74.3.725

Ford, T., Vizard, T., Sadler, K., et al. (2020). Data resource profile: The mental health of children and young people surveys (MHCYP). *International Journal of Epidemiology*, 49(2), 363–364. https://doi.org/10.1093/ije/dyz259

Foster, C., & Frieden, J. (2017). Crisis of trust: Socio-economic determinants of Europeans' confidence in government. *European Union Politics*, 18(4), 511–535.

Fragale, A. R., & Heath, C. (2016). Evolving informational credentials: The (mis) attribution of believable facts to credible sources. *Personality and Social Psychology Bulletin*. https://doi.org/10.1177/0146167203259933

Fraley, R. C. (2019). Attachment in adulthood: Recent developments, emerging debates, and future direction. *Annual Review of Psychology*, 70, 401–422.

Frances, M., Payne, J. W., & Bettman, J. R. (1999). Emotional trade-off difficulty and choice. *Journal of Marketing Research*, 36, 143–159.

Fredrickson, B. (1998). What good are positive emotions? *Review of General Psychology*, 2, 300-319.

Frey, B. S., & Meier, S. (2004). Social comparisons and pro-social behavior: Testing "conditional cooperation" in a field experiment. *American Economic Review*, 94(5), 1717–1722.

120   *Individuals, Groups, and Society in Pandemics*

Frey, B. S., & Torgler, B. (2007). Tax morale and conditional cooperation. *Journal of Comparative Economics*, 35(1), 136–159.

Frijda, N. H. (1986). *Studies in Emotion and Social Interaction. The Emotions*. Cambridge University Press.

Furnham, A. (1988). *Lay Theories: Everyday Understanding of Problems in the Social Sciences*. Oxford: Pergamon Press.

Gächter, S., Herrmann, B., & Thöni, C. (2004). Trust, voluntary cooperation, and socio-economic background: Survey and experimental evidence. *Journal of Economic Behavior & Organization*, 55(4), 505–531.

Gaddy, M. A., & Ingram, R. E. (2014). A meta-analytic review of mood-congruent implicit memory in depressed mood. *Clinical Psychology Review*, 34(5), 402–416.

Gailliot, M. T., Schmeichel, B. J., & Baumeister, R. F. (2006). Self-regulatory processes defend against the threat of death: Effects of self-control depletion and trait self-control on thoughts and fears of dying. *Journal of Personality and Social Psychology*, 91(1), 49–62. https://doi.org/10.1037/0022-3514.91.1.49

Gailliot, M. T., Stillman, T. F., Schmeichel, B. J., Maner, J. K., & Plant, E. A. (2008). Mortality salience increases adherence to salient norms and values. *Personality and Social Psychology Bulletin*, 34(7), 993–1003. https://doi.org/10.1177/0146167208316791

Gaines, B. J., Kuklinski, J. H., Quirk, P. J., Peyton, B., & Verkuilen, J. (2007). Same facts, different interpretations: Partisan motivation and opinion on Iraq. *The Journal of Politics*, 69(4), 957–974.

Galesic, M., & Garcia-Retamero, R. (2011). Do low-numeracy people avoid shared decision making? *Health Psychology*, 30(3), 336–341.

Garcia-Retamero, R., & Cokely, E. T. (2013). Communicating health risks with visual aids. *Current Directions in Psychological Science*, 22(5), 392–399.

Garcia-Retamero, R., & Cokely, E. T. (2017). Designing visual aids that promote risk literacy: A systematic review of health research and evidence-based design heuristics. *Human Factors*, 59(4), 582–627.

Gardner, B. (2020). NHS volunteer army of 750,000 has been given fewer than 20,000 tasks, data reveals. *The Telegraph*. https://www.telegraph.co.uk/news/2020/04/16/least730000-volunteers-nhs-scheme-yet-deployed-care-home-bosses/

Gasiorowska, A., & Zaleskiewicz, T. (2020). Trading in search of structure: Market relationships as a compensatory control tool. *Journal of Personality and Social Psychology*, 120(2), 300–334. https://doi.org/10.1037/pspi0000246

Gasiorowska, A., Zaleskiewicz, T., & Kesebir, P. (2018). Money as an existential anxiety buffer: Exposure to money prevents mortality reminders from leading to increased death thoughts. *Journal of Experimental Social Psychology*, 79, 394–409. https://doi.org/10.1016/j.jesp.2018.09.004

Gazeta Prawna. (2020). Coronavirus. There is a fine of 5,000 PLN for breaking the quarantine. (March 10). https://www.gazetaprawna.pl/artykuly/1458695,-koronawirus-kwarantanna-jaka-kara.html

Gerber, M. M., & Jackson, J. (2017). Justifying violence: Legitimacy, ideology and public support for police use of force. *Psychology, Crime & Law*, 23(1), 79–95.

Gerber, T. P., & Mayorova, O. (2010). Getting personal: Networks and stratification in the Russian labor market, 1985–2001. *American Journal of Sociology*, 116(3), 855–908.

Gerend, M. A., & Sias, T. (2009). Message framing and color priming: How subtle threat cues affect persuasion. *Journal of Experimental Social Psychology*, 45(4), 999–1002.

Gesthuizen, M., Van der Meer, T., & Scheepers, P. (2009). Ethnic diversity and social capital in Europe: Tests of Putnam's thesis in European countries. *Scandinavian Political Studies*, 32(2), 121–142.

Gigerenzer, G. (2008a). *Rationality For Mortals: How People Cope With Uncertainty.* Oxford University Press.

Gigerenzer, G. (2008b). *Gut Feelings.* London: Penguin Books.

Gigerenzer, G. (2011). What are natural frequencies? *British Medical Journal*, 343, d6386.

Gigerenzer, G. (2015). *Calculated Risks: How to Know When Numbers Deceive You.* New York: Simon and Schuster.

Gigerenzer, G. (2018). The bias bias in behavioral economics. *Review of Behavioral Economics*, 5, 303–336.

Gigerenzer, G., Gaissmaier, W., Kurz-Milcke, E., Schwartz, L. M., & Woloshin, S. (2007). Helping doctors and patients make sense of health statistics. *Psychological Science in the Public Interest: A Journal of the American Psychological Society*, 8(2), 53–96. https://doi.org/10.1111/j.1539-6053.2008.00033.x

Gilovich, T., Griffin, D. W., & Kahneman, D. (Eds.) (2002). *Heuristics and Biases: The Psychology of Intuitive Judgment.* Cambridge University Press.

Glanville, J. L., & Paxton, P. (2007). How do we learn to trust? A confirmatory tetrad analysis of the sources of generalized trust. *Social Psychology Quarterly*, 70(3), 230–242.

Goertzel, T. (1994). Belief in conspiracy theories. *Political Psychology*, 15(4), 731–742.

Goldenberg, J. L., Pyszczynski, T., Greenberg, J., & Solomon, S. (2000). Fleeing the body: A terror management perspective on the problem of human corporeality. *Personality and Social Psychology Review*, 4(3), 200–218. https://doi.org/10.1207/S15327957PSPR0403_1

Gollust, S. E., Nagler, R. H., & Fowler, E. F. (2020). The emergence of COVID-19 in the US: A public health and political communication crisis. *Journal of Health Politics, Policy and Law*, 45(6), 967–981.

Goodwin, R., Gaines, S. 0., Myers, L., & Neto, F. (2009). Initial psychological reactions to swine flu. *International Journal of Behavioral Medicine*, 18, 88–92.

Gordon-Hecker, T., Rosensaft-Eshel, D., Pittarello, A., Shalvi, S., & Bereby-Meyer, Y. (2017). Not taking responsibility: Equity trumps efficiency in allocation decisions. *Journal of Experimental Psychology: General*, 146(6), 771–775.

Granovetter, M. (1983). The strength of weak ties: A network theory revisited. *Sociological Theory*, 1, 201–233.

Gray, J. R. (1999). A bias toward short-term thinking in threat-related negative emotional states. *Personality and Social Psychology Bulletin*, 25(1), 65–75.

Greenaway, K. H., Haslam, S. A., Cruwys, T., Branscombe, N. R., Ysseldyk, R., & Heldreth, C. (2015). From "we" to "me": Group identification enhances perceived personal control with consequences for health and well-being. *Journal of Personality and Social Psychology*, 109(1), 53–74. https://doi.org/10.1037/pspi0000019

Greenberg, J., Pyszczynski, T., & Solomon S. (1986). The causes and consequences of a need for self-esteem: A terror management theory. In R. F. Baumeister (Ed.), *Public Self and Private Self* (pp. 189–212). Springer Series in Social Psychology. New York: Springer.

Greenberg, J., Simon, L., Pyszczynski, T., Solomon, S., & Chatel, D. (1992). Terror management and tolerance: Does mortality salience always intensify negative reactions to others who threaten one's worldview? *Journal of Personality and Social Psychology*, 63(2), 212–220. https://doi.org/10.1037/0022-3514.63.2.212

Greenberg, J., Solomon, S., & Arndt, J. (2008). A basic but uniquely human motivation: Terror management. In J. Y. Shah, & W. L. Gardner (Eds.), *Handbook of Motivation Science* (pp. 114–134). The Guilford Press.

Greenhalgh, T., Schmid, M. B., Czypionka, T., Bassler, D., & Gruer, L. (2020). Face masks for the public during the Covid-19 crisis. *BMJ*, 369.

Grimes, M. (2006). Organizing consent: The role of procedural fairness in political trust and compliance. *European Journal of Political Research*, 45(2), 285–315.

Grootelaar, H. A., & van den Bos, K. (2018). How litigants in Dutch courtrooms come to trust judges: The role of perceived procedural justice, outcome favorability, and other sociolegal moderators. *Law & Society Review*, 52(1), 234–268.

Grupe, D. W., & Nitschke, J. B. (2013). Uncertainty and anticipation in anxiety: An integrated neurobiological and psychological perspective. *Nature Reviews Neuroscience*, 14(7), 488–501.

Guerino, P., Harrison, P. M., & Sabol, W. J. (2011). *Prisoners in 2010*. Washington, DC: Bureau of Justice Statistics.

Guess, A. M., Lerner, M., Lyons, B., Montgomery, J. M., Nyhan, B., Reifler, J., & Sircar, N. (2020). A digital media literacy intervention increases discernment between mainstream and false news in the United States and India. *Proceedings of the National Academy of Sciences*, 117(27), 15536–15545. https://doi.org/10.1073/pnas.1920498117

Guardian News (2020). Jacinda Ardern: New coronavirus cases are "unacceptable failure of the system." (June 17). https://www.youtube.com/watch?v=9keqVcx77TA

Habibov, N., & Afandi, E. (2015). Pre-and post-crisis life-satisfaction and social trust in transitional countries: An initial assessment. *Social Indicators Research*, 121(2), 503–524.

Hagger, M. S., Koch, S., Chatzisarantis, N. L. D., & Orbell, S. (2017). The common sense model of self-regulation: Meta-analysis and test of a process model. *Psychological Bulletin*, 143, 1117–1154.

Hahn, U., Lagnado, D., Lewandowsky, S., & Chater, N. (2020). Crisis knowledge management: Reconfiguring the behavioural science community for rapid responding in the Covid-19 crisis. (March 21). https://doi.org/10.31234/osf.io/hsxdk

Haidt, J. (2012). *The Righteous Mind: Why Good People Are Divided by Politics and Religion*. New York: Pantheon/Random House.

Halawa, M., & Olcon-Kubicka, M. (2018). Digital householding: Calculating and moralizing domestic life through homemade spreadsheets. *Journal of Cultural Economy*, 11, 514–534.

Hamer, K., McFarland, S., & Penczek, M. (2019). What lies beneath? Predictors of identification with all humanity. *Personality and Individual Differences*, 141, 258–267. https://doi.org/10.1016/j.paid.2018.12.019

Hammen, C. (2005). Stress and depression. *Annual Review of Clinical Psychology*, 1, 293–319.

Hammer, J. C., Fisher, J. D., Fitzgerald, P., & Fisher, W. A. (1996). When two heads aren't better than one: AIDS risk behavior in college-age couples. *Journal of Applied Social Psychology*, 26, 375–397.

Han, S., Lerner, J. S., & Keltner, D. (2007). Feelings and consumer decision making: The appraisal-tendency framework. *Journal of Consumer Psychology*, 17(3), 158–168.

References 123

Han, Z., Lu, X., Hörhager, E. I., & Yan, J. (2017). The effects of trust in government on earthquake survivors' risk perception and preparedness in China. *Natural Hazards*, 86(1), 437–452.

Hansford, T. G., & Gomez, B. T. (2015). Reevaluating the sociotropic economic voting hypothesis. *Electoral Studies*, 39, 15–25.

Harel, A., & Porat, A. (2011). Commensurability and agency: Two yet-to-be-met challenges for law and economics. *Cornell Law Review*, 749. http://scholarship.law.cornell.edu/clr/vol96/iss4/22

Harmon-Jones, E., & Harmon-Jones, C. (2016). In L. Feldman Barrett, M. Lewis, & J. M. Haviland-Jones (Eds.), *Handbook of Emotions* (pp. 774–791). New York: The Guilford Press.

Harper, C. A., Satchell, L., Fido, D., & Latzman, R. (2020). Functional fear predicts public health compliance in the COVID-19 pandemic. (April 1). https://doi.org/10.31234/osf.io/jkfu3

Hartner, M., Kirchler, E., Poschalko, A., & Rechberger, S. (2010). Taxpayers' compliance by procedural and interactional fairness perceptions and social identity. *Journal of Psychology & Economics*, 3, 12–31.

Haslam, N., Bastian, B., & Bissett, M. (2004). Essentialist beliefs about personality and their implications. *Personality and Social Psychology Bulletin*, 30(12), 1661–1673. https://doi.org/10.1177/0146167204271182

Haslam, S. A., & Reicher, S. D. (2017). 50 years of "obedience to authority": From blind conformity to engaged followership. *Annual Review of Law and Social Science*, 13, 59–78.

Haslam, S. A., & Turner, J. C. (1992). Context-dependent variation in social stereotyping 2: The relationship between frame of reference, self-categorization and accentuation. *European Journal of Social Psychology*, 22, 251–277.

Haslam, S. A., Jetten, J., Postmes, T., & Haslam, C. (2009). Social identity, health and well-being: An emerging agenda for applied psychology. *Applied Psychology: An International Review*, 58(1), 1–23. https://doi.org/10.1111/j.1464-0597.2008.00379.x

Haslam, S. A., Jetten, J., Reicher, S., & Cruwys, T. (2020) *Together apart: The psychology of COVID-19*. New York: Sage.

Haslam, S. A., McMahon, C., Cruwys, T., Haslam, C., Greenaway, K. H., Jetten, J., & Steffens, N. K. (2018). Social cure, what social cure? The propensity to underestimate the importance of social factors for health. *Social Science & Medicine*, 198, 14–21.

Haslam, S. A., Reicher, S., & Levine, M. (2012). When other people are heaven, when other people are hell: How social identity determines the nature and impact of social support. In J. Jetten, C. Haslam, & S. A. Haslam (Eds.), *The Social Cure: Identity, Health, and Well-being*. London & New York: Psychology Press.

Haslam, S. A., Reicher, S. D., and Platow, M. J. (2020). *The New Psychology of Leadership: Identity, Influence and Power*. New York: Routledge.

Hawkins, R. L., & Maurer, K. (2010). Bonding, bridging and linking: How social capital operated in New Orleans following Hurricane Katrina. *British Journal of Social Work*, 40(6), 1777–1793.

Hays, J. (2005). *Epidemics and Pandemics: Their Impacts on Human History*. Santa Barbara, Denver, Oxford: ABC CLIO.

Hays, N., & Blader, S. (2017). To give or not to give? Interactive effects of status and legitimacy on generosity. *Journal of Personality and Social Psychology*, 112, 17–38.

124 *Individuals, Groups, and Society in Pandemics*

Hedman, E., Lekander, M., Karshikoff, B., Ljótsson, B., Axelsson, E., & Axelsson, J. (2016). Health anxiety in a disease-avoidance framework: Investigation of anxiety, disgust and disease perception in response to sickness cues. *Journal of Abnormal Psychology*, 125(7), 868–878.

Heflick, N. A., Goldenberg, J. L., Keroack, L. J., & Cooper, D. P. (2011). *Grim Reaping Psychological Well-being: Repeated Death Contemplation, Intrinsic Motivation, and Depression*. Unpublished manuscript, University of South Florida.

Heidegger, M. (1982). *Being and Time*. New York: Harper & Row. (Original work published 1926)

Helliwell, J., & Huang, H. (2008). How's your government? International evidence linking good government and well-being. *British Journal of Political Science*, 38, 595–619.

Helliwell, J. F., Huang, H., & Wang, S. (2014). Social capital and well-being in times of crisis. *Journal of Happiness Studies*, 15(1), 145–162.

Hernandez, E. M., Pullen, E., & Brauer, J. (2019). Social networks and the emergence of health inequalities following a medical advance: Examining prenatal H1N1 vaccination decisions. *Social Networks*, 58, 156–167.

Hetherington, M. J., & Husser, J. A. (2012). How trust matters: The changing political relevance of political trust. *American Journal of Political Science*, 56(2), 312–325.

Hetherington, M. J., & Nelson, M. (2003). Anatomy of a rally effect: George W. Bush and the war on terrorism. *PS: Political Science & Politics*, 36(1), 37–42.

Hetherington, M. J., & Rudolph, T. J. (2008). Priming, performance, and the dynamics of political trust. *The Journal of Politics*, 70(2), 498–512.

Hetherington, M. J., & Rudolph, T. J. (2015). *Why Washington Won't Work: Polarization, Political Trust, and the Governing Crisis*. University of Chicago Press.

Hetherington, M., & Weiler, J. (2015). Authoritarianism and polarization in American politics, still? In J. Thurber, & A. Yoshinaka (Eds.), *American Gridlock: The Sources, Character, and Impact of Political Polarization* (pp. 86–112). Cambridge University Press. doi:10.1017/CBO9781316287002.006

Hewitt, J. P. (2009). The social construction of self-esteem. In C. R. Snyder, & S. Lopez (Eds.), *Oxford Handbook of Positive Psychology* (pp. 217–224). Oxford University Press.

Hibbing, J. R., & Alford, J. R. (2004). Accepting authoritative decisions: Humans as wary cooperators. *American Journal of Political Science*, 48(1), 62–76.

Hibbing, J. R., & Theiss-Morse, E. (2002). *Stealth Democracy: Americans' Beliefs About How Government Should Work*. Cambridge University Press.

Hirsch, C. R., & Holmes, E. A. (2007). Mental imagery in anxiety disorders. *Psychiatry*, 6, 161–165.

Hoffrage, U., & Gigerenzer, G. (1998). Using natural frequencies to improve diagnostic inferences. *Academic Medicine*, 73(5), 538–540.

Hofstede, G. H. (2001). *Culture's Consequences: Comparing Values, Behaviors, Institutions and Organizations Across Nations*. Thousand Oaks, CA: Sage Publications.

Hofstede, G., Hofstede, G. J., & Minkov, M. (2010). *Cultures and Organizations: Software of the Mind* (Rev. 3rd ed.). New York: McGraw-Hill.

Holmes, E. A., & Mathews, A. (2005). Mental imagery and emotion: A special relationship? *Emotion*, 5, 489–497.

Holmes, E. A., & Mathews, A. (2010). Mental imagery in emotion and emotional disorders. *Clinical Psychology Review*, 30(3), 349–362. https://doi.org/10.1016/j.cpr.2010.01.001

Holmes, E. A., Mathews, A., Dalgleish, T., & Mackintosh, B. (2006). Positive interpretation training: Effects of mental imagery versus verbal training on positive mood. *Behavior Therapy*, 37, 237–247.

Holmes, E. A., Mathews, A., Mackintosh, B., & Dalgleish, T. (2008). The causal effect of mental imagery on emotion assessed using picture-word cues. *Emotion*, 8, 395–409.

Holmes, E. A., O'Connor, R. C., Perry, V. H., et al. (2020). Multidisciplinary research priorities for the COVID-19 pandemic: A call for action for mental health science. *The Lancet Psychiatry*, 7(6), 547–560. https://doi.org/10.1016/S2215-0366(20)30168-1

Holtgrave, D. R., & Weber, E. U. (1993). Dimensions of risk perception for financial and health risks. *Risk Analysis*, 13(5), 553–558.

Holtzworth-Munroe, A., & Clements, K. (2007). The association between anger and male perpetration of intimate partner violence. In T. A. Cavell, & K. T. Malcolm (Eds.), *Anger, Aggression and Interventions for Interpersonal Violence* (pp. 313–348). London: Lawrence Erlbaum Associates Publishers.

Honigsbaum, M. (2009). *Living with Enza: The Forgotten Story of Britain and the Great Flu Pandemic of 1918*. London: Macmillan.

Hoorens, V. (1993). Self-enhancement and superiority biases in social comparison. In W. Stroebe, & M. Hewstone (Eds.), *European Review of Social Psychology* (Vol. 4, pp. 113–139). Chichester: Wiley.

Hopf, H., Krief, A., Mehta, G., & Matlin, S. A. (2019). Fake science and the knowledge crisis: Ignorance can be fatal. *Royal Society Open Science*, 6, 190161.

Hopkins, N., Reicher, S., Stevenson, C., Pandey, K., Shankar, S., & Tewari, S. (2019). Social relations in crowds: Recognition, validation and solidarity. *European Journal of Social Psychology*, 49, 1283–1297.

Hornsey, M., Harris, J., & Fielding, K. (2018). The psychological roots of anti-vaccination attitudes: A 24-nation investigation. *Health Psychology*, 37, 307–315. http://dx.doi.org/10.1037/hea0000586

Hough, M., Jackson, J., Bradford, B., Myhill, A., & Quinton, P. (2010). Procedural justice, trust, and institutional legitimacy. *Policing: A Journal of Policy and Practice*, 4(3), 203–210.

Hsee, C. K. (2000). Attribute evaluability and its implications for joint-separate evaluation reversals and beyond. In D. Kahneman, & A. Tversky (Eds.), *Choices, Values and Frames*. Cambridge University Press.

Hung, A., Parker, A. M., & Yoong, J. (2009). *Defining and Measuring Financial Literacy*. RAND Working Paper Series WR-708. https://ssrn.com/abstract=1498674 or http://dx.doi.org/10.2139/ssrn.1498674

Hussain, A., Ali, S., Ahmed, M., & Hussain, S. (2018). The anti-vaccination movement: A regression in modern medicine. *Cureus*, 10, e2919. https://doi.org/10.7759/cureus.2919

Huston, S. J. (2010). Measuring financial literacy. *The Journal of Consumer Affairs*, 44(2), 296–316.

Iglič, H., Rözer, J., & Volker, B. G. (2020). Economic crisis and social capital in European societies: The role of politics in understanding short-term changes in social capital. *European Societies*, 23(2), 195–231.

IJzerman, H., Lewis, N. A., Jr., Weinstein, N., et al. (2020). Is Social and Behavioural Science Evidence Ready for Application and Dissemination? (April 27). https://doi.org/10.31234/osf.io/whds4

126 *Individuals, Groups, and Society in Pandemics*

Illiashenko, P. (2019). "Tough guy" vs. "Cushion" hypothesis: How does individualism affect risk-taking? *Journal of Behavioral and Experimental Finance*, 24, 100212. https://doi.org/10.1016/j.jbef.2019.04.005

International Food Policy Research Institute. (2020). How much will poverty increase because of COVID-19? (March 20). https://www.ifpri.org/blog/how-much-will-global-poverty-increase-because-covid-19 (accessed March 23, 2020).

Ioannidis, J. P. (2020). A fiasco in the making? As the coronavirus pandemic takes hold, we are making decisions without reliable data. (March 17). STAT. https://www.statnews.com/2020/03/17/a-fiasco-in-the-making-as-the-coronavirus-pandemic-takes-hold-we-are-making-decisions-without-reliable-data/

Islam, M. K., Merlo, J., Kawachi, I., Lindström, M., & Gerdtham, U. G. (2006). Social capital and health: Does egalitarianism matter? A literature review. *International Journal for Equity in Health*, 5(1), 3.

Izard, C. E. (1977). *Human Emotions*. New York: Plenum Press.

James, S. L., Abate, D., Abate, K. H., et al. (2018). Global, regional, and national incidence, prevalence, and years lived with disability for 354 diseases and injuries for 195 countries and territories, 1990–2017: A systematic analysis for the Global Burden of Disease Study 2017. *The Lancet*, 392(10159), 1789–1858.

Jaśko, K., & Kossowska, M. (2013). The impact of superordinate identification on the justification of intergroup inequalities. *European Journal of Social Psychology*, 43, 255–262.

Jetten, J., & Peters, K. (Eds.). (2019). *The Social Psychology of Inequality*. Cham, Switzerland: Springer.

Jetten, J., Bentley, S. V., Crimston, C. R., Selvanathan, H. P., Steffens, N. K., Haslam, C., Haslam, S. A., & Cruwys, T. (2020). *How COVID-19 affects our social life*. Unpublished data: The University of Queensland.

Jetten, J., Branscombe, N. R., Haslam, S. A., et al. (2015). Correction: Having a lot of a good thing: Multiple important group memberships as a source of self-esteem. *PLOS ONE*, 10(6), e0131035. https://doi.org/10.1371/journal.pone.0131035

Jetten, J., Haslam, C., & Haslam, S. A. (Eds.). (2012). *The Social Cure: Identity, Health and Well-being*. New York: Psychology Press.

Jetten, J., Mols, F., Healy, N., & Spears, R. (2017). "Fear of falling": Economic instability enhances collective angst among societies' wealthy class. *Journal of Social Issues*, 73(1), 61–79. https://doi.org/10.1111/josi.12204

Jiang, Y., Chen, Z., & Wyer Jr., R. (2014). Impact of money on emotional expression. *Journal of Experimental Social Psychology*, 55, 228–233.

Ji, J. L., Heyes, S. B., MacLeod, C., & Holmes, E. A. (2016). Emotional mental imagery as simulation of reality: Fear and beyond – A tribute to Peter Lang. *Behavior Therapy*, 47(5), 702–719. https://doi.org/10.1016/j.beth.2015.11.004

Ji, L.-J., Zhang, Z., Usborne, E., & Guan, Y. (2004). Optimism across cultures: In response to the severe acute respiratory syndrome outbreak. *Asian Journal of Social Psychology*, 7, 25–34.

Jilke, S. (2018). Citizen satisfaction under changing political leadership: The role of partisan motivated reasoning. *Governance*, 31(3), 515–533.

Johnson, S., & Mitton, T. (2003). Cronyism and capital controls: Evidence from Malaysia. *Journal of Financial Economics*, 67(2), 351–382.

Jonas, E., Martens, A., Niesta Kayser, D., Fritsche, I., Sullivan, D., & Greenberg, J. (2008). Focus theory of normative conduct and terror-management theory: The interactive impact of mortality salience and norm salience on social judgment. *Journal of Personality and Social Psychology*, 95(6), 1239–1251.

References 127

Josef, A. K., Richter, D., Samanez-Larkin, G. R., Wagner, G. G., Hertwig, R., & Mata, R. (2016). Stability and change in risk-taking propensity across the adult life span. *Journal of Personality and Social Psychology*, 111(3), 430.

Jung, M., Lin, L., & Viswanath, K. (2013). Associations between health communication behaviors, neighborhood social capital, vaccine knowledge, and parents' H1N1 vaccination of their children. *Vaccine*, 31(42), 4860–4866.

Kahan, D. M. (2017). *Misconceptions, Misinformation, and the Logic of Identity-Protective Cognition*. (May 24). Cultural Cognition Project Working Paper Series No. 164; Yale Law School, Public Law Research Paper No. 605; Yale Law & Economics Research Paper No. 575. https://ssrn.com/abstract=2973067 or http://dx.doi.org/10.2139/ssrn.2973067

Kahneman, D. (2003). A perspective on judgment and choice: Mapping bounded rationality. *American Psychologist*, 58, 697–720.

Kahneman, D., & Thaler, R. H. (2006). Anomalies: Utility maximization and experienced utility. *Journal of Economic Perspectives*, 20, 221–234.

Kanadiya, M. K., & Sallar, A. M. (2011). Preventive behaviors, beliefs, and anxieties in relation to the swine flu outbreak among college students aged 18–24 years. *Journal of Public Health*, 19, 139–145.

Kasser, T., & Sheldon, K. M. (2000). Of wealth and death: Materialism, mortality salience, and consumption behavior. *Psychological Science*, 11(4), 348–351. https://doi.org/10.1111/1467-9280.00269

Kaustia, M., Laukkanen, H., & Puttonen, V. (2009). Should good stocks have high prices or high returns? *Financial Analysts Journal*, 65, 55–62.

Kawachi, I., Kennedy, B. P., & Glass, R. (1999). Social capital and self-rated health: A contextual analysis. *American Journal of Public Health*, 89(8), 1187–1193.

Kawakami, K., & Dion, K. L. (1995). Social identity and affect as determinants of collective action: Toward an integration of relative deprivation and social identity theories. *Theory & Psychology*, 5(4), 551–577. https://doi.org/10.1177/0959354395054005

Keane, M. P., & Thorp, S. (2016). Complex decision making: The roles of cognitive limitations, cognitive decline, and aging. In J. Piggott, & A. Woodland (Eds.), *Handbook of the Economics of Population Aging* (Vol. 1, pp. 661–709). North-Holland: Elsevier.

Keele, L. (2005). The authorities really do matter: Party control and trust in government. *The Journal of Politics*, 67(3), 873–886.

Keeney, R. L., Raiffa, H., & Meyer, R. F. (1993). *Decisions with Multiple Objectives: Preferences and Value Trade-offs*. Cambridge University Press.

Keinan, G. (1987). Decision making under stress: Scanning of alternatives under controllable and uncontrollable threats. *Journal of Personality and Social Psychology*, 52(3), 639.

Keltner, D., Tracy, J., Sauter, D. A., Cordaro, D. C., & McNeil, G. (2016). Expression of emotion. In L. Feldman Barrett, M. Lewis, & J. M. Haviland-Jones (Eds.), *Handbook of Emotions* (pp. 467–482). New York: The Guilford Press.

Kilgo, D., Yoo, J., & Johnson, T. (2019). Spreading Ebola panic: Newspaper and social media coverage of the 2014 Ebola health crisis. *Health Communication*, 34(8), 811–817. https://doi.org/10.1080/10410236.2018.1437524

Kim, H. K., & Niederdeppe, J. (2013). Exploring optimistic bias and the integrative model of behavioral prediction in the context of a campus influenza outbreak. *Journal of Health Communication*, 18, 206–222.

Kim, J., & Oh, S. S. (2015). Confidence, knowledge, and compliance with emergency evacuation. *Journal of Risk Research*, 18(1), 111–126.

Kirby, T. (2020). Evidence mounts on the disproportionate effect of COVID-19 on ethnic minorities. *The Lancet Respiratory Medicine*, 8, 547–548. https://doi.org/10.1016/S2213-2600(20)30228-9

Klandermans, B. (2000). Identity and protest: How group identification helps to overcome collective action dilemmas. In M. Van Vugt, M. Snyder, T. R. Tyler, & A. Biel (Eds.), *Cooperation in Modern Society: Promoting the Welfare of Communities, States and Organizations* (pp. 162–183). London, UK: Routledge.

Klandermans, B. (2002). How group identification helps to overcome the dilemma of collective action. *American Behavioral Scientist*, 45, 887–900.

Klapper, L., Lusardi, A., & van Oudheusden P. (2015). *Financial Literacy around the World: Insights from Standard & Poor's Ratings Services Global Financial Literacy Survey.* http://gflec.org/wp-content/uploads/2015/11/3313-Finlit_Report_FINAL-5.11.16.pdf?x28148

Klein, C., & Helweg-Larsen, M. (2002). Perceived control and the optimistic bias: A meta-analytic review. *Psychology & Health*, 17, 437–446.

Koole, S. L., & Van den Berg, A. E. (2004). *Paradise lost and reclaimed: A motivational analysis of human-nature relations*. In J. Greenberg, S. L. Koole, & T. Pyszczynski (Eds.), *Handbook of Experimental Existential Psychology* (p. 86–103). Guilford Press.

Kosloff, S., & Greenberg, J. (2009). Pearls in the desert: Death reminders provoke immediate derogation of extrinsic goals, but delayed inflation. *Journal of Experimental Social Psychology*, 45(1), 197–203. https://doi.org/10.1016/j.jesp.2008.08.022

Kosslyn, S. M., Ganis, G., & Thompson, W. L. (2001). Neural foundations of imagery. *Nature Reviews. Neuroscience*, 2, 635–642.

Kossowska, M. (2005). *Umysł niezmienny...: Poznawcze mechanizmy sztywności*. Wydawnictwo Uniwersytetu Jagiellońskiego.

Kossowska, M., Szumowska, E., & Szwed, P. (2020). *The Psychology of Tolerance in Times of Uncertainty*. London: Routledge.

Kossowska, M., Szwed, P., & Czarnek, G. (2020). Ideologically motivated perception: The role of political context and active open-mindedness. (November 11). https://psyarxiv.com/2bstm/

Kossowska, M., Szwed, P., & Czarnek, G. (2021). Ideology shapes trust in scientists and attitudes towards vaccines during the COVID-19 pandemic. *Group Processes & Intergroup Relations*, 24(5), 720–737. doi:10.1177/13684302211001946

Kossowska, M., Szumowska, E., Dragon, P., Jaśko, K., & Kruglanski, A. W. (2018). Disparate roads to certainty processing strategy choices under need for closure. *European Review of Social Psychology*, 29(1), 161–211. https://doi.org/10.1080/1046 3283.2018.1493066

Koster, E. H., De Raedt, R., Goeleven, E., Franck, E., & Crombez, G. (2005). Mood-congruent attentional bias in dysphoria: Maintained attention to and impaired disengagement from negative information. *Emotion*, 5(4), 446.

Kraft-Todd, G., Yoeli, E., Bhanot, S., & Rand, D. (2015). Promoting cooperation in the field. *Current Opinion in Behavioral Sciences*, 3, 96–101. https://doi.org/10.1016/j.cobeha.2015.02.006

Kramer, A. D. I., Guillory, J. E., & Hancock, J. T. (2014). Experimental evidence of massive-scale emotional contagion through social networks. *Proceedings of the National Academy of Sciences of the United States of America*, 111, 8788–8790.

Kraus, M. W., Rucker, J. M., & Richeson, J. A. (2017). Americans misperceive racial economic equality. *Proceedings of the National Academy of Sciences*, 114(39), 10324–10331. https://doi.org/10.1073/pnas.1707719114

References 129

Kruglanski, A. W. (1989a). *Lay Epistemics and Human Knowledge: Cognitive and Motivational Bases*. New York: Springer Science+Business Media.

Kruglanski, A. W. (1989b). The psychology of being "right": The problem of accuracy in social perception and cognition. *Psychological Bulletin*, 106(3), 395–409. https://doi.org/10.1037/0033-2909.106.3.395

Kruglanski, A. W. (2012). Lay epistemic theory. In P. A. M. Van Lange, A. W. Kruglanski, & E. T. Higgins (Eds.), *Handbook of Theories of Social Psychology (Vol. 1)* (pp. 460–482). Thousand Oaks, CA: Sage.

Kruglanski, A. W., & Webster, D. M. (1996). Motivated closing of the mind: "Seizing" and "freezing." *Psychological Review*, 103(2), 263.

Kubzansky, L. D., & Winning, A. (2016). Emotions and health. In L. Feldman Barrett, M. Lewis, & J. M. Haviland-Jones (Eds.), *Handbook of Emotions* (pp. 751–773). New York: The Guilford Press.

Kunda, Z. (1987). Motivated inference: Self-serving generation and evaluation of causal theories. *Journal of Personality and Social Psychology*, 53, 636–647.

Kunda, Z. (1990). The case for motivated reasoning. *Psychological Bulletin*, 108(3), 480–498. https://doi.org/10.1037/0033-2909.108.3.480

Kuniecki, M., Pilarczyk, J., & Wichary, S. (2015). The color red attracts attention in an emotional context. An ERP study. *Frontiers in Human Neuroscience*, 9, 212.

Kurer, O. (2005). Corruption: An alternative approach to its definition and measurement. *Political Studies*, 53(1), 222–239: 230.

LaBar, K. S. (2016). Fear and anxiety. In L. Feldman Barrett, M. Lewis, & J. M. Haviland-Jones (Eds.), *Handbook of Emotions* (pp. 613–633). New York: The Guilford Press.

Lahad, M., Cohen, R., Fanaras, S., Leykin, D., & Apostolopoulou, P. (2018). Resiliency and adjustment in times of crisis, the case of the Greek economic crisis from a psycho-social and community perspective. *Social Indicators Research*, 135(1), 333–356.

Lai, G., Lin, N., & Leung, S. Y. (1998). Network resources, contact resources, and status attainment. *Social Networks*, 20(2), 159–178.

Lai, J. C. L., & Cheng, S.-T. (2004). Health beliefs, optimism, and health-related decisions: A study with Hong Kong Chinese. *International Journal of Psychology*, 39, 179–189.

Lai, J., Ma, S., Wang, Y., et al. (2020). Factors associated with mental health outcomes among health care workers exposed to coronavirus disease 2019. *JAMA Network Open*, 3, Article e203976.

Lambert, J. (2019). Measles cases mount in Pacific Northwest outbreak. (February 8). *NPR*. https://www.npr.org/sections/healthshots/2019/02/08/692665531/measles-cases-mount-in -pacificnorthwest-outbreak

Landy, J. F., & Goodwin, G. P. (2015). Does incidental disgust amplify moral judgment? A meta-analytic review of experimental evidence. *Perspectives on Psychological Science*, 10(4), 518–536.

Lange, T. (2015). Social capital and job satisfaction: The case of Europe in times of economic crisis. *European Journal of Industrial Relations*, 21(3), 275–290.

Larson, H., Cooper, L., Eskola, J., Katz, S., & Ratzan, S. (2011). Addressing the vaccine confidence gap. *Lancet*, 378, 526–535.

Larson, H. J., Jarrett, C., Eckersberger, E., Smith, D. M. D., & Paterson, P. (2014). Understanding vaccine hesitancy around vaccines and vaccination from a global perspective: A systematic review of published literature, 2007–2012. *Vaccine*, 32(19), 2150–2159. https://doi.org/10.1016/j.vaccine.2014.01.081

130   *Individuals, Groups, and Society in Pandemics*

Lattie, E. G., Nicholas, J., Knapp, A. A., Skerl, J. J., Kaiser, S. M., & Mohr, D. C. (2020). Opportunities for and tensions surrounding the use of technology-enabled mental health services in community mental health care. *Administration and Policy in Mental Health and Mental Health Services Research*, 47, 138–149. https://doi.org/10.1007/s10488-019-00979-2

Lauriola, M., Panno, A., Levin, I. P., & Lejuez, C. W. (2014). Individual differences in risky decision making: A meta-analysis of sensation seeking and impulsivity with the balloon analogue risk task. *Journal of Behavioral Decision Making*, 27(1), 20–36.

Lazarus, R. S. (1991). Progress on a cognitive-motivational-relational theory of emotion. *American Psychologist*, 46(8), 819–834.

Le Bon, G. (2009). *Psychology of Crowds*. London: Sparkling Books.

LeDoux, J. (2012a). Rethinking the emotional brain. *Neuron*, 73(4), 653–676. https://doi.org/10.1016/j.neuron.2012.02.004

LeDoux, J. E. (2012b). Evolution of human emotion: A view through fear. *Progress in Brain Research*, 195, 431–442.

LeDoux, J. E. (2020). *Lęk. Neuronauka na tropie źródeł leku i strachu*. Kraków: Copernicus Center Press.

Lee, D., Stajkovic, A. D., & Cho, B. (2011). Interpersonal trust and emotion as antecedents of cooperation: Evidence from Korea. *Journal of Applied Social Psychology*, 41(7), 1603–1631.

Leiser, D., & Shemesh, Y. S. (2018). *How we Misunderstand Economics and Why it Matters: The Psychology of Bias, Distortion and Conspiracy*. London: Routledge.

Leiserowitz, A. (2005). American risk perceptions: Is climate change dangerous? *Risk Analysis*, 25, 1433–1442.

Lempert, K. M., & Phelps, E. A. (2013). Neuroeconomics of emotion and decision making. In P. Glimcher, & E. Fehr (Eds.), *Neuroeconomics: Decision Making and the Brain* (2nd ed.) (pp. 219–236). Oxford: Academic Press.

Lempert, K. M., & Phelps, E. A. (2016). The malleability of intertemporal choice. *Trends in Cognitive Sciences*, 20(1), 64–74.

Lerner, J. S., & Keltner, D. (2000). Beyond valence: Toward a model of emotion-specific influences on judgement and choice. *Cognition and Emotion*, 14(4), 473–493.

Lerner, J. S., & Keltner, D. (2001). Fear, anger, and risk. *Journal of Personality and Social Psychology*, 81(1), 146–159.

Lerner, J. S., Li, Y., Valdesolo, P., & Kassam, K. S. (2015). Emotion and decision making. *Annual Review of Psychology*, 66(1), 799–823.

Letki, N. (2006). Investigating the roots of civic morality: Trust, social capital, and institutional performance. *Political Behavior*, 28(4), 305–325.

Letki, N., & Mieriņa, I. (2015). Getting support in polarized societies: Income, social networks, and socioeconomic context. *Social Science Research*, 49, 217–233.

Łętowska, E., & Sobczak, K. (2012). *Rzeźbienie państwa prawa: 20 lat później*. Warszawa: Wolters Kluwer Polska.

Leuker, C., Samartzidis, L., Hertwig, R., & Pleskac, T. J. (2020). When money talks: Judging risk and coercion in high-paying clinical trials. *PLoS ONE*, 15(1), e0227898.

Leung, K., Jit, M., Lau, E. H., & Wu, J. T. (2017). Social contact patterns relevant to the spread of respiratory infectious diseases in Hong Kong. *Scientific Reports*, 7(1), 1–12.

References 131

Leventhal, H., Diefenbach, M., & Leventhal, E. A. (1992). Illness cognition: Using common sense to understand treatment adherence and affect cognition interactions. *Cognitive Therapy and Research*, 16(2), 143–163.

Levi, M., & Sacks, A. (2009). Legitimating beliefs: Sources and indicators. *Regulation & Governance*, 3(4), 311–333.

Levy, S. R., Plaks, J. E., & Dweck, C. S. (1999). Modes of social thought: Implicit theories and social understanding. In S. Chaiken & Y. Trope (Eds.), *Dual-process Theories in Social Psychology* (pp. 179–202). Guilford Press.

Lewandowsky, S., Gignac, G. E., & Oberauer, K. (2015). Correction: The role of conspiracist ideation and worldviews in predicting rejection of science. *PLoS ONE*, 10, e0134773. https://doi.org/10.1371/journal.pone.0134773

Lewinsohn, S., & Mano, H. (1993). Multi-attribute choice and affect: The influence of naturally occurring and manipulated moods on choice processes. *Journal of Behavioral Decision Making*, 6(1), 33–51.

Li, J., Yang, A., Dou, K., & Cheung, R. Y. M. (2020). Self-control moderates the association between perceived severity of the coronavirus disease 2019 (COVID-19) and mental health problems among the Chinese public. (March 11). https://doi.org/10.31234/osf.io/2xadq

Lighthall, N. R., Mather, M., & Gorlick, M. A. (2009). Acute stress increases sex differences in risk seeking in the balloon analogue risk task. *PLoS ONE*, 4(7), e6002.

Lillard, D., Burkhauser, R., Hahn, M., & Wilkins, R. (2015). Does early-life income inequality predict self-reported health in later life? Evidence from the United States. *Social Science & Medicine*, 128, 347–355.

Lin, N. (2000). Inequality in social capital. *Contemporary Sociology*, 29(6), 785–795.

Lindström, M., & Giordano, G. N. (2016). The 2008 financial crisis: Changes in social capital and its association with psychological wellbeing in the United Kingdom – A panel study. *Social Science & Medicine*, 153, 71–80.

Lipkus, I. M., Samsa, G., & Rimer, B. K. (2001). General performance on a numeracy scale among highly educated samples. *Medical Decision Making*, 21(1), 37–44.

Liu, J. H., & Hilton, D. J. (2005). How the past weighs on the present: Social representations of history and their role in identity politics. *British Journal of Social Psychology*, 44, 537–556. https://doi.org/10.1348/014466605X27162

Liu, Y., Yan, L.-M., Wan, L., et al. (2020). Viral dynamics in mild and severe cases of COVID-19. *The Lancet Infectious Diseases*, 20(6), pp. 656–657. https://doi.org/10.1016/S1473-3099(20)30232-2

Lodder, P., Ong, H. H., Grasman, R. P. P. P., & Wicherts, J. M. (2019). A comprehensive meta-analysis of money priming. *Journal of Experimental Psychology: General*, 148(4), 688–712.

Loewenstein, G. F., Weber, E. U., Hsee, C. K., & Welch, N. (2001). Risk as feelings. *Psychological Bulletin*, 127(2), 267.

Lopez, S. V., & Leffingwell, T. R. (2020). The role of unrealistic optimism in college student risky sexual behavior. *American Journal of Sexuality Education*, 15, 201–217.

Lord, C. S., Ross, L., & Lepper, M. (1979). Biased assimilation and attitude polarization: The effects of prior theories on subsequently considered evidence. *Journal of Personality and Social Psychology*, 37, 2098–2109.

Luce, M. F., Payne, J. W., & Bettman, J. R. (1999). Emotional trade-off difficulty and choice. *Journal of Marketing Research*, 36(2), 143–159.

Luce, M. F., Payne, J. W., & Bettman, J. R. (2001). The impact of emotional tradeoff difficulty on decision behavior. In E. U. Weber, J. Baron, & G. Loomes (Eds.), *Conflict and Tradeoffs in Decision Making* (pp. 86–109). Cambridge University Press.

Lundgren, R. E., & McMakin, A. H. (Eds.) (2018). *Risk Communication: A Handbook for Communicating Environmental, Safety, and Health Risks*. Hoboken, NJ: Wiley.

Lundgren, S. R., & Prislin, R. (1998). Motivated cognitive processing and attitude change. *Personality and Social Psychology Bulletin*, 24, 715–726.

Lunn, P. D., Belton, C. A., Lavin, C., McGowan, F. P., Timmons, S., & Robertson, D. A. (2020). Using behavioral science to help fight the coronavirus. *Journal of Behavioral Public Administration*, 3(1). https://doi.org/10.30636/jbpa.31.147

Lusardi, A., & Mitchell, O. S. (2014). The economic importance of financial literacy: Theory and evidence. *Journal of Economic Literature*, 52, 5–44.

Luszczynska, A., Gutiérrez-Doña, B., & Schwarzer, R. (2005). General self-efficacy in various domains of human functioning: Evidence from five countries. *International Journal of Psychology*, 40, 80–89.

Lykins, E. L. B., Segerstrom, S. C., Averill, A. J., Evans, D. R., & Kemeny, M. E. (2007). Goal shifts following reminders of mortality: Reconciling posttraumatic growth and terror management theory. *Personality and Social Psychology Bulletin*, 33(8), 1088–1099. https://doi.org/10.1177/0146167207303015

Macias, T. (2015). Risks, trust, and sacrifice: Social structural motivators for environmental change. *Social Science Quarterly*, 96(5), 1264–1276.

Maier, J. (2011). The impact of political scandals on political support: An experimental test of two theories. *International Political Science Review*, 32(3), 283–302.

Maier, S. F., & Seligman, M. E. (2016). Learned helplessness at fifty: Insights from neuroscience. *Psychological Review*, 123(4), 349–367.

Ma-Kellams, C., & Blascovich, J. (2013). "Culturally divergent responses to mortality salience": Corrigendum. *Psychological Science*, 24(5), 813.

Makridakis, S., & Moleskis, A. (2015). The costs and benefits of positive illusions. *Frontiers in Psychology*, 6, 859.

Malhotra, N., & Kuo, A. G. (2008). Attributing blame: The public's response to Hurricane Katrina. *The Journal of Politics*, 70(1), 120–135.

Maltezou, H., Theodoridou, K., Ledda, C., Rapisarda, V., & Theodoridou, M. (2018). Vaccination of healthcare workers: Is mandatory vaccination needed? *Expert Review of Vaccines*, 18(1) 5–13. https://doi.org/10.1080/14760584.2019.1552141

Mano, H. (1992). Judgments under distress: Assessing the role of unpleasantness and arousal in judgment formation. *Organizational Behavior and Human Decision Processes*, 52(2), 216–245.

March, J. G. (1997). Understanding how decisions happen in organizations. In Z. Shapira (ed.), *Organizational Decision Making* (pp. 9–32). Cambridge University Press.

Marien, S., & Hooghe, M. (2011). Does political trust matter? An empirical investigation into the relation between political trust and support for law compliance. *European Journal of Political Research*, 50(2), 267–291.

Marris, C., Langford, I. H., Saunderson, T., & O'Riordan, T. (1997). Exploring the "psychometric paradigm": Comparisons between aggregate and individual analyses. *Risk Analysis*, 17, 3303–3312.

Mata, R., Josef, A. K., & Hertwig, R. (2016). Propensity for risk taking across the life span and around the globe. *Psychological Science*, 27(2), 231–243.

References 133

Mata, R., Josef, A. K., Samanez-Larkin, G. R., & Hertwig, R. (2011). Age differences in risky choice: A meta-analysis. *Annals of the New York Academy of Sciences*, 1235, 18.

Mata, R., Schooler, L. J., & Rieskamp, J. (2007). The aging decision maker: Cognitive aging and the adaptive selection of decision strategies. *Psychology and Aging*, 22(4), 796.

Mather, M., Gorlick, M. A., & Lighthall, N. R. (2009). To brake or accelerate when the light turns yellow? Stress reduces older adults' risk taking in a driving game. *Psychological Science*, 20(2), 174–176.

Mathes, B. M., Norr, A. M., Allan, N. P., Albanese, B. J., & Schmidt, N. B. (2018). Cyberchondria: Overlap with health anxiety and unique relations with impairment, quality of life, and service utilization. *Psychiatry Research*, 261, 204–211.

Matt, G. E., Vázquez, C., & Campbell, W. K. (1992). Mood-congruent recall of affectively toned stimuli: A meta-analytic review. *Clinical Psychology Review*, 12(2), 227–255.

Mazerolle, L., Antrobus, E., Bennett, S., & Tyler, T. R. (2013). Shaping citizen perceptions of police legitimacy: A randomized field trial of procedural justice. *Criminology*, 51(1), 33–63.

Mazerolle, L., Bennett, S., Davis, J., Sargeant, E., & Manning, M. (2013). Procedural justice and police legitimacy: A systematic review of the research evidence. *Journal of Experimental Criminology*, 9(3), 245–274.

Mazure, C. M. (1998). Life stressors as risk factors in depression. *Clinical Psychology: Science and Practice*, 5, 291–313.

McFarland, S., Hackett, J., Hamer, K., Katzarska-Miller, I., Malsch, A., Reese, G., & Reysen, S. (2019). Global human identification and citizenship: A review of psychological studies. *Political Psychology*, 40, 141–171. https://doi.org/10.1111/pops.12572

McGregor, I., Haji, R., Nash, K., & Teper, R. (2008) Religious zeal and the uncertain self. *Basic and Applied Social Psychology*, 30(2), 183–188. https://doi.org/10.1080/01973530802209251

McGregor, I., Nash, K., Mann, N., & Phills, C. E. (2010). Anxious uncertainty and reactive approach motivation (RAM). *Journal of Personality and Social Psychology*, 99(1), 133–147. https://doi.org/10.1037/a0019701

McGregor, I., Prentice, M., & Nash, K. A. (2013). Reactive approach motivation (RAM) for religious, idealistic, and lifestyle extremes. *Journal of Social Issues*, 69, 537–563.

McKay, B. (2020). Lockdown blunder costs NZ Health Minister. *The Canberra Times*. (April7). www.canberratimes.com.au/story/6714105/lockdown-blunder-costs-nz-health-minister/?cs=14232

McPhail, C. (2017). *The Myth of the Madding Crowd*. London: Routledge.

McPherson, M., Smith-Lovin, L., & Cook, J. M. (2001). Birds of a feather: Homophily in social networks. *Annual Review of Sociology*, 27(1), 415–444.

Mead, N. L., & Stuppy, A. (2014). Two sides of the same coin: Money can promote and hinder interpersonal processes. In E. H. Bijleveld, & H. Aarts (Eds.), *The Psychological Science of Money* (pp. 243–262). New York: Springer.

Meier, B. P., D'agostino, P. R., Elliot, A. J., Maier, M. A., & Wilkowski, B. M. (2012). Color in context: Psychological context moderates the influence of red on approach- and avoidance-motivated behavior. *PloS ONE*, 7(7).

Mercier, H., & Sperber, D. (2011). Why do humans reason? Arguments for an argumentative theory. *Behavioral and Brain Sciences*, 34, 57–111.

Michel-Kerjan, E., & Slovic, P. (Eds.). (2010). *The Irrational Economist: Making Decisions in a Dangerous World*. New York: Public Affairs Books.

Mikulincer, M., & Shaver, P. R. (2017). *Attachment in Adulthood. Structure, Dynamics, and Change*. New York: The Guilford Press.

Mikulincer, M., Florian, V., & Hirschberger, G. (2003). The existential function of close relationships: Introducing death into the science of love. *Personality and Social Psychology Review*, 7(1), 20–40. https://doi.org/10.1207/S15327957PSPR0701_2

Milgram S. (1974). *Obedience to Authority: An Experimental View*. New York: Harper & Row.

Miner, A. S., Laranjo, L., & Kocaballi, A. B. (2020). Chatbots in the fight against the COVID-19 pandemic. *npj Digital Medicine*, 3, 65. https://doi.org/10.1038/s41746-020-0280-0

Mohnen, S. M., Groenewegen, P. P., Völker, B., & Flap, H. (2011). Neighborhood social capital and individual health. *Social Science & Medicine*, 72(5), 660–667.

Mohr, P. N. C., Biele, G., & Heekeren, H. R. (2010). Neural processing of risk. *Journal of Neuroscience*, 30(19), 6613–6619.

Molden, D. C., & Higgins, E. T. (2005). Motivated thinking. In K. Holyoak & B. Morrison (Eds.) *Handbook of Thinking and Reasoning* (pp. 295–320). New York: Cambridge University Press.

Molinsky, A. L., Grant, A. M., & Margolis, J. D. (2012). The bedside manner of homo economicus: How and why priming an economic schema reduces compassion. *Organizational Behavior and Human Decision Processes*, 119(1), 27–37.

Mols, F., Haslam, S. A., Jetten, J., & Steffens, N. K. (2015). Why a nudge is not enough: A social identity critique of governance by stealth. *European Journal of Political Research*, 54, 81–98.

Moran, T. P. (2016). Anxiety and working memory capacity: A meta-analysis and narrative review. *Psychological Bulletin*, 142(8), 831.

Mossong, J., Hens, N., Jit, M., et al. (2008). Social contacts and mixing patterns relevant to the spread of infectious diseases. *PLoS Medicine*, 5(3), e74.

Moulding, R., Nix-Carnell, S., Schnabel, A., Nedeljkovic, M., Burnside, E. E., Lentini, A. F., & Mehzabin, N. (2016). Better the devil you know than a world you don't? Intolerance of uncertainty and worldview explanations for belief in conspiracy theories. *Personality and Individual Differences*, 98, 345–354.

Moulton, S. T., & Kosslyn, S. M. (2009). Imagining predictions: Mental imagery as mental emulation. *Philosophical Transactions of the Royal Society B: Biological Sciences*, 364, 1273–1280.

Muldoon, O. T., Haslam, S. A., Haslam, C., Cruwys, T., Kearns, M., & Jetten, J. (2019). The social psychology of responses to trauma: Social identity pathways associated with divergent traumatic responses. *European Review of Social Psychology*, 30, 311–348.

Murphy, D. (2020). We've been responding to the rapidly developing situation with #Covid_19 but I've tried to step back & map out the many areas where psychology & psychologists can contribute to coping with the pandemic. Here's my VERY rough 1st draft [Tweet]. (March 21). https://twitter.com/ClinPsychDavid/status/1241449772382388228/

Murphy, K., Mazerolle, L., & Bennett, S. (2014). Promoting trust in police: Findings from a randomised experimental field trial of procedural justice policing. *Policing and Society*, 24(4), 405–424.

References 135

Myers, L. (2020). *Adherance to Treatment in Medical Conditions.* London: CRC Press.

Nadarevic, L., & Aßfalg, A. (2017). Unveiling the truth: Warnings reduce the repetition-based truth effect. *Psychological Research*, 81(4), 814–826. https://doi.org/10.1007/s00426-016-0777-y

Nagaoka, K., Fujiwara, T., & Ito, J. (2012). Do income inequality and social capital associate with measles-containing vaccine coverage rate? *Vaccine*, 30(52), 7481–7488.

Narayan, D. (1999). *Bonds and Bridges: Social Capital and Poverty* (Vol. 2167). Washington DC: World Bank, Poverty Reduction and Economic Management Network, Poverty Division.

Nash, K., Schiller, B., Gianotti, L. R., Baumgartner, T., & Knoch, D. (2013). Electro physiological indices of response inhibition in a Go/NoGo task predict self-control in a social context. *PloS ONE*, 8(11), e79462.

Nes, L. S., & Segerstrom, S. C. (2006). Dispositional optimism and coping: A meta-analytic review. *Personality and Social Psychology Review*, 10, 235–251.

Neuberg, S. L., Kenrick, D. T., & Schaller, M. (2011). Human threat management systems: Self-protection and disease avoidance. *Neuroscience & Biobehavioral Reviews*, 35(4), 1042–1051.

Neville, F. G., & Reicher, S. D. (2018). Crowds, social identities, and the shaping of everyday social relations. In C. J. Hewer, & E. Lyons (Eds.), *Political Psychology: A Social Psychological Approach* (pp. 231–252). Chichester, UK: Wiley-Blackwell.

Newton, K., D. Stolle, & S. Zmerli (2018). Social and political trust. *The Oxford Handbook of Social and Political Trust.* Oxford University Press.

Ngan, H. F., & Tze-Ngai Vong, L. (2018). Hospitality employees' unrealistic optimism in promotion perception: Myth or reality? *Journal of Human Resources in Hospitality & Tourism*, 18, 172–193. https://doi.org/10.1080/15332845.2019.1558480

Nickerson, R. S. (1998). Confirmation bias: A ubiquitous phenomenon in many guises. *Review of General Psychology*, 2, 175–220. http://dx.doi.org/10.1037/1089-2680.2.2.175

Nielsen, R., Fletcher, R., Newman, N., Brennen, S., & Howard, P. (2020). *Navigating the 'infodemic': How People in Six Countries Access and Rate News and Information about Coronavirus.* Published by the Reuters Institute for the Study of Journalism as part of the Oxford Martin Programme on Misinformation, Science and Media, a three-year research collaboration between the Reuters Institute, the Oxford Internet Institute, and the Oxford Martin School.

Nishi, A., Shirado, H., Rand, D., & Christakis, N. (2015). Inequality and visibility of wealth in experimental social networks. *Nature*, 526, 426–429.

Nix, J., Wolfe, S. E., Rojek, J., & Kaminski, R. J. (2015). Trust in the police: The influence of procedural justice and perceived collective efficacy. *Crime & Delinquency*, 61(4), 610–640.

Norris, F. H., Stevens, S. P., Pfefferbaum, B., Wyche, K. F., & Pfefferbaum, R. L. (2008). Community resilience as a metaphor, theory, set of capacities, and strategy for disaster readiness. *American Journal of Community Psychology*, 41(1–2), 127–150.

Norton, M., & Ariely, D. (2011). Building a better America – one wealth quintile at a time. *Perspectives on Psychological Science*, 6, 9–12.

Novelli, D., Drury, J., & Reicher, S. (2010). Come together: Two studies concerning the impact of group relations on "personal space." *British Journal of Social Psychology*, 49, 223–236.

Nowak, M. A. (2006). Five rules for the evolution of cooperation. *Science*, 314(5805), 1560–1563. https://doi.org/10.1126/science.1133755

136 *Individuals, Groups, and Society in Pandemics*

O'Brien, W. H., VanEgeren, L., & Mumby, P. B. (1995). Predicting health behaviors using measures of optimism and perceived risk. *Health Values: The Journal of Health Behavior, Education & Promotion*, 19, 21–28.

O'Connor, D. B., Thayer, J. F., & Vedhara, K. (2020). Stress and health: A review of psychobiological processes. *Annual Review of Psychology*, 72.

O'Sullivan, S., Healy, A. E., & Breen, M. J. (2014). Political legitimacy in Ireland during economic crisis: Insights from the European social survey. *Irish Political Studies*, 29(4), 547–572.

Oakes, P. J., Haslam, S. A., & Turner, J. C. (1994). *Stereotyping and Social Reality*. Oxford: Blackwell Publishing.

Oberauer, K., Farrell, S., Jarrold, C., & Lewandowsky, S. (2016). What limits working memory capacity? *Psychological Bulletin*, 142(7), 758.

OECD (2020). Combatting COVID-19 disinformation on online platforms. OECD Paris. https://www.oecd.org/coronavirus/policy-responses/combatting-covid-19-disinformation-on-online-platforms-d854ec48/

Oishi, S., Kesebir, S., & Diener, E. (2011). Income inequality and happiness. *Psychological Science*, 22, 1095–1100.

Okan, Y., Garcia-Retamero, R., Cokely, E. T., & Maldonado, A. (2012). Individual differences in graph literacy: Overcoming denominator neglect in risk comprehension. *Journal of Behavioral Decision Making*, 25(4), 390–401.

Opel, D., Mangione-Smith, R., Taylor, J., Korfiatis, C., Wiese, C., Catz, S., & Martin, D. P. (2011). Development of a survey to identify vaccine-hesitant parents: The parent attitudes about childhood vaccines survey. *Human Vaccines*, 7, 419–425.

Orr, M., & West, D. (2007). Citizen evaluations of local police: Personal experience or symbolic attitudes? *Administration & Society*, 38(6), 649–668.

Pachur, T., Hertwig, R., & Wolkewitz, R. (2014). The affect gap in risky choice: Affect-rich outcomes attenuate attention to probability information. *Decision*, 1(1), 64–78.

Paldam, M. (2000). Social capital: One or many? Definition and measurement. *Journal of Economic Surveys*, 14(5), 629–653.

Pandey, K., Stevenson, C., Shankar, S., Hopkins, N. P., & Reicher, S. D. (2013). Cold comfort at the Magh Mela: Social identity processes and physical hardship. *The British Journal of Social Psychology*, 53, 675–690.

Pariser, E. (2011). *The Filter Bubble: What The Internet Is Hiding From You*. UK: Penguin.

Parker-Stephen, E. (2013). Tides of disagreement: How reality facilitates (and inhibits) partisan public opinion. *The Journal of Politics*, 75(4), 1077–1088.

Parrott, W. G. (2017). Role of emotions in risk perception. In G. Emilien, R. Weitkunat, & F. Lüdicke (Eds.), *Consumer Perception of Product Risks and Benefits* (pp. 221–232). Cham, Switzerland: Springer.

Payne, J. W., & Bettman, J. R. (2004). Walking with the scarecrow: The information-processing approach to decision research. In D. J. Koehler, & N. Harvey (Eds.), *Blackwell Handbook of Judgment and Decision Making* (pp. 110–132). Hoboken, NJ: Blackwell.

Peng, L., Tan, J., Lin, L., & Xu, D. (2019). Understanding sustainable disaster mitigation of stakeholder engagement: Risk perception, trust in public institutions, and disaster insurance. *Sustainable Development*, 27(5), 885–897.

Pennycook, G., & Rand, D. G. (2019). Fighting misinformation on social media using crowdsourced judgments of news source quality. *Proceedings of the*

References 137

National Academy of Sciences, 116(7), 2521–2526. https://doi.org/10.1073/pnas.1806781116

Pennycook, G., Cannon, T. D., & Rand, D. G. (2018). Prior exposure increases perceived accuracy of fake news. *Journal of Experimental Psychology. General*, 147(12), 1865–1880. https://doi.org/10.1037/xge0000465

Pennycook, G., McPhetres, J., Zhang, Y., Lu, J. G., & Rand, D. G. (2020). Fighting COVID-19 misinformation on social media: Experimental evidence for a scalable accuracy nudge intervention. (March 17). https://doi.org/10.31234/osf.io/uhbk9

Peters, E. (2020). Is Obsessing Over Daily Coronavirus Statistics Counterproductive? (March 12). *The New York Times*. https://www.nytimes.com/2020/03/12/opinion/sunday/coronavirus-statistics.html

Peters, E., & Bjalkebring, P. (2015). Multiple numeric competencies: When a number is not just a number. *Journal of Personality and Social Psychology*, 108(5), 802–822.

Peters, E., Västfjäll, D., Gärling, T., & Slovic, P. (2006). Affect and decision making: A "hot" topic. *Journal of Behavioral Decision Making*, 19(2), 79–85.

Peterson, C., & Seligman, M. E. P. (2003). Character strengths before and after September 11. *Psychological Science*, 14(4), 381–384. https://doi.org/10.1111/1467-9280.24482

Petrova, D., & Garcia-Retamero R. (2018). How to effectively communicate risks to diverse consumers. *Health Risk Analysis*, 4, 114–119.

Petrova, D., Garcia-Retamero, R., Catena, A., & van der Pligt, J. (2016). To screen or not to screen: What factors influence complex screening decisions? *Journal of Experimental Psychology: Applied*, 22(2), 247–260. https://doi.org/10.1037/xap0000086

Pettigrew, E. (1983). *The Silent Enemy: Canada and the Deadly Flu of 1918*. Saskatoon, SK: Western Producer Praire Books.

Pfister, H.-R., & Böhm, G. (2008). The multiplicity of emotions: A framework of emotional functions in decision making. *Judgment and Decision Making*, 3(1), 5–17.

Pichler, F., & Wallace, C. (2009). Social capital and social class in Europe: The role of social networks in social stratification. *European Sociological Review*, 25(3), 319–332.

Pirisi, A. (2000). Low health literacy prevents equal access to care. *The Lancet, 356*, 1828.

Plaks, J. E., Levy, S. R., & Dweck, C. S. (2009). Lay theories of personality: Cornerstones of meaning in social cognition. *Social and Personality Psychology Compass*, 3(6), 1069–1081.

Plutchik, R. (2002). *Emotions and Life: Perspectives from Psychology, Biology, and Evolution*. Washington, D.C.: American Psychological Association.

Poortinga, W. (2012). Community resilience and health: The role of bonding, bridging, and linking aspects of social capital. *Health & Place*, 18(2), 286–295.

Popova, L., Owusu, D., Weaver, S. R., Kemp, C. B., Mertz, C. K., Pechacek, T. F., & Slovic, P. (2018). Affect, risk perception, and the use of cigarettes and e-cigarettes: A population study of U.S. adults. *BMC Public Health*, 18, 395.

Poppa, T., & Bechara, A. (2018). The somatic marker hypothesis: Revisiting the role of the 'body-loop' in decision-making. *Current Opinion in Behavioral Sciences*, 19, 61–66.

Portes, A. (1998). Social capital: Its origins and applications in modern sociology. *Annual Review of Sociology*, 24(1), 1–24.

Prati, G., Pietrantoni, L., & Zani, B. (2011). Compliance with recommendations for pandemic influenza H1N1 2009: The role of trust and personal beliefs. *Health Education Research*, 26(5), 761–769.

138 *Individuals, Groups, and Society in Pandemics*

Procopio, C. H., & Procopio, S. T. (2007). Do you know what it means to miss New Orleans? Internet communication, geographic community, and social capital in crisis. *Journal of Applied Communication Research*, 35(1), 67–87.

Pronin, E., Gilovich, T., & Ross, L. (2004). Objectivity in the eye of the beholder: Divergent perceptions of bias in self versus others. *Psychological Review*, 111, 781–799.

Putnam, R. D. (2000). *Bowling alone: The collapse and revival of American community.* New York: Simon and Schuster.

Pyszczynski, T., & Kesebir, P. (2011). Anxiety buffer disruption theory: A terror management account of posttraumatic stress disorder. *Anxiety, Stress & Coping*, 24(1), 3–26. https://doi.org/10.1080/10615806.2010.517524

Pyszczynski, T., Greenberg, J., & Solomon, S. (1999). A dual-process model of defense against conscious and unconscious death-related thoughts: An extension of terror management theory. *Psychological Review*, 106(4), 835–845. https://doi.org/10.1037/0033-295X.106.4.835

Pyszczynski, T., Greenberg, J., Solomon, S., Arndt, J., & Schimel, J. (2004). Converging toward an integrated theory of self-esteem: Reply to Crocker and Nuer (2004), Ryan and Deci (2004), and Leary (2004). *Psychological Bulletin*, 130(3), 483–488. https://doi.org/10.1037/0033-2909.130.3.483

Radcliffe, N. M., & Klein, W. M. P. (2002). Dispositional, unrealistic, and comparative optimism: Differential relations with the knowledge and processing of risk information and beliefs about personal risk. *Personality and Social Psychology Bulletin*, 28, 836–846.

Radke, H. R. M., Hornsey, M. J., & Barlow, F. K. (2016). Barriers to women engaging in collective action to overcome sexism. *American Psychologist*, 71, 863–874.

Rai, T. S., & Fiske, A. P. (2011). Moral psychology is relationship regulation: Moral motives for unity, hierarchy, equality, and proportionality. *Psychological Review*, 118(1), 57–75.

Rand, D. G., & Nowak, M. A. (2013). Human cooperation. *Trends in Cognitive Sciences*, 17, 413–425.

Rasmussen, H. N., Scheier, M. F., & Greenhouse, J. B. (2009). Optimism and physical health: A meta-analytic review. *Annals of Behavioral Medicine*, 37, 239–256.

Raviv, A., Bar-Tal, D., Raviv, A., & Abin, R. (1993). Measuring epistemic authority: Studies of politicians and professors. *European Journal of Personality*, 7, 119–138.

Read, D. (2007). Experienced utility: Utility theory from Jeremy Bentham to Daniel Kahneman. *Thinking & Reasoning*, 13(1), 45–61. https://doi.org/10.1080/13546780600872627

Redelmeier, D. A., Katz, J., & Kahneman, D. (2003). Memories of colonoscopy: A randomized trial. *Pain*, 104(1–2), 187–194.

Reeskens, T., & van Oorschot, W. (2014). European feelings of deprivation amidst the financial crisis: Effects of welfare state effort and informal social relations. *Acta Sociologica*, 57(3), 191–206.

Reicher, S. D. (1984). The St. Pauls' riot: An explanation of the limits of crowd action in terms of a social identity model. *European Journal of Social Psychology*, 14, 1–21.

Reicher, S. D. (1987). Crowd behaviour as social action. In J. C. Turner, M. A. Hogg, P. J. Oakes, S. D. Reicher, & M. S. Wetherell, *Rediscovering the Social Group: A Self-categorization Theory* (pp. 171–202). Oxford: Blackwell.

References 139

Reicher, S. D. (2001). The psychology of crowd dynamics. In M. A. Hogg, & R. S. Tindale (Eds.), *Blackwell Handbook of Social Psychology: Group Processes* (pp. 182–208). Oxford: Blackwell Publishers.

Reicher, S. (2021). For psychologists, the pandemic has shown people's capacity for cooperation. (January 2). *The Guardian*. https://www.theguardian.com/commentisfree/2021/jan/02/psychologists-pandemic-cooperation-government-public-britain

Reicher, S. D., Haslam, S. A., & Hopkins, N. (2005). Social identity and the dynamics of leadership: Leaders and followers as collaborative agents in the transformation of social reality. *The Leadership Quarterly*, 16, 547–568.

Reinhardt, G. Y. (2015). First-hand experience and second-hand information: Changing trust across three levels of government. *Review of Policy Research*, 32(3), 345–364.

Renner, B., Gamp, M., Schmälzle, R., & Schupp, H. T. (2015). Health risk perception. In J. D. Wright (Ed.) *International Encyclopedia of the Social & Behavioral Sciences* (2nd ed.) (pp. 702–709). Oxford: Elsevier.

Reysen, S., & Katzarska-Miller, I. (2013). A model of global citizenship: Antecedents and outcomes. *International Journal of Psychology*, 48, 858–870. https://doi.org/10.1080/00207594.2012.701749

Robb, K. A., Simon, A. E., & Wardle, J. (2009). Socioeconomic disparities in optimism and pessimism. *International Journal of Behavioral Medicine*, 16, 331–338.

Rönnerstrand, B. (2014). Social capital and immunization against the 2009 A (H1N1) pandemic in the American States. *Public Health*, 128(8), 709–715.

Roozenbeek, J., & van der Linden, S. (2019). Fake news game confers psychological resistance against online misinformation. *Palgrave Communications*, 5(1), 1–10. https://doi.org/10.1057/s41599-019-0279-9

Roth, A. E. (2007). Repugnance as a constraint on markets. *Journal of Economic Perspectives*, 21(3), 37–58. https://doi.org/10.1257/jep.21.3.37

Roth, A. E. (2015). *Who Gets What and Why: The Hidden World of Matchmaking and Market Design*. London: William Collins.

Rothstein, B., & Stolle, D. (2003). Social capital, impartiality and the welfare state: An institutional approach. In M. Hooghe & D. Stolle (Eds.), *Generating Social Capital* (pp. 191–209). New York: Palgrave Macmillan.

Rottenstreich, Y., & Hsee, C. K. (2001). Money, kisses, and electric shocks: On the affective psychology of risk. *Psychological Science*, 12(3), 185–190.

Routledge, C., & Juhl, J. (2010). When death thoughts lead to death fears: Mortality salience increases death anxiety for individuals who lack meaning in life. *Cognition and Emotion*, 24(5), 848–854. https://doi.org/10.1080/02699930902847144

Routledge, C., Arndt, J., & Goldenberg, J. L. (2004). A time to tan: Proximal and distal effects of mortality salience on sun exposure intentions. *Personality and Social Psychology Bulletin*, 30(10), 1347–1358. https://doi.org/10.1177/0146167204264056

Rubin, G. J., Amlot, R., Page, L., & Wessely, S. (2009). Public perceptions, anxiety, and behaviour change in relation to the swine flu outbreak: Cross sectional telephone survey. *BMJ*, 339, b2651.

Rudisill, C. (2013). How do we handle new health risks? Risk perception, optimism, and behaviors regarding the H1N1 virus. *Journal of Risk Research*, 16(8), 959–980.

Rudolph, T. J. (2003a). Institutional context and the assignment of political responsibility. *The Journal of Politics*, 65(1), 190–215.

Rudolph, T. J. (2003b). Who's responsible for the economy? The formation and consequences of responsibility attributions. *American Journal of Political Science*, 47(4), 698–713.

Rutjens, B. T., Heine, S. J., Sutton, R. M., & van Harreveld, F. (2018). Attitudes towards science. In E. S. P. Olson (Ed.), *Advances in Experimental Psychology* (Vol. 57, pp. 125–165). Academic Press. https://doi.org/10.1016/bs.aesp.2017.08.001

Sachdeva, S., Iliev, R., & Medin, D. L. (2009). Sinning saints and saintly sinners: The paradox of moral self-regulation. *Psychological Science*, 20(4), 523–528. https://doi.org/10.1111/j.1467-9280.2009.02326.x

Salthouse, T. A. (2011). Neuroanatomical substrates of age-related cognitive decline. *Psychological Bulletin*, 137(5), 753.

Sani, F. (2008). Schism in groups: A social psychological account. *Social and Personality Psychology Compass*, 2, 718–732.

Satchell, L. P., Bacon, A. M., Firth, J. L., & Corr, P. J. (2018). Risk as reward: Reinforcement sensitivity theory and psychopathic personality perspectives on everyday risk-taking. *Personality and Individual Differences*, 128, 162–169. https://doi.org/10.1016/j.paid.2018.02.039

Saxena, H. (2018). Are anxious patients causing the flu vax shortage by having two shots? *Pharmacy News*. https://www.ausdoc.com.au/news/are-anxious-patients-causing-flu-vax-shortage-having-two-shots

Schaller, M. (2016). The behavioral immune system. In D. M. Buss (Ed.), *The Handbook of Evolutionary Psychology* (2nd ed.) (pp. 206–224). New York: Wiley.

Scheier, M. F., & Carver, C. S. (1992). Effects of optimism on psychological and physical well-being: Theoretical overview and empirical update. *Cognitive Therapy and Research*, 16, 201–228.

Schnall, S., & Roper, J. (2012). Elevation puts moral values into action. *Social Psychological and Personality Science*, 3, 373–378.

Schnall, S., Haidt, J., Clore, G. L., & Jordan, A. H. (2008). Disgust as embodied moral judgment. *Personality and Social Psychology Bulletin*, 34(8), 1096–1109. https://doi.org/10.1177/0146167208317771

Schneider, C. R., Fehrenbacher, D. D., & Weber, E. U. (2017). Catch me if I fall: Cross-national differences in willingness to take financial risks as a function of social and state 'cushioning'. *International Bussiness Review*, 26, 1023–1033.

Scholz, J. T., & Lubell, M. (1989). Trust and taxpaying: Testing the heuristic approach to collective action. *American Journal of Political Science*, 42(2), 398–417.

Schraff, D. (2020). Political trust during the COVID-19 pandemic: Rally around the flag or lockdown effects? *European Journal of Political Research*, 60(4), 1007–1017.

Schreiber, C. A., & Kahneman, D. (2000). Determinants of the remembered utility of aversive sounds. *Journal of Experimental Psychology. General*, 129(1), 27–42.

Schumpe, B. M., Brizi, A., Giacomantonio, M., Panno, A., Kopetz, C., Kosta, M., & Mannetti, L. (2017). Need for Cognitive Closure decreases risk taking and motivates discounting of delayed rewards. *Personality and Individual Differences*, 107, 66–71.

Schutte, J. W., Valerio, J. K., & Carrillo, V. (1996). Optimism and socioeconomic status: A cross-cultural study. *Social Behavior and Personality: An International Journal*, 24, 9–18.

Schwarz, N. (2001). Feelings as information: Implications for affective influences on information processing. In L. L. Martin, & G. L. Clore (Eds.), *Theories of Mood and Cognition: A User's Handbook* (pp. 159–176). Mahwah, NJ: Erlbaum.

References 141

Schwarz, N., Bless, H., Strack, F., Klumpp, G., Rittenauer-Schatka, H., & Simons, A. (1991). Ease of retrieval as information: Another look at the availability heuristic. *Journal of Personality and Social Psychology*, 61, 195–202.

Scopelliti, I., Morewedge, C. K., McCormick, E., Min, H. L., Lebrecht, S., & Kassam, K. S. (2015). Bias blind spot: Structure, measurement, and consequences. *Management Science*, 61, 2468–2486.

Segerstrom, S. C. (2007). Optimism and resources: Effects on each other and on health over 10 years. *Journal of Research in Personality*, 41, 772–786.

Seibt, B., Schubert, T. W., Zickfeld, J. H., et al. (2018). Kama Muta: Similar emotional responses to touching videos across the United States, Norway, China, Israel, and Portugal. *Journal of Cross-Cultural Psychology*, 49(3), 418–435. https://doi. org/10.1177/0022022117746240

Seligman, M. E., & Maier, S. F. (1967). Failure to escape traumatic shock. *Journal of Experimental Psychology*, 74(1), 1–9.

Senderecka, M., Szewczyk, J., Wichary, S., & Kossowska, M. (2018). Individual differences in decisiveness: ERP correlates of response inhibition and error monitoring. *Psychophysiology*, 55(10), e13198.

Shanteau, J. (1992). Competence in experts: The role of task characteristics. *Organizational Behavior and Human Decision Processes*, 53, 252–266.

Shariff, A., Wiwad, D., & Aknin, L. (2016). Income mobility breeds tolerance for income inequality: Cross-national and experimental evidence. *Perspectives on Psychological Science*, 11, 373–380.

Sharma, M., Yadav, K., Yadav, N., & Ferdinand, K. (2017). Zika virus pandemic – analysis of Facebook as a social media health information platform. *American Journal of Infection Control*, 45, 301–302.

Sharot, T. (2011). *The Optimism Bias: A Tour of the Irrationally Positive Brain*. Pantheon/Random House.

Sheeran, P., & Webb, T. L. (2016). The intention–behavior gap. *Social and Personality Psychology Compass*, 10(9), 503–518.

Sheeran, P., Harris, P. R., & Epton, T. (2014). Does heightening risk appraisals change people's intentions and behavior? A meta-analysis of experimental studies. *Psychological Bulletin*, 140(2), 511–543.

Shefrin, H. (2014). Investors' judgments, asset pricing factors and sentiment. *European Financial Management*, 21, 205–221.

Shepperd, J. A., Pogge, G., & Howell, J. L. (2016). Assessing the consequences of unrealistic optimism: Challenges and recommendations. *Consciousness and Cognition*, 50, 69–78.

Shepperd, J. A., Waters, E. A., Weinstein, N. D., & Klein, W. M. P. (2015). A primer on unrealistic optimism. *Current Directions in Psychological Science*, 24(3), 232–237. https://doi.org/10.1177/0963721414568341

Sherrieb, K., Norris, F. H., & Galea, S. (2010). Measuring capacities for community resilience. *Social Indicators Research*, 99, 227–247. https://doi.org/10.1007/s11205-010-9576-9

Shin, J., & Thorson, K. (2017). Partisan selective sharing: The biased diffusion of fact-checking messages on social media. *Journal of Communication*, 67(2), 233–255.

Shoji, K., Cieslak, R., Smoktunowicz, E., Rogala, A., Benight, C. C., & Luszczynska, A. (2016). Associations between job burnout and self-efficacy: A meta-analysis. *Anxiety, Stress, & Coping*, 29(4), 367–386.

142   *Individuals, Groups, and Society in Pandemics*

Shor, E., Roelfs, D. J., & Yogev, T. (2013). The strength of family ties: A meta-analysis and meta-regression of self-reported social support and mortality. *Social Networks*, 35(4), 626–638.

Siałkowski, K., & Krawczyk, D. (2020). Protest przedsiębiorców. Policja otoczyła ich kordonem, wylegitymowała. Paweł Tanajno zatrzymany. (May 23). *Wyborcza.pl.* https://warszawa.wyborcza.pl/warszawa/7,54420,25968735,protest-przedsiebiorcow.html

Siegrist, M., Keller, C., & Kiers, H. A. L. (2005). A new look at the psychometric paradigm of perception of hazards. *Risk Analysis*, 25, 211–222.

Simon, B., & Klandermans, B. (2001). Politicized collective identity: A social psychological analysis. *American Psychologist*, 56(4), 319–331. https://doi.org/10. 1037/0003-066X.56.4.319

Simons-Morton, B. G., Bingham, C. R., Falk, E. B., Li, K., & Pradhan, A. K. (2014). Experimental effects of injunctive norms on simulated risky driving among teenage males. *Health Psychology*, 33, 616–627.

Sjöberg, L. (2000). Factors in risk perception. *Risk Analysis*, 20, 1–11.

Sjöberg, L. (2001). Political decisions and public risk perception. *Reliability Engineering & System Safety*, 72, 115–123.

Slovic, P. (1987). Perception of risk. *Science*, 236(4799), 280–285.

Slovic, P. (Ed.). (2000). *The perception of risk*. Earthscan Publications.

Slovic, P. (2001). Cigarette smokers: Rational actors or rational fools? In P. Slovic (Ed.), *Smoking: Risk, Perception, & Policy* (pp. 97–124). Thousand Oaks, CA: Sage Publications.

Slovic, P., & Peters, E. (2006). Risk perception and affect. *Current Directions in Psychological Science*, 15(6), 322–325.

Slovic, P., Finucane, M. L., Peters, E., & MacGregor, D. G. (2004). Risk as analysis and risk as feelings: Some thoughts about affect, reason, risk, and rationality. *Risk Analysis*, 24, 311–322.

Slovic, P., Fischhoff, B., & Lichtenstein, S. (1986). The psychometric study of risk perception. In V. T. Covello, J. Menkes, & J. Mumpower (eds), *Risk Evaluation and Management. Contemporary Issues in Risk Analysis* (1st ed.). Boston, MA: Springer.

Smith, H. J., Pettigrew, T. F., Pippin, G. M., & Bialosiewicz, S. (2012). Relative deprivation: A theoretical and meta-analytic review. *Personality and Social Psychology Review*, 16(3), 203–232. https://doi.org/10.1177/1088868311430825

Sniezek, J. A., Schrah, G. E., & Dalal, R. S. (2004). Improving judgement with prepaid expert advice. *Journal of Behavioral Decision Making*, 17, 173–190.

Sobkow, A., Traczyk, J., & Zaleskiewicz, T. (2016). The affective bases of risk perception: Negative feelings and stress mediate the relationship between mental imagery and risk perception. *Frontiers in Psychology*, 7, 932.

Sobkow, A., Zaleskiewicz, T., Petrova, D., Garcia-Retamero, R., & Traczyk, J. (2020). Worry, risk perception, and controllability predict intentions toward COVID-19 preventive behaviors. *Frontiers in Psychology*, 11, 582720. https://doi.org/10.3389/fpsyg.2020.582720

Sokolowska, J., & Zaleskiewicz, T. (2020). Willingness to bear economic costs in the fight against the COVID-19 pandemic. *Frontiers in Psychology*, 11, 588910. https://doi.org/10.3389/fpsyg.2020.588910

Soll, J. B., & Larrick, R. P. (2009). Strategies of revising judgment: How (and how well) people use others' opinions. *Journal of Experimental Psychology: Learning, Memory and Cognition*, 35, 780–805.

References   143

Sønderskov, K. M. (2009). Different goods, different effects: Exploring the effects of generalized social trust in large-N collective action. *Public Choice*, 140(1–2), 145–160.

Sønderskov, K. M. (2011). Explaining large-N cooperation: Generalized social trust and the social exchange heuristic. *Rationality and Society*, 23(1), 51–74.

Soroka, S. (2006). Good news and bad news: Asymmetric responses to economic information. *The Journal of Politics*, 68, 372–385.

Sparkman, D., & Eidelman, S. (2018). We are the "human family". Multicultural experiences predict less prejudice and greater concern for human rights through identification with humanity. *Social Psychology*, 49, 135–153. https://doi.org/10.1027/1864-9335/a000337

Sparkman, G., & Walton, G. M. (2017). Dynamic norms promote sustainable behavior, even if it is counternormative. *Psychological Science*, 28(11), 1663–1674. https://doi.org/10.1177/0956797617719950

Srivastava, S., McGonigal, K. M., Richards, J. M., Butler, E. A., & Gross, J. J. (2006). Optimism in close relationships: How seeing things in a positive light makes them so. *Journal of Personality and Social Psychology*, 91, 143–153.

Stanton-Salazar, R. D., & Dornbusch, S. M. (1995). Social capital and the reproduction of inequality: Information networks among Mexican-origin high school students. *Sociology of Education*, 68(2), 116–135.

Statman, M., Fisher, K., & Anginer, D. (2008). Affect in a behavioral asset-pricing model. *Financial Analysts Journal*, 64(2), 20–29.

Steffens, N. K., Haslam, S. A., Jetten, J., & Mols, F. (2018). Our followers are lions, theirs are sheep: How social identity shapes theories about followership and social influence. *Political Psychology*, 39, 23–42.

Stoffels, P. (2020). What you need to know about the latest on the coronavirus – and a potential preventive vaccine. (January 28). Johnson & Johnson. https://www.jnj.com/latest-news/what-you-need-to-know-about-coronavirus-and-a-potential-johnson-johnson-vaccine

Strachan, E., Schimel, J., Arndt, J., Williams, T., Solomon, S., Pyszczynski, T., & Greenberg, J. (2007). Terror mismanagement: Evidence that mortality salience exacerbates phobic and compulsive behaviors. *Personality and Social Psychology Bulletin*, 33(8), 1137–1151.

Sturmer, S., & Simon, B. (2004). Collective action: Towards a dual-pathway model. *European Review of Social Psychology*, 15, 59–99.

Su, Y., Sun, X. P., & Zhao, F. (2017). Trust and its effects on the public's perception of flood risk: A social science investigation of the middle and lower reaches of the Yangtze River. *Journal of Flood Risk Management*, 10(4), 487–498.

Subašić, E., Schmitt, M. T., & Reynolds, K. J. (2011). Are we all in this together? Co-victimization, inclusive social identity and collective action in solidarity with the disadvantaged. *British Journal of Social Psychology*, 50, 707–725.10.1111/j.2044-8309.2011.02073.x

Suddendorf, T., & Corballis, M. C. (2007). The evolution of foresight: What is mental time travel, and is it unique to humans? *Behavioral and Brain Sciences*, 30, 299–313.

Sunshine, J., & Tyler, T. R. (2003) The role of procedural justice and legitimacy in public support for policing. *Law and Society Review*, 37, 3, 513–548.

Sunstein, C. R. (2018). *#Republic: Divided Democracy in the Age of Social Media*. Princeton University Press.

144 *Individuals, Groups, and Society in Pandemics*

Szreter, S., & Woolcock, M. (2004). Health by association? Social capital, social theory, and the political economy of public health. *International Journal of Epidemiology*, 33(4), 650–667.

Tabibnia, G., & Lieberman, M. D. (2007). Fairness and cooperation are rewarding: Evidence from social cognitive neuroscience. *Annals of the New York Academy of Sciences*, 1118(1), 90–101.

Tabri, N., Hollingshead, S., & Wohl, M. J. A. (2020). Framing COVID-19 as an existential threat predicts anxious arousal and prejudice towards Chinese people. (March 31). https://doi.org/10.31234/osf.io/mpbtr

Taha, S. A., Matheson, K., & Anisman, H. (2013). The 2009 H1N1 influenza pandemic: The role of threat, coping, and media trust on vaccination intentions in Canada. *Journal of Health Communication*, 18, 278–290.

Tajfel, H. (1972). Social categorization. English manuscript of La categorisa- tion sociale. In S. Moscovici (Ed.), *Introduction à la psychologie sociale* (Vol. 1, pp. 272–302). Paris: Larousse.

Tajfel, H., & Turner, J. C. (1979). An integrative theory of intergroup conflict. In W. G. Austin & S. Worchel (Eds.), *The Social Psychology of Intergroup Relations* (pp. 33–48). Monterey, CA: Brooks/Cole.

Tausch, N., Becker, J. C., Spears, R., Christ, O., Saab, R., Singh, P., & Siddiqui, R. N. (2011). Explaining radical group behavior: Developing emotion and efficacy routes to normative and nonnormative collective action. *Journal of Personality and Social Psychology*, 101(1), 129–148. https://doi.org/10.1037/a0022728

Taylor, S. (2019). *The Psychology of Pandemics*. Cambridge Scholar Publishing.

Taylor, S. E., & Brown, J. D. (1988). Illusion and well-being: A social psychological perspective on mental health. *Psychological Bulletin*, 103, 193–210.

Taylor, S. E., & Brown, J. D. (1994). Positive illusions and well-being revisited: Separating fact from fiction. *Psychological Bulletin*, 116, 21–27.

Taylor, S., Asmundson, G. J. G., & Coons, M. J. (2005). Current directions in the treatment of hypochondriasis. *Journal of Cognitive Psychotherapy*, 19, 285–304.

Terpstra, T. (2011). Emotions, trust, and perceived risk: Affective and cognitive routes to flood preparedness behavior. *Risk Analysis: An International Journal*, 31(10), 1658–1675.

Tetlock, P. E. (2003). Thinking the unthinkable: Sacred values and taboo cognitions. *Trends in Cognitive Sciences*, 7, 320–324.

Tetlock, P. E. & Gardner, D. (2015). *Superforecasting: The Art and Science of Prediction*. New York: Crown Publishers/Random House.

Tetlock, P. E., Kristel, O. V., Elson, S. B., Green, M. C., & Lerner, J. S. (2000). The psychology of the unthinkable: Taboo trade-offs, forbidden base rates, and heretical counterfactuals. *Journal of Personality and Social Psycholology*, 78, 853–870.

Thaler, R., & Sunstein, C. (2003). Libertarian paternalism. *American Economic Review*, 93, 175–179.

Thaler, R. H., & Sunstein, C. R. (2009). *Nudge: Improving Decisions About Health, Wealth, and Happiness*. New York: Penguin.

Thøgersen, J. (2008). Social norms and cooperation in real-life social dilemmas. *Journal of Economic Psychology*, 29, 458–472.

Thompson, N., Wang, X., & Daya, P. (2020). Determinants of news sharing behavior on social media. *Journal of Computer Information Systems*, 60(6), 593–601. https://doi.org/10.1080/08874417.2019.1566803

References   145

Tinghög, G., & Västfjäll, D. (2018). Why people hate health economics – two psychological explanations. *LiU Working Papers in Economics*, 6.

Traczyk, J., & Zaleskiewicz, T. (2015). Implicit attitudes toward risk: The construction and validation of the measurement method. *Journal of Risk Research*, 19, 632–644. https://doi.org/10.1080/13669877.2014.1003957

Traczyk, J., Sobkow, A., & Zaleskiewicz, T. (2015). Affect-laden imagery and risk taking: The mediating role of stress and risk perception. *PloS ONE*, 10(3).

Tu, J. (2020). How female Prime Ministers are leading in this time of crisis. (March 18). *Women's Agenda*. https://womensagenda.com.au/latest/how-female-prime-ministers-are-leading-in-this-time-of-crisis/

Turner, J. C. (1982). Towards a redefinition of the social group. In H. Tajfel (Ed.), *Social Identity and Intergroup Relations* (pp. 15–40). Cambridge University Press.

Turner, J. C. (1991). *Social Influence*. Milton Keynes, UK: Open University Press.

Turner, J. C., Hogg, M. A., Oakes, P. J., Reicher, S. D., & Wetherell, M. S. (1987). *Rediscovering the Social Group: A Self-categorization Theory*. Oxford: Basil Blackwell.

Tversky, A., & Kahneman, D. (1974). Judgment under uncertainty: Heuristics and biases. *Science*, 185(4157), 1124–1131.

TVN24. (2020). Despite a lot of disturbing information regarding the spread of the new coronavirus, the isolation of society also has its positive sides. Environmental pollution is reduced and people unite in difficult times. (March 23). https://tvnmeteo.tvn24.pl/informacje-pogoda/ciekawostki,49/czystsze-powietrze-solidarnosc-i-nie-tylko-co-dobrego-daje-swiatu-pandemia-covid-19,318108,1,0.html

Tyler, T. (2011). Procedural justice shapes evaluations of income inequality: Commentary on Norton and Ariely (2011). *Perspectives on Psychological Science*, 6, 15–16.

Tyler, T. R. (2021). *Why People Obey the Law*. Princeton University Press.

Tyler, T. R., & Blader, S. L. (2003). The group engagement model: Procedural justice, social identity, and cooperative behavior. *Personality and Social Psychology Review*, 7(4), 349–361. https://doi.org/10.1207/S15327957PSPR0704_07

Tyler, T. R., & Huo, Y. J. (2002). Trust in the law: Encouraging public cooperation with the police and courts. New York: Russell Sage Foundation.

Uhl-Bien, M., Riggio, R. E., Lowe, K. B., & Carsten, M. K. (2014). Followership theory: A review and research agenda. *The Leadership Quarterly*, 25, 83–104.

Umberson, D., & Karas Montez, J. (2010). Social relationships and health: A flashpoint for health policy. *Journal of Health and Social Behavior*, 51(1_suppl), S54–S66.

Umberson, D., Crosnoe, R., & Reczek, C. (2010). Social relationships and health behavior across the life course. *Annual Review of Sociology*, 36, 139–157.

Unsworth, N., & Robison, M. K. (2017). A locus coeruleus-norepinephrine account of individual differences in working memory capacity and attention control. *Psychonomic Bulletin & Review*, 24(4), 1282–1311.

Uslaner, E. M. (2002). *The Moral Foundations of Trust*. Cambridge University Press.

Uslaner, E. (2018). The study of trust. *The Oxford Handbook of Social and Political Trust*. Oxford University Press.

Uslaner, E., & Brown, M. (2005). Inequality, trust, and civic engagement. *American Politics Research*, 33, 868–894.

Vail, K., Arndt, J., Motyl, M., & Pyszczynski, T. (2009). Compassionate values and presidential politics: Mortality salience, compassionate values, and support for Barack Obama and John Mccain in the 2008 Presidential Election (February, 18 2011). *Analyses of Social Issues and Public Policy*, 9, 255–268. https://ssrn.com/abstract=1763545

146 Individuals, Groups, and Society in Pandemics

Vail, K. E., Juhl, J., Arndt, J., Vess, M., Routledge, C., & Rutjens, B. T. (2012). When death is good for life: Considering the positive trajectories of terror management. *Personality and Social Psychology Review*, 16(4), 303–329. https://doi.org/10.1177/1088868312440046

Valentino, N. A., Banks, A. J., Hutchings, V. L., & Davis, A. K. (2009). Selective exposure in the internet age: The interaction between anxiety and information utility. *Political Psychology*, 30(4), 591–613.

Vallone, R. P., Ross, L., & Lepper, M. R. (1985). The hostile media phenomenon: Biased perception and perceptions of media bias in coverage of the Beirut massacre. *Journal of Personality and Social Psychology*, 49(3), 577–585.

Van Bavel, J. J., & Pereira, A. (2018). The partisan brain: An identity-based model of political belief. *Trends in Cognitive Sciences*, 22(3), 213–224. https://doi.org/10.1016/j.tics.2018.01.004

Van Bavel, J. J., Baicker, K., Boggio, P. S., et al. (2020). Using social and behavioural science to support COVID-19 pandemic response. *Nature Human Behaviour*, 4, 460–471.

van den Bos, R., Homberg, J., & de Visser, L. (2013). A critical review of sex differences in decision-making tasks: Focus on the Iowa Gambling Task. *Behavioural Brain Research*, 238, 95–108.

van der Does, R., Kantorowicz, J., Kuipers, S., & Liem, M. (2019). Does terrorism dominate citizens' hearts or minds? The relationship between fear of terrorism and trust in government. *Terrorism and Political Violence*, 33(6), 1276–1294.

van der Linden, S. (2015). The social-psychological determinants of climate change risk perceptions: Towards a comprehensive model. *Journal of Environmental Psychology*, 41, 112–124. https://doi.org/10.1016/j.jenvp.2014.11.012

van der Linden, S. (2017). Determinants and measurement of climate change risk perception, worry, and concern. In M. C. Nisbet, M. Schafer, E. Markowitz, S. Ho, S. O'Neill, & J. Thaker (Eds.), *The Oxford Encyclopedia of Climate Change Communication*. Oxford University Press.

van der Meer, T., & Hakhverdian, A. (2017). Political trust as the evaluation of process and performance: A cross-national study of 42 European countries. *Political Studies*, 65(1), 81–102.

van der Weerd, W., Timmermans, D. R., Beaujean, D. J., Oudhoff, J., & van Steenbergen, J. E. (2011). Monitoring the level of government trust, risk perception and intention of the general public to adopt protective measures during the influenza A (H1N1) pandemic in the Netherlands. *BMC Public Health*, 11(1), 575.

Van de Walle, S., & Bouckaert, G. (2003). Public service performance and trust in government: The problem of causality. *International Journal of Public Administration*, 26(8–9), 891–913.

Van Lange, P. A. M., Joireman, J., & Milinski, M. (2018). Climate change: What psychology can offer in terms of insights and solutions. *Current Directions in Psychological Science*, 27(4), 269–274. https://doi.org/10.1177/0963721417753945

van Prooijen, J.-W. (2017). Why education predicts decreased belief in conspiracy theories. *Applied Cognitive Psychology*, 31, 50–58.

van Prooijen, J.-W. (2019). Belief in conspiracy theories: Gullibility or rational skepticism? In J. P. Forgas, & R. F. Baumeister (Eds.), *The Social Psychology of Gullibility: Fake News, Conspiracy Theories and Irrational Beliefs* (pp. 319–332). London: Taylor & Francis.

References 147

Van Ryzin, G. G. (2011). Outcomes, process, and trust of civil servants. *Journal of Public Administration Research and Theory*, 21(4), 745–760.

van Teunenbroek, C., & Bekkers, R. (2020). Follow the crowd: Social information and crowdfunding donations in a large field experiment. *Journal of Behavioral Public Administration*, 3(1). https://doi.org/10.30636/jbpa.31.87

van Zomeren, M., Postmes, T., & Spears, R. (2008). Toward an integrative social identity model of collective action: A quantitative research synthesis of three socio-psychological perspectives. *Psychological Bulletin*, 134(4), 504–535. https://doi.org/10.1037/0033-2909.134.4.504

Verboon, P., & van Dijke, M. (2011). When do severe sanctions enhance compliance? The role of procedural fairness. *Journal of Economic Psychology*, 32(1), 120–130.

Villoria, M., Van Ryzin, G. G., & Lavena, C. F. (2013). Social and political consequences of administrative corruption: A study of public perceptions in Spain. *Public Administration Review*, 73(1), 85–94.

Visschers, V. H. M., & Siegrist, M. (2018). Differences in risk perception between hazards and between individuals. In M. Raue, E. Lermer, & B. Streicher (Eds.), *Psychological Perspectives on Risk and Risk Analysis* (pp. 63–80). New York: Springer.

Vohs, K. D. (2015). Money priming can change people's thoughts, feelings, motivations, and behaviors: An update on 10 years of experiments. *Journal of Experimental Psychology: General*, 144(4), e86–e93.

Vollhardt, J. R. (2015). Inclusive victim consciousness in advocacy, social movements, and intergroup relations: Promises and pitfalls. *Social Issues and Policy Review*, 9, 89–120.

Vollmann, M., Antoniw, K., Hartung, F., & Renner, B. (2011). Social support as mediator of the stress buffering effect of optimism: The importance of differentiating the recipients' and providers' perspective. *European Journal of Personality*, 25(2), 146–154. https://doi.org/10.1002/per.803

von Dawans, B., Trueg, A., Kirschbaum, C., Fischbacher, U., & Heinrichs, M. (2018). Acute social and physical stress interact to influence social behavior: The role of social anxiety. *PloS ONE*, 13(10).

Vosoughi, S., Roy, D., & Aral, S. (2018). The spread of true and false news online. *Science*, 359(6380), 1146–1151. https://doi.org/10.1126/science.aap9559

Wallace, C., & Latcheva, R. (2006). Economic transformation outside the law: Corruption, trust in public institutions and the informal economy in transition countries of Central and Eastern Europe. *Europe-Asia Studies*, 58(1), 81–102.

Walter, N., & Murphy, S. T. (2018). How to unring the bell: A meta-analytic approach to correction of misinformation. *Communication Monographs*, 85(3), 423–441. https://doi.org/10.1080/03637751.2018.1467564

Wang, X., McKee, M., Torbica, A., & Stuckler, D. (2019). Systematic literature review on the spread of health-related misinformation on social media. *Social Science & Medicine*, 240, 112–552.

Washer, P. (2004). Representations of SARS in the British newspapers. *Social Science and Medicine*, 59, 2561–2571. https://doi.org/10.1016/j.socscimed.2004.03.038

Weber, E. U. (2017). Understanding public risk perception and responses to changes in perceived risk. In E. J. Balleisen, L. S. Bennear, K. D. Krawiec, & J. B. Wiener (Eds.), *Policy Shock: Regulatory Responses to Oil Spills, Nuclear Accidents, and Financial Crashes* (pp. 82–106). Cambridge University Press.

148 *Individuals, Groups, and Society in Pandemics*

Weber E. U., & Hsee, C. K. (1999). Models and mosaics: Investigating cross-cultural differences in risk perception and risk preference. *Psychonomic Bulletin & Review,* 6, 611–617.

Weber, E. U., & Hsee, C. K. (2000). Culture and individual decision-making. *Applied Psychology: An International Journal,* 49, 32–61.

Weber, E. U., & Stern, P. C. (2011). Public understanding of climate change in the United States. *American Psychologist,* 66(4), 315–328.

Weber, E. U., Baron, J., & Loomes, G. (Eds.) (2001). *Conflict and Tradeoffs in Decision Making.* Cambridge University Press.

Webster, D. M., & Kruglanski, A. W. (1994). Individual differences in need for cognitive closure. *Journal of Personality and Social Psychology,* 67(6), 1049.

Wegner, D., & Smart, L. (1997). Deep cognitive activation: A new approach to the unconscious. *Journal of Consulting and Clinical Psychology,* 65, 984–995.

Weigmann, K. (2018). The genesis of a conspiracy theory: Why do people believe in scientific conspiracy theories and how do they spread? *EMBO Reports,* 19, https://doi.org/10.15252/embr.201845935

Weinstein, N. D. (1980). Unrealistic optimism about future life events. *Journal of Personality and Social Psychology,* 39, 806–820.

Weinstein, N. D. (1989). Optimistic biases about personal risks. *Science,* 246, 1232–1233.

Weinstein, N. D. (2001). Smokers' recognition of their vulnerability to harm. In P. Slovic (Ed.), *Smoking: Risk, Perception, & Policy* (pp. 81–96). Thousand Oaks, CA: Sage.

Weinstein, N. D., & Klein, W. M. (1996). Unrealistic optimism: Present and future. *Journal of Social and Clinical Psychology,* 15, 1–8.

Weller, J. A., Levin, I. P., Shiv, B., & Bechara, A. (2009). The effects of insula damage on decision-making for risky gains and losses. *Social Neuroscience,* 4(4), 347–358.

Wenzel, M. (2004). The social side of sanctions: Personal and social norms as moderators of deterrence. *Law and Human Behavior,* 28, 547–567. https://doi.org/10.1023/B:LAHU.0000046433.57588.71

Wetterberg, A. (2007). Crisis, connections, and class: How social ties affect household welfare. *World Development,* 35(4), 585–606.

Wheaton, M. G., Abramowitz, J. S., Berman, N. C., Fabricant, L. E., & Olatunji, 8. O. (2012). Psychological predictors of anxiety in response to the HINl (swine flu) pandemic. *Cognitive Therapy and Research,* 36, 210–218. doi:l0.l007/s10608-011-9353-3

Wheaton, M. G., Berman, N. C., Franklin, J. C., & Abramowitz, J. S. (2010). Health anxiety: Latent structure and associations with anxiety-related psychological processes in a student sample. *Journal of Psychopathology and Behavioral Assessment,* 32(4), 565–574.

White, M. D., Mulvey, P., & Dario, L. M. (2016). Arrestees' perceptions of the police: Exploring procedural justice, legitimacy, and willingness to cooperate with police across offender types. *Criminal Justice and Behavior,* 43(3), 343–364.

WHO. (2019). Ten threats to global health in 2019. https://www.who.int/news-room/spotlight/ten-threats-to-global-health-in-2019

Wiadomości Onet (2020). (March 24). https://wiadomosci.onet.pl/kraj/koronawirus-w-polsce-rzad-wprowadza-nowe-restrykcje-co-oznaczaja/b6rrhbv

Wichary, S., Kossowska, M., Orzechowski, J., Ślifierz, S., & Marković, J. (2008). Individual differences in decisiveness: Pre-decisional information search and decision strategy use. *Polish Psychological Bulletin,* 39(1), 47–53.

Wichary, S., Mata, R., & Rieskamp, J. (2016). Probabilistic inferences under emotional stress: How arousal affects decision processes. *Journal of Behavioral Decision Making*, 29(5), 525–538.

Wilkinson, R., & Pickett, K. (2010). *The Spirit Level: Why Equality is Better for Everyone*. UK: Penguin.

Williams, L., Rasmussen, S., Maharaj, S., Kleczkowski, A., & Cairns, N. (2015). Protection motivation theory and social distancing behaviour in response to a simulated infectious disease epidemic. *Psychology, Health and Medicine*, 20(7), 832–837.

Williams, R., & Drury, J. (2009). Psychosocial resilience and its influence on managing mass emergencies and disasters. *Psychiatry*, 8, 293–296.

Wisman, A., & Koole, S. L. (2003). Hiding in the crowd: Can mortality salience promote affiliation with others who oppose one's worldviews? *Journal of Personality and Social Psychology*, 84(3), 511–526. https://doi.org/10.1037/0022-3514.84.3.511

Witteman, H. O., Chipenda Dansokho, S., Exe, N., Dupuis, A., Provencher, T., & Zikmund-Fisher, B. J. (2015). Risk communication, values clarification, and vaccination decisions. *Risk Analysis*, 35, 1801–1819.

Wohl, M. J. A., Hornsey, M. J., & Bennett, S. H. (2012). Why group apologies succeed and fail: Intergroup forgiveness and the role of primary and secondary emotions. *Journal of Personality and Social Psychology*, 102(2), 306–322. https://doi.org/10.1037/a0024838

Woolcock, M. (2001). The place of social capital in understanding social and economic outcomes. *Canadian Journal of Policy Research*, 2(1), 11–17.

World Bank. (2020). COVID-19 to plunge global economy into worst recession since World War II. (June 8). https://www.worldbank.org/en/news/press-release/2020/06/08/covid-19-to-plunge-global-economy-into-worst-recession-since-world-war-ii

Wroe, A. (2016). Economic insecurity and political trust in the United States. *American Politics Research*, 44(1), 131–163.

Xie, W., Campbell, S., & Zhang, W. (2020). Working memory capacity predicts individual differences in social distancing compliance during the COVID-19 pandemic in the US. *Proceedings of the National Academy of Sciences of the USA*, 117, 17667–17674.

Yalom, I. (1980). *Existential Psychotherapy*. New York: Basic Books.

Yamagishi, T. (1986). The provision of a sanctioning system as a public good. *Journal of Personality and Social Psychology*, 51(1), 110–116. https://doi.org/10.1037/0022-3514.51.1.110

Yang, K., & Holzer, M. (2006). The performance–trust link: Implications for performance measurement. *Public Administration Review*, 66(1), 114–126.

Yaniv, I. (2004). Receiving other people's advice: Influence and benefit. *Organizational Behavior and Human Decision Processes*, 93, 1–13.

Yaniv, I., & Kleinberger, E. (2000). Advice taking in decision making: Egocentric discounting and reputation formation. *Organizational Behavior and Human Decision Processes*, 83, 260–281.

Yaniv, I., & Milyavsky, M. (2007). Using advice from multiple sources to revise and improve judgment. *Organizational Behavior and Human Decision Processes*, 103, 104–120.

Yaqub, O., Castle-Clarke, S., Sevdalis, N., & Chataway, J. (2014). Attitudes to vaccination: A critical review. *Social Science & Medicine*, 112, 1–11. https://doi.org/10.1016/j.socscimed.2014.04.018

Yiend, J. (2010). The effects of emotion on attention: A review of attentional processing of emotional information. *Cognition and Emotion*, 24(1), 3–47.

Yu, R. (2016). Stress potentiates decision biases: A stress induced deliberation-to-intuition (SIDI) model. *Neurobiology of Stress*, 3, 83–95.

Zaleskiewicz, T. (2006). Behavioral finance. In M. Altman (Ed.), *Handbook of Contemporary Behavioral Economics. Foundations and Developments* (pp. 706–728). New York: Routledge.

Zaleskiewicz, T., & Gasiorowska, A. (2018). Tell me what I wanted to hear: Confirmation effect in lay evaluations of financial expert authority. *Applied Psychology: An International Review*, 67, 686–722.

Zaleskiewicz, T., & Gasiorowska, A. (2021). Evaluating experts serves psychological needs: Self-esteem, bias blind spot, and processing fluency explain confirmation effect in assessing financial advisors' authority. *Journal of Experimental Psychology: Applied*, 27(1), 27–45.

Zaleskiewicz, T., & Traczyk, J. (2020). Emotions and financial decision making. In T. Zaleskiewicz, & J. Traczyk (Eds.), *Psychological Perspectives on Financial Decision Making* (pp. 109–136). New York: Springer.

Zaleskiewicz, T., Bernady, A., & Traczyk, J. (2020). Entrepreneurial risk taking is related to mental imagery: A fresh look at the old issue of entrepreneurship and risk. *Applied Psychology: An International Review*, 69(4), 1438–1469. https://doi.org/10.1111/apps.12226

Zaleskiewicz, T., Gasiorowska, A., & Kesebir, P. (2015). The Scrooge effect revisited: Mortality salience increases the satisfaction derived from prosocial behavior. *Journal of Experimental Social Psychology*, 59, 67–76. https://doi.org/10.1016/j.jesp.2015.03.005

Zaleskiewicz, T., Gasiorowska, A., & Vohs, K. D. (2017). The psychological meaning of money. In R. Ranyard (Ed.), *Economic Psychology* (pp. 107–122). London: Wiley.

Zaleskiewicz, T., Gasiorowska, A., Kesebir, P., Luszczynska, A., & Pyszczynski, T. (2013). Money and the fear of death: The symbolic power of money as an existential anxiety buffer. *Journal of Economic Psychology*, 36, 55–67. https://doi.org/10.1016/j.joep.2013.02.008

Zaleskiewicz, T., Gasiorowska, A., Kuzminska, A., Korotusz, P., & Tomczak, P. (2020). Market mindset impacts moral decisions: The exposure to market relationships makes moral choices more utilitarian by means of proportional thinking. *European Journal of Social Psychology*, 50(7), 1500–1522. https://doi.org/10.1002/ejsp.2701

Zaleskiewicz, T., Gasiorowska, A., Stasiuk, K., Maksymiuk, R., & Bar-Tal, Y. (2016). Lay evaluation of financial experts: The action advice effect and confirmation bias. *Frontiers in Psychology*, 7, 1476. https://doi.org/10.3389/fpsyg.2016.01476

Zaleskiewicz, T., Piskorz, Z., & Borkowska, A. (2002). Fear or money? Decisions on insuring oneself against flood. *Risk, Decision, and Policy*, 7, 221–233.

Zion, S. R., Schapira, L., & Crum, A. J. (2019). Targeting mindsets, not just tumors. *Trends in Cancer*, 5(10), 573–576.

Ziv, I., & Leiser, D. (2013). The need for central resources in answering questions in different domains: Folk psychology, biology, and economics. *Journal of Cognitive Psychology*, 25(7), 816–832.

PART 2

CULTURE AND POLICY IN TIMES OF PANDEMICS

CASE STUDIES

Edited by:
Małgorzata Kossowska, Natalia Letki, Tomasz Zaleskiewicz,
and Szymon Wichary

6 THE COVID-19 EPIDEMIC IN POLAND, AS OF SUMMER 2021[1]

Jerzy Duszyński

The sudden appearance of an atypical form of severe pneumonia in December 2019 took healthcare providers by surprise, first in Wuhan, a city of nearly 9 million residents in the Chinese province of Hubei, and soon afterwards in the entire province, with its population of 58.4 million. An extremely intense period of research began, aiming to identify the pathogen causing the mysterious disease, scrambling for ways to curb its transmission, and ultimately to reduce, as rapidly as possible, the number of deaths caused by the new disease and its profound impact on economies across the world. To demonstrate the intensity of research in this seemingly narrow field of study, we need merely note that, between January 1, 2020 and July 5, 2021, the biomedical database PubMed recorded 153,380 new publications that included the terms "COVID-19" or "SARS-CoV-2" in their titles or abstracts, which translates into an average of 280 new publications a day over the past 18 months.

These mind-boggling numbers reflect an unprecedented global research effort devoted to the problem. As a reminder, the atypical respiratory disease, first observed in December 2019, was officially named COVID-19 on February 11, 2020 (as announced by the World Health Organization), and three days later, the virus causing the disease was labelled SARS-CoV-2. Remarkable progress has been made in elucidating the new disease in the brief time since its discovery: scientists have identified the SARS-CoV-2 virus that causes COVID-19, sequenced its genetic material, established the pace at which the virus mutates, and explained how it enters the body and its cells. Moreover, specific tests have been developed to detect the virus in infected people – both molecular tests for the presence of SARS-CoV-2 RNA, and serological ones detecting antibodies specific to proteins in the viral envelope. The course of COVID-19 is now quite well understood, and groups of patients at the highest risk of severe illness have been pinpointed. Intensive work on developing COVID-19 drugs is still under way and several types of vaccine have been produced. Effective means of curtailing the epidemic by minimizing the risk of infection have been identified. The course of the epidemic and the appearance of new variants of SARS-CoV-2

DOI: 10.4324/9781003254133-9

are being monitored, and the new variants' epidemic characteristics have been studied.

Now, by way of contrast, let us compare the current situation to 1981, when the first cases of a new disease (today known as AIDS) were reported. Reliable tests for AIDS (only serological ones at that time) were not available before 1986, and the debate about whether the disease was really caused by the Human Immunodeficiency Virus (HIV) raged until 1994. Another disease, severe acute respiratory syndrome (SARS), emerged in 2002. This time it took just a few months to identify the pathogen (SARS-CoV) and develop reliable tests. A revolution in molecular biology has occurred since that time, resulting from, in particular, the implementation of the polymerase chain reaction technique (commonly known as PCR) as a basic diagnostic tool.

Further refinements of this technique made it possible to identify SARS-CoV-2 as the casual factor of COVID-19 within mere weeks, between December 2019 and January 2020. China officially reported cases of a new type of pneumonia at the end of December 2019. On January 10, 2020, Australian scientists shared the first sequences of the viral genome, and as early as January 13, the Charité Hospital in Berlin made a test for SARS-CoV-2 available. Thus, what had taken researchers several years in the case of AIDS, and a few months in the case of SARS, required no more than a couple of weeks when COVID-19 appeared. This attests to the tremendous strides in scientific progress we have seen in recent years.

The COVID-19 pandemic has become the focus of public attention worldwide, allowing the general public to take a closer look at how science works. More people now realize that we are in the midst of a dynamic process of exploration of the new virus, in which breakthroughs are frequent, so that what is true one day may no longer be valid the next. This is how science works. In the field of public health, the key to success is evidence-based medicine. The pandemic has precipitated a medical, social, and economic crisis, but also taught a salutary lesson to all of us. Hopefully, the opportunity to observe how science is developed and how it influences everyday life will lead to increased rationality in social life, and higher public acceptance of rational means of knowledge acquisition. The public has never been so close to the scientific process, with its twists and turns, leaps forward, and unprecedented successes.

But we also can't help but notice a growing resistance to evidence-based rationality. Groups that promote irrational ideas, or, on occasion, even deny the very existence of the pandemic, are becoming ever more active. A large proportion of society stands somewhere in between these two viewpoints: the rational and irrational, somewhat bewildered and overwhelmed by the flood of inconsistent information (which has been termed an "infodemic"). The role of scientists and the media is to expose irrational thinking and to set it apart from the revision of ideas and the clash of hypotheses, which are inevitable in the process of gaining knowledge in science.

The first case of COVID-19 in Poland was formally diagnosed on March 4, 2020, and the first death caused by the disease was reported on March 12.

The ongoing COVID-19 epidemic has not only affected (and continues to affect) people's general health status and the functioning of healthcare in Poland, it also has significant economic, social, and psychological repercussions. Every nation on Earth was transfixed when, on March 11, 2020, the World Health Organization declared the COVID-19 outbreak a pandemic – defined as an epidemic occurring globally. By the time of writing this (July 5, 2021), COVID-19 cases have been reported in every country in the world; their overall number is 183,204,313, while the total number of deaths, globally, is 3,966,232 (according to Dong et al, 2020). Poland has had 2,880,107 COVID-19 cases and 75,065 deaths caused by the disease (again, see Dong et al., 2020). What should be added to these grim figures is the tragic toll of excess mortality linked to the inefficiency of the healthcare system as well as significant delays in treatment procedures for conditions other than COVID-19. Suffice to say, every year 170,000 people in Poland die of cardiovascular diseases, 110,000 of cancer, 30,000 of dementia, 17,000 of gastrointestinal diseases, and 7,000 of diabetes. Not surprisingly, the accompanying partial discontinuation or delay in their treatment has led to dramatic outcomes, equal to those directly attributable to the pandemic.

One might assume that, having endured 18 months of the COVID-19 epidemic in Poland, an average Pole would have come to realize the severity of the epidemic threat. Many people have friends or family members who have lost their health or lives to the epidemic. Moreover, many have been hit hard by COVID-19 lockdowns, which crippled particular areas of the economy, such as the hospitality sector, the beauty industry, and the arts, depriving people of their earning capacity for months on end.

The pandemic forced schools to move classes online for an indefinite time. Cut off from direct contact with their teachers and peers, students can also be seen as victims of the pandemic because, despite their lower risk of infection, the psychological and educational effects of lockdown can be very severe for this group, possibly extending for much longer than the pandemic itself. Research suggests young people experience particularly high levels of stress related to the COVID-19 epidemic, which results from factors including a destabilized family life, isolation from peers, and having to change their habits and safe daily routines. Their fear and uncertainty are aggravated by intensive exposure to negative information about the pandemic and its effects. All these factors add to the stress associated with natural developmental changes, both biological and psychosocial, including qualitative changes in how young people feel and think.

Research shows that home confinement has a particularly negative impact on young people's psychological wellbeing, as it not only condemns them to inactivity and isolation from peers, but also, in many cases, deprives them of the privacy and intimacy which they need so desperately at this stage of development. Moreover, home confinement can cause children and young people to start spending inordinate and unhealthy amounts of time online. Young people, especially those on the brink of adulthood, may also be concerned about their potentially poorer prospects for the future: The pandemic may well shatter their dreams, thwart their desires, and dash their hopes of future success. In addition, at a time when many parents and caregivers struggle with serious difficulties, young people may fall victim to verbal, psychological, or physical abuse, experienced directly or indirectly.

Another group hit hard by the COVID-19 pandemic is minorities. The pandemic has greatly affected people with disabilities, those living in residential care, refugees, migrants, and those experiencing homelessness. Several other groups have also felt the far-reaching impact of the pandemic. These include problem drug users, patients of various types of treatment facilities, residents in nursing homes and residential care facilities, victims of domestic violence, and non-heteronormative people (LGBTQI+). The pandemic has impaired the functioning of facilities that typically provide help for these groups. The better prepared these facilities are to deliver services during the pandemic, the lower the material, psychological, and health costs are for those using their services, not to mention the staff. Non-heteronormative individuals face the additional problem of prolonged confinement in a potentially hostile family environment, and possibly exposure to violence. Adding fuel to the fire, LGBTQI+ persons have become a target of political attacks and hate speech during the current pandemic. All of the above has exacerbated their distress and led to a host of psychological issues, which now constitutes a major social problem, affecting, in total, more than 20% of Polish society.

Given all this, the rapidity of change in public mood around the pandemic can often be astounding. Periods of relatively high vigilance and utmost caution are followed by periods of conspicuous laxity and flagrant carelessness. One reason why the COVID-19 epidemic has been treated quite lightly by a section of Polish society is the fact that COVID-19 restrictions were first introduced at a time when the epidemic was virtually invisible in Poland, even though in other countries it had already put people's life and limb in serious jeopardy. What is now referred to as the first wave of the epidemic in Europe, which clearly occurred in Germany in late March and early April 2020, was virtually imperceptible to Polish society, since it was exactly at that time, on March 16, 2020, when the first lockdown was imposed in Poland (see Figure 6.1 and Figure 6.2).

Such was the effectiveness of the measures brought in that Polish society was (and continues to be) susceptible to various conspiracy theories about the pandemic. In the spring of 2020, people in Poland experienced a kind of cognitive dissonance, whereby information about how grave the situation was, conveyed by the media and by decision makers, was starkly at odds with people's everyday lived experience. During the first wave, Polish citizens were quite unlikely to see the disease among their family, friends, or even acquaintances. Yet, tight restrictions were imposed on social life. Then came the second and third waves of the pandemic (beginning in October 2020 and February 2021, respectively), which took a horrendous toll in Poland. But the initial doubts about the actual reality of the pandemic in spring 2020

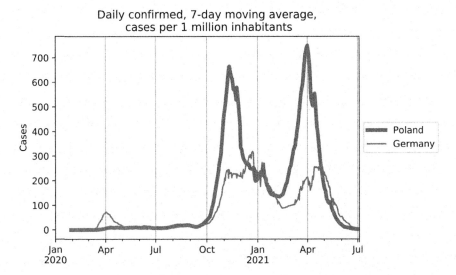

Figure 6.1 Comparison of Poland's and Germany's daily confirmed cases per 1 million habitants, 7-day moving average.
Based on Dong et al. (2020)

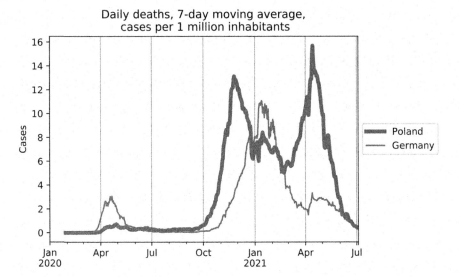

Figure 6.2 Comparison of Poland's and Germany's daily deaths per 1 million habitants, 7-day moving average.
Based on Dong et al. (2020)

may have been the reason why the commonly experienced tragic outcomes of the subsequent epidemic waves in Poland, and the related self-discipline in following appropriate hygiene rules, were later so easily replaced by a general loosening of standards. The consequences of this were not slow in coming, as Poland's third wave of COVID-19 proved extremely treacherous.

This was quite a contrast to the situation in Germany (Figures 6.1 and 6.2), where society, mindful of the devastating aftermath of the previous two waves, continued to maintain strict hygiene discipline and follow the DDM (distancing, disinfection, masks) rule. These rules were also followed quite consistently by people in many other European countries, who had vivid memories of the dreadful periods when the epidemic swept certain regions (such as Lombardy in Italy) or the entire country (for example, Spain), inflicting large swathes of casualties.

One dramatic example is the superspreading event in Bergamo, Italy. It all started in high spirits. On February 19, 2020, the San Siro Stadium in Milan hosted a Champions League match between Atalanta Bergamo of Italy and Valencia CF of Spain. Flocking to the stadium were 45,000 spectators, including 35,000 Atalanta fans and 2,500 Valencia supporters, who packed the venue to watch the game. Despite being played two days before the first case of COVID-19 was detected in Italy, many asymptomatic carriers existed in the country, unbeknownst to anyone. In early February 2020, no one in Italy was on the lookout for people who had been in contact with those coming from countries where the epidemic was already on the rampage. As a result, several people infected with SARS-CoV-2 were among the fans at San Siro. The game ended 4:1 in favour of the Italian team. After each goal, people fell into each other's arms, patted each other, hugged, and cheered with excitement. And, as it turned out later, in doing so, they were transmitting the deadly virus on a massive scale.

The San Siro match of February 19 is now described as a "biological bomb," which exploded a few weeks later. By mid-March, Bergamo had run out of coffins, and bodies were being transported from the city in military trucks. The traumatic events of that time were seared into the memories of the people of Lombardy, and all of Italy, preventing them from taking the COVID-19 epidemic lightly, or denying its existence. Similar horrific abiding memories are present in the collective consciousness of those living in Valencia, Barcelona, New York, and many other cities, regions, and countries around the world. For people in Poland, however, who are lacking such firsthand experience, the epidemic has been treated more heedlessly.

The world's large economies are experiencing seismic convulsions. In developed countries, some major sectors of the economy (such as the travel, aviation, and automotive industries) are being decimated by the COVID-19 pandemic. Looking to the future, a deep global recession seems to be on the horizon, and COVID-19 seems to be the first falling domino sparking severe disruption. The media present catastrophic forecasts about inevitable record unemployment rates, imminent social turmoil, and impending political crises in many countries.

That being said, despite an 18-month struggle with the disease, attitudes ignoring or downplaying the dangers of COVID-19 are widespread in Poland. Indeed, we have seen the prevailing view of the COVID-19 epidemic swing wildly from negative to positive, from times when a wave sweeps the country to those times when all seems well again, usually as a result of restrictions on social life. These wide disparities in outlook result in conflicting cues and feelings, in cognitive dissonance, and ineffective information policies. This dissonance is particularly salient in Poland, the only society among 22 countries surveyed by YouGov in which friends and family are more trusted than healthcare professionals. To make matters worse, Poles currently have exceptionally low levels of trust in the media and politicians, leading some people to believe that the response of the body politic and the fifth estate to COVID-19 is grossly exaggerated. Still others take matters further and claim the whole thing is a conspiracy that has nothing to do with any genuine concern for public health but rather represents an attempt to take full control of society. The mechanisms underlying such attitudes toward COVID-19 and their spread in society ought to become a focus of psychological research.

Since mid-May 2021, the third epidemic wave has been tapering off in Poland. The numbers of COVID-19 cases, hospitalizations, and deaths have substantially declined. This has been achieved not only by imposing strict social restrictions but also as a result of the growing number of vaccinated people, plus the relatively high number already infected by COVID-19 who have developed immunity to the disease. As of July 3, 2021, the number of fully vaccinated people in Poland was 13,854,142, that is, 36.5% of the population. By comparison, as of the same day, the proportions of fully vaccinated people were 37.9% in Germany, 31.4% in France, 50.1% in the UK, 39.3% in Spain, and 32.8% in Italy. At the time of writing, the weather is another factor helping to suppress the epidemic: The warmer weather means people spend more time outdoors and ventilate their homes more frequently. In July 2021, social and economic life has largely returned to normal: Schools, restaurants, sports facilities, and cultural centres have been re-opened, and maximum numbers of participants in weddings, funerals, and other special events are now very high.

By mid-June 2021, Poles were already starting to hope that the abatement of the pandemic could be permanent. However, we should be prepared for a much gloomier scenario, as a fourth wave of the pandemic struck in the fall of 2021. What may contribute to another COVID-19 surge and a huge fourth wave is the current re-opening of the economy in Poland and the return of social life to its previous norms, combined with an insufficient vaccination rate and the appearance of a new, more infectious variant of the virus. Such a new, more infectious, variant – known as the Delta variant, first identified in India – is already dominant in the UK, and will no doubt become so across the Polish population. In the light of data that suggests the Delta variant is most likely to attack unvaccinated people, the fourth wave will be particularly perilous for populations with low vaccination rates (such as eastern and south-eastern parts of Poland).

160 *Culture and Policy in Pandemics: Case Studies*

How the COVID-19 epidemic will unfold in Poland, Europe, and throughout the whole world is anyone's guess. What seems most likely, though, is that the SARS-CoV-2 virus may stay with us for years. With that in mind, the lessons to be learnt from our experience so far, which may be applied in future pandemics, are these: First of all, we need strong and independent institutions to be more effective in combatting future epidemics, which are likely just around the corner. Therefore, it would be prudent to invest in a modern healthcare system; build professional, independent institutions in the field of public health; make data available to experts; and, last but not least, invest in science and education. Of crucial importance is an effective information policy from the government, which would build trust in independent scientific and expert institutions who ought to be tasked with informing the public about the epidemic. Their representatives should be promoted in the media, with statements by "pop experts" or "pop scientists," who lack credentials from reputable scientific and expert institutions, limited to the minimum.

Equally important in the fight against epidemics is the promotion of social solidarity. Thus, it would be advisable to build trust and cooperation in society, and foster a belief that steps taken for the common good are beneficial to all. During the current pandemic, we have learned how much depends on our own behaviour, especially when institutions are operating in a suboptimal manner. Risks and uncertainty can be greatly mitigated by strict adherence to safety guidelines, primarily those included in the simple DDM (distancing, disinfection, masks) rule. But we need to stand in solidarity with one another. Solidarity is not just in the best interests of the community but also in the best interests of each of us, individually. In this respect, free riding is an anathema to solidarity: Thinking that it suffices that others are vaccinated for us to be safe will mean that everyone will be put in jeopardy. We need to bear in mind that no one will be fully safe from the COVID-19 threat until we are all safe, that is, fully vaccinated.

Note

1 The chapter is based on statements and reports developed by the COVID-19 Advisory Team to the President of the Polish Academy of Sciences (PAS) (https://institution.pan.pl/index.php/covid-19-advisory-team). The team is led by Prof. Jerzy Duszyński, President of the Polish Academy of Sciences, with Prof. Krzysztof Pyrć (Jagiellonian University) performing the role of the Deputy Team Leader. Anna Plater-Zyberek, PhD (Polish Academy of Sciences), is the Team's Secretary. Other members include: Aneta Afelt, PhD (University of Warsaw), Prof. Małgorzata Kossowska (Jagiellonian University), Prof. Radosław Owczuk (Medical University of Gdańsk), Anna Ochab-Marcinek, PhD (dr hab.) (Institute of Physical Chemistry PAS), Wojciech Paczos, PhD (Institute of Economics PAS and Cardiff University), Magdalena Rosińska, PhD (dr hab.) (National Institute of Public Health – National Institute of Hygiene), Prof. Andrzej Rychard (Institute of Philosophy and Sociology PAS), Tomasz Smiatacz, PhD (dr hab.) (Medical University of Gdańsk).

7 PANDEMIC AND CULTURAL DIFFERENCES
EXAMPLES FROM ISLAM AND HINDUISM

Piotr Kłodkowski and Anna Siewierska-Chmaj

By definition, being a global phenomenon, a pandemic can take a terrible toll all around the world. Still, we know now that fatality rates vary significantly across continents and countries. And while symptoms of the disease, its course, and medical consequences are likely to be virtually the same worldwide, as are the recommended treatments and pharmaceuticals, other factors can differ to a remarkable degree. These include the means of communicating risk, the reasons provided to justify government measures, and even people's responses to the pandemic. These variations depend on the cultural milieu because, while cultural differences do enrich our world, they also – as emphasized by Hofstede – create barriers in the communication process, which may (or may not) lead to unexpected consequences (Hofstede, 2004). Thus, being aware of those differences aids in the design of appropriate messages for a selected target group, which may constitute a greater or lesser proportion in societies characterized by cultural and religious heterogeneity. The effectiveness of the measures taken and their justifications in a specific cultural environment can also depend (especially in the long run) on the context of messages being too low or too high, as suggested by Edward T. Hall, who pointed to significant communication problems between a sender and a receiver arising from a high-context culture and a low-context culture, respectively (Hall, 1990). In relation to a pandemic, of particular relevance here is his research on proxemics, or culturally determined interpersonal space. The accepted (that is, not anger- or aggression-inducing) amount of space between various individuals in different situations is dissimilar in the US, France, India, and China. Given these considerations, we can understand why universal, externally imposed rules of social distancing are more easily accepted and internalized in Nordic countries than, for example, in South Asia.

Let us emphasize, however, an important fact that is not always recognized: Cultural differences do not necessarily correspond with religious differences, just as religious diversity does not necessarily translate into significant cultural diversity. For example, a Muslim from Kerala, one of India's states, will share many customs with a Hindu living in the same area, will speak the same language, and use a similar cultural code (Tharoor, 2007). The religious

DOI: 10.4324/9781003254133-10

162   *Culture and Policy in Pandemics: Case Studies*

difference between them certainly imposes different patterns of behaviour and perceptions of the world but does not eliminate their common areas of daily functioning. On the other hand, a Muslim from Kashmir, Morocco, or Indonesia may share a number of religious practices (such as prayer, fasting, and pilgrimage) with their fellow believer in Kerala but does not necessarily share a similar cultural code, which would enable relatively harmonious co-existence. A case in point is that of the Polish Tatars who are Muslims and have lived in Poland for hundreds of years (currently Poland's ambassador to Kazakhstan has a Tartar ethnic background, an exceptional occurrence in a religiously homogenous nation such as Poland). This group uses a cultural code that is completely different from the one used in Egypt or Malaysia, despite belonging to the same *umma* (community of believers).

Still, in many regions of the world, religion continues to determine the local culture and has a strong influence on cultures separated by thousands of kilometers. The cultural substrate of Saudi Arabia, Turkey, Pakistan, Jordan, or Iraq cannot be correctly analyzed without referring to the Islamic civilization. Although they speak different languages (or different dialects of Arabic) and have different customs and behaviours, their shared religion imposes similar, if not identical, legal, moral, and political norms. It is particularly important in countries where Muslims constitute the substantial majority of the population. The same is true for the Buddhist world in countries such as Thailand, Sri Lanka, or Myanmar, which have founded their cultures on Buddhism, a religion that continues to define the identities of the vast majority of their inhabitants. In India, the same is true for Hinduism, which is practiced by more than 80% of India's citizens, determining their ways of thinking, functioning, and responding to various threats and challenges. Even the existence of secular law and religiously neutral public institutions in India does not mean the role of religion in social and political life is reduced by any means.

If we were to provide an illustrative working model of the relationship between culture and religion around the world, we could use two circles, representing culture and religion respectively. For the sake of simplicity, culture would be defined locally or regionally, and religion globally (Christianity, Islam, Buddhism, and, to a lesser degree, Hinduism). Without delving into the various definitions of culture, let us define culture as broadly as possible: as societies' material and mental activity, and its products.

In the broadly understood Euro-Atlantic civilization, there would be just a slight overlap between the two circles; this would certainly apply, for example, to France, the Netherlands, the Nordic countries, the Czech Republic, and the UK, where the Enlightenment legacy, and thus the philosophy of a secular state and the declining influence of institutional religion on people's daily lives, are uncontested actualities. The diagram representing the same relationship in Eastern and Central Europe, including Poland, but also in Greece, would look quite different: The overlap between the two circles would be significantly larger than in the previous version. In most countries in which Muslims constitute more than 80% of the population, the two circles – religion and culture – would almost completely overlap, even though there would be some regional differences, for example between Saudi Arabia and Tunisia. Buddhist countries would be closer to the second diagram, with the two circles overlapping to a larger extent than in the first example but far less than in the Islamic civilization. India would be located somewhere between the countries of the Buddhist and Muslim world: The overlap would take more than three quarters of both circles. We believe countries of East Asia (China, South Korea, and Vietnam) would be the best illustration of the intermediate variant, provided Confucianism is not defined as a religion.[1]

This way of representing the relationship between religion and culture is not a purely academic exercise. On the contrary, it has considerable practical implications that encompass message design concerning risk and its consequences. The relationship also affects rules of behaviour, which depend on how the recipients of messages perceive the world and interpret various phenomena. When culture is not, to any great degree, determined by religion (i.e., when there is tiny overlap between the two circles), the content of messages conveying key information does not need to refer to any metaphysical elements at all. In such circumstances, the drama of events and the measures taken are not elucidated by citing quotes from religious texts or their specific interpretations. If, however, culture is largely determined by the dominant religion (the two circles overlap to a great extent or almost completely), messages, especially those concerning human health and life, are designed differently. References to strictly religious concepts or the use of themes from a specific religion may be not only a necessary precondition for the effectiveness of future actions, but also an important explication of their meaning in a broader metaphysical context. If the ultimate goal is to reach the recipients and persuade them to engage in recommended behaviours, then explaining the meaning of these behaviours in a way acceptable to believers is a must.

We will not focus on differences within the European or, more broadly, Euro-Atlantic civilization, assuming these are better understood thanks to abundant media coverage. Instead, we will concentrate on two key regions of the world: the civilizations of Islam (about 1.8 billion believers) and Hinduism (1.1 billion believers), the world's third largest religion (Lipka, 2017; Hackett, 2017). Obviously, it is impossible to provide a detailed description of the entire geographical variety of responses on the part of Muslims and Hindus to the COVID-19 pandemic in a single chapter. Nonetheless, the selected examples may serve as illustrations of a more general phenomenon.

7.1 MUSLIMS AND THE PANDEMIC

The Islamic world is devoid of any single "headquarters" making decisions about faith and religious practices that would be binding for all believers, especially given that the majority of all Muslims, Sunnis, acknowledge different religious and legal authorities than the minority, Shias (or Shiites). All the same, there are institutions which are globally acknowledged, such as the Supreme

164 *Culture and Policy in Pandemics: Case Studies*

Ulema Council at the Al-Azhar University in Cairo, and some regional or national boards of Muslim scholars whose legal opinions on religious issues (fatwas) are commonly respected. For example, as early as in March 2020, the Supreme Council issued a fatwa banning collective prayers in mosques to prevent the spread of COVID-19. Detailed guidelines on how to behave in times of a health threat and explanations of these, based on Islamic law and the truths of Islamic faith, were developed by various Muslim organizations around the world, in dozens of languages. A prime example is the "Guidance on safe religious practice for Muslim communities during the coronavirus pandemic," developed by Islamic Relief Worldwide, one of the largest international humanitarian aid organizations, established by a group of Muslims in the UK. The specific guidelines on religious practices during the pandemic were developed in cooperation with the British Board of Scholars and Imams, after careful consideration of the legal opinions issued by Al-Ahzar. In practice, they can be followed by all Sunni Muslims, but they should also be known to healthcare professionals, state administration employees, and representatives of aid organizations who do not practice Islam but still work with Muslims. All the information about the activities, goals, and principles of the organization itself is published both in English and in Arabic (Islamic Relief Worldwide, 2020).

Notably, instead of the vague term "recommendations," used in European countries, the authors of the Guidance chose a much stronger word, "obligation," invoking legal opinions on Islamic law (fatwas) and the authority of the major schools of Islamic jurisprudence (*fiqh*). Information provided by the Guidance includes the religious grounds for closing mosques during the epidemic, the religiously justified obligation to self-isolate (*wajib*) if you have symptoms of COVID-19 or suspect you may have had contact with someone infected with the coronavirus, and the arrangement of traditional Islamic burial practices in ways ensuring the protection of the organizers and attendees. The authors of the Guidance emphasize that even though the pandemic and the related restrictions have greatly impacted the religious life of Muslims around the world (cancelled Friday prayers, closed madrasas, bans or severe restrictions on mass gatherings, etc.), all believers are obliged to fully comply with the measures and guidelines, issued both by government bodies and by religious institutions. Each point is supported by health-based justifications (the opinions of WHO and other health experts), social considerations (one's responsibility for the whole of the community's health), and strictly religious arguments, that is, quotes from the Hadith (reports of statements of Prophet Muhammad), which is the second main source of Islamic tradition after the Quran. More specifically:

- The ban on forwarding unconfirmed news reports about SARS-CoV-2 and the attendant disease, especially on social media, is supported by a quote from a hadith by Muslim ibn al-Hajjaj:

  Sufficient for a person to be considered a liar
  is that they spread news without confirming it.

- The obligation to come to the aid of the sick and those who have self-isolated, including spiritual and moral support via the phone, digital communication channels such as WhatsApp, and social networking sites, is backed up by a quote from the same source:

Allah assists His servants as long
as His servants are assisting their fellow man.

Additionally, the Guidance provides practical advice on, for example, using hand sanitizers containing alcohol, a substance that is considered religiously impure. The authors assure all devout Muslims that ritual ablutions before prayers will remove any impurity, including the effects of using an alcohol-based sanitizer. The appropriate sequence has to be maintained, though: the ritual wash of water should always follow sanitizing.

Detailed guidance is also provided on Muslim funerary rites, targeted both at imams, and at funeral workers and families of the deceased. The authors emphasize that cremation is forbidden in Islam as it is inconsistent with the special status bestowed by God upon all human beings (as they explain). Islam regards the human body as a gift (*amana*) from Allah, so any violation of bodily integrity, including cremation, is strictly forbidden (*haram*). At the same time, the authors realize that during the pandemic Muslims living in some non-Muslim countries may encounter this funeral practice, sometimes performed without any consent from the family of a COVID-19 victim. Should this happen, imams are advised to comfort family members by assuring them that they are not to blame and "that Allah can make the cremated body whole again for resurrection." This theological explication is supported by quotes from a hadith by Al-Bukhari and Muslim:

The one who dies in a plague …
dies as a martyr in the path of Allah.

The Guidance developed by Islamic Relief Worldwide, in partnership with an association of imams and Muslim scholars, provides practical, detailed sanitary advice combined with strictly religious arguments. There can be no doubt that the purpose of this publication, apart from the most obvious one, that is, promoting safe religious practices, is to provide spiritual and psychological support for believers. It stresses the role of community and emphasizes the strength of the Muslim community during a serious crisis, clarifying any concerns about non-standard measures (from the perspective of the Islamic tradition) based on selected quotes from the Hadith and the Quran.

In this context, it is worth citing an opinion by two female Saudi researchers: an Islamic scholar and a psychologist respectively, Nawal A. Al Eid and Boshra A. Arnout, who have interpreted the content of the Quran and hadiths in the context of the current pandemic. In their view, there is an "Islamic model of crisis management," based on appropriately organized teamwork (which is a moral obligation of the faith community), with a responsible leader playing a key role in the process. The authors emphasize the importance of a Muslim's positive attitude in the face of a crisis, which should arise from the right interpretation of Islamic teachings. "A Muslim must not view the crisis as all evil, as a negative view impedes proper thinking that facilitates the attainment of an appropriate solution" (Al Eid and Arnout, 2020). The authors cite Surah 24 of the Quran, which mentions the story of the flood and Noah (regarded as a prophet by Muslims), who was saved by God together with his companions, and Surah 9 (*The Repentance*), which describes Prophet Muhammad's struggles with natural hardships and enemies of the religious community. They conclude that Muslims have always had to face various hazards, which required them to develop a specific Islamic model of crisis management – one which can now be applied in times of pandemic.

The responses of Muslims around the world to COVID-19 lockdowns, and the phases of restrictions that followed are interesting to see. At the beginning of the pandemic, numerous conspiracy theories emerged about the origins of the virus, or even the alleged political motivations of donor countries (such as China or the US), which were offering medical aid to countries in more trying economic conditions. At that time, no accurate data was available on the scale of the pandemic or the number of cases and deaths, which certainly had an effect on people's trust in government and, as a consequence, on the perception of official messages. The vast majority of countries defined as Muslim (where far more than half of the population practice Islam) are classified by Freedom House as "not free" or "partly free," and their authoritarian or semi-authoritarian governments are thought to engage in censorship or manipulate information.[2] In Iran, hardest hit by the pandemic among Middle East countries, the government's initial responses were feeble and poorly coordinated. In March 2020, during the Nowruz holiday (or the Persian New Year), millions of Iranians travelled around the country (despite the pandemic-related restrictions imposed), contributing to the rapid spread of SARS-CoV-2, even despite the fact that in February 2020 a number of respected clerics died from COVID-19 in Qom, a Shia religious centre. The officially reported numbers of infections and deaths were soon questioned by foreign observers and mistrusted by Iranians themselves.[3] At the same time, Iranian officials, including the country's Health Minister Saeed Namaki, complained about the lack of social discipline (failure to wear masks, insufficient social distancing in public places) in the face of risks to citizens' life and health (Takeyh, 2020).

Iran is officially an Islamic Republic, which means that religion plays a crucial role in the nation's social and political life. The Shia clergy work closely with the government, even though many clerics do not fully support official policy.[4] The pandemic required radical and previously unseen measures. Ayatollah Hossein Mousavi Tabrizi, professor at the prestigious Qom Seminary and secretary of the Assembly of Qom Seminary Scholars and Researchers, together with numerous other respected clerics, for the first time in the country's history accepted the closure of shrines, seminaries, mosques, and the cancellation of Friday prayers. According to analysts, it was the clergy's cooperation with the government and the immediate acceptance of the closure of places of worship that helped to subdue, at least partly, the spread of the coronavirus in Iran, which could otherwise have reached catastrophic levels (Bozorgmehr, 2020). "Under the Islamic decrees, protecting your life and saving others is the most important religious duty for which you can stop carrying out an obligation like daily prayers, or commit a forbidden act such as a man touching a naked woman if she is drowning," explained Hossein Mousavi Tabrizi to justify the Shia clergy's decision. He added that some senior clerics may not want to go online, while others are open to exploring online teaching in order to stay in touch with their students. "If the second wave comes, I may consider holding online classes, despite my feelings of isolation. In today's world, social distancing does not mean you cut off all your communications" (Bozorgmehr, 2020). It should be emphasized that such decisions and their justifications constitute an important precedent in the history of Shia Islam.

Of course, not all Muslims around the world are willing to strictly comply with pandemic-related bans and requirements. In most Islamic countries, governments, supported by religious leaders, closed or significantly reduced access to mosques, a measure which was generally accepted by their societies. In some places, however, local religious leaders refused to acknowledge government decisions, even though the authorities invoked the unequivocal fatwa issued by the Supreme Ulema Council at the Al-Azhar University in Cairo. These leaders regarded the prolonged restrictions on religious schools and mosques as attempts to undermine their authority and status in the society. Pakistan's government, headed by Prime Minister Imran Khan, yielded to pressure from religious leaders, led by Hanif Jalandhari – one of Pakistan's most influential Muslim leaders, general secretary of a federation controlling more than 10,000 seminaries and 23,000 madrasas – and lifted restrictions on traditional religious and educational practices at the end of April 2020, a move which was heavily criticized by the medical community.[5] As a result, the daily number of new cases began to grow exponentially (Hashim, 2020). Ahsan Butt explains why Pakistan is a unique case: "It's a state built on [the idea of] Muslim nationalism, so Islam and Muslim identity are crucial to the state and the wider society, and the conception of the collective self" (Hashim, 2020). Muslim leaders and institutions have great influence and social power but are not explicitly a part of the state, unlike in Saudi Arabia, where religious leaders are integrally linked to political authority. Even the military, which plays a central role in Pakistan, has been clearly theocratic at least since the late 1970s, and has to take account of common religious sentiments. Hence, in contrast to the Pakistani setting, Saudi Arabia was able to control its religious institutions during the coronavirus outbreak, shutting down or restricting people's access to places of worship, including Islam's holiest site, the Kaaba. The difference between the countries is also related to the fact that Pakistan's political system meets some minimum democratic standards and, unlike the Saud dynasty, the government's mandate is granted through general elections. In addition, religious leaders in each province have

168 *Culture and Policy in Pandemics: Case Studies*

considerable autonomy and enjoy a high social status, a state of affairs which would be hardly imaginable in fully authoritarian countries. In Pakistan, however, this may (or may not) have a negative effect on social discipline during the pandemic, at a point when temporary restrictions on religious practices are necessary for curtailing the spread of SARS-CoV-2.

The meaning of the pandemic is completely different for supporters of radical Islam, which is often hostile to many governments. Pierre Boussel notes how the Islamic State (IS) designs messages to its supporters. In IS communications, the current health crisis is just another chapter in the history of war against enemies of Islam, and the fight is compared to the original clash of Prophet Mohammad and the first Muslim community with their opponents in Mecca in the 7th century (Boussel, 2020). Thus, the current set of circumstances are nothing but a novel version of the eternal battle between good and evil. The Islamic State's official newsletter, *Al-Naba*, instructs the following: "Muslims should not pity the disbelievers and apostates, but should use the current opportunities to continue working to free Muslim prisoners from the camps in which they face subjugation and disease, and should intensify the pressure on them however they can. They should also remember that obedience to God – the most beloved form of which is jihad – turns away the torment and wrath of God" (i.e., performing jihad is the best guarantee of protecting yourself from the epidemic) (Al-Tamimi, 2020). It is emphasized that the pandemic is "the wrath of God" and "the worst nightmare of the Crusaders," a statement which may be understood as a call for more radical or even criminal actions. The communist government in Beijing plays a sinister role in the Islamic State's extremist propaganda whereby the Chinese origins of the virus are presented as punishment for the persecution of Uighur Muslims in the province of Xinjiang.

Meanwhile, Aboubakar Shekau, the leader of West Africa's Boko Haram militia group linked to the IS, officially thanked God for the pandemic that was weakening "the reign of Trump," and forbade his militants to conform to sanitary rules, claiming that true believers were immune to the virus (Boussel, 2020). Radical propaganda focuses on the idea that the epidemic is "a message from God," designed to strengthen Muslims' faith and to oppress both unbelievers and "those Muslims who have diverted from true Islam." The mass graves of COVID-19 victims on New York City's Hart Island were depicted as the ultimate proof of America's barbarity and the weakness of the United States. It was never mentioned, of course, that Hart Island had an over 150-year-long history as a graveyard for New Yorkers during epidemics when bodies were not claimed by family members.

Emphasizing the huge differences in wealth among victims of the global pandemic is a significant ideological element of radical propaganda. SARS-CoV-2 is depicted as the virus of wealthy countries, seen to be disbursing billions of dollars to save their economies, even though no money was expended by the same countries to support the fight against Ebola, seen as the virus of poverty-stricken countries (Boussel, 2020). Initially, such allegations may have been convincing even to moderate Muslims, who are far from accepting the IS or Al-Qaida's ideologies. However, the rapid spread of the pandemic in poor countries, such as Bangladesh or Pakistan, has certainly undermined those claims. Still, new interpretations of the social aspect of COVID-19 may well contribute to designing similar propaganda messages in the future.

It should be emphasized that all these conspiracy theories and extreme interpretations of events are not merely an end in themselves, but rather are employed to recruit new volunteers from around the world, especially those who cannot accept the injustice (as they perceive it) existing in current North–South relations. These messages provide ideological fuel for potential volunteers and justify their possible sacrifices in the future. Clearly, today neither the Islamic State nor al-Qaida (or rather its remaining fragmented structures) have the same power they had in past times. In the foreseeable future, these entities are also unlikely to be able to build a strong regional organization that would threaten the stability of the entire Greater Middle East and South Asia. That being said, during a pandemic, people tend to ask themselves existential and ideological questions, which help to build prospective recruitment networks, so it is hard to predict what consequences this global crisis may have in the future.

Not all radical groups share the same view on the principles regulating people's behaviour during the pandemic. Various versions of the standard conspiracy theories may go hand in hand with measures recommended by the WHO. The Taliban in Afghanistan may see the coronavirus as "punishment from God" or "a sign from God," but this is where the similarity to radicals from the Islamic State or Boko Haram ends. According to analyses by Roshni Kapur and Chayaniki Saxena: "The Taliban has made moves to assist both domestic and international efforts to limit the spread of the virus in areas under its control" (Kapur and Saxena, 2020). According to the two researchers from the National University of Singapore, the Taliban responded promptly to the risks posed by the pandemic, implementing a seven-step plan:

- they declared a ceasefire in their controlled areas;
- they conducted workshops for local residents to raise their awareness of the need to use gloves and face masks, wash hands with soap, and practise social distancing;
- they distributed medical equipment, including surgical masks and protective gloves, as well as brochures on health precautions and COVID-19 prevention;
- they set up quarantine centres to isolate those suspected of carrying the virus and residents coming from other provinces;
- they cancelled public (including religious) events, and instructed people to pray at home instead of visiting mosques;
- they employed the available technology and communication tools (such as WhatsApp) to inform local residents about where and when government health officials would be distributing soap and face masks; and
- they lifted the ban on World Health Organization (WHO) and Red Cross activity in areas under their control, and guaranteed the security of aid and health workers providing assistance in those territories.

170   *Culture and Policy in Pandemics: Case Studies*

Thus, not only did the Taliban go along with the pandemic-related sanitary measures, they also established institutional cooperation with the WHO and other international organizations to provide more effective help for local residents, a policy that was officially declared on Twitter on March 16, 2020, by the Taliban's spokesman Suhail Shaheen.[6] This is a rather surprising turn of events, in view of the fact that foreign aid workers were previously treated as Western spies, were not allowed to work freely, and had even been physically attacked. Ironically, the Taliban themselves did not follow the pandemic-related restrictions, which led to a wave of infections and deaths among their top leadership (O'Donnell and Khan, 2020). Apart from its apparent intention to protect the local populace, this type of behaviour may result from a simple political calculation. At the time, the Taliban controlled large swathes of the country, fighting against the government in Kabul. Now that they have taken full control of Afghanistan, their decisions on sanitary rules are perceived as actions taken by responsible political players, whose concern about local residents can easily fit into selected interpretations of Islam. By contrast, radical groups such as IS or al-Qaida have little chance of seizing stable, widely accepted power, and this is what allows them to promote extremist ideologies and ignore universal sanitary rules for which they have minimal or no responsibility.

Today's Islamic world is so politically, linguistically, and culturally diverse that we cannot really talk about a single unified policy against the pandemic. Let us emphasize, however, one important aspect, which seems to be common to all Muslim authorities (barring extremist organizations): The imposed or recommended sanitary rules may be practically identical to other parts of the world, but their justifications and explanations are firmly grounded in Islam. In other words, hygiene and human health or life cannot be considered in isolation from faith, and from all its implications.

7.2 THE COVID-19 PANDEMIC AND HINDUISM: SELECTED EXAMPLES

A similar argument about hygiene and human health and life being closely linked to religion applies to Hinduism. This religion does not have a single doctrine shared by all believers, but rather could be figuratively described as being like many different rivers flowing into one ocean. There is an intellectually sophisticated and philosophically elaborate version of Hinduism, but in everyday life, a popular or folk version is applied, filled with rich mythological iconography (Kłodkowski, 2015). Vivid representations of Hindu gods can be seen both in temples across the country and in home shrines. More or less complicated religious rituals constitute an integral, ubiquitous part of human existence in India, give meaning to people's lives, and, frequently, ensure a healthy balance between the individual and the communal. On the other hand, mythological images help to represent the complex truths of faith to those who are less adept at philosophical speculations, or even those who feel comfortable at both levels of religious experience. Needless to say, during a crisis, these rituals and complex mythology play a special role, both individually and socially (Tharoor, 2018).

One interesting example in the context of COVID-19 is the use of female deities, for centuries associated with diseases and epidemics that plagued India. These goddesses, popular especially in the folk version of Hinduism, were supposed to protect believers from dangerous diseases, and their temples were built all over the country. Their images did not necessarily reflect a nurturing mother goddess; instead, they were depicted as formidable figures with multiple arms, ready to protect people from pestilence but also to punish them with disease for their faults. During a fatal epidemic they were offered animal sacrifices, while convalescents engaged in different forms of mortification. The most popular goddess in South India is Mariamman (in Tamil *Mari* means "rain," and *Amman*, "mother"), depicted with a curved sword for killing the demons of diseases and epidemics. In the North, people worship Shitala (which literally means "one who cools" in Sanskrit, that is, one who cures fever), a goddess holding a pot full of healing water, a broom to dust off dirt, a twig of a neem tree (*Asadirachta indica*) – an alleged cure for skin diseases and respiratory distress – and a jug of amrita, the elixir of immortality.

Tulasi Srinivas provides interesting examples of how images of deities have been used in wide-reaching awareness-raising campaigns on disease prevention. On World AIDS Day in 1997, an image of a new goddess was introduced, AIDSAmma, resembling Mariamman, of course, and drawing on the latter's popularity. This artistic and religious project was not intended to generate the divine power to cure the disease, but rather to present measures to prevent AIDS. The narrative around the new image of an old goddess was designed to effectively get through to worshipers strongly attached to the centuries-old tradition (Srinivas, 2020). During the COVID-19 pandemic, which has devastated India as one of its most tragic victims, an artist, Sandhya Kumari, presented her rendering of Mother-India (Bhārat Mātā/Maa Bharati) fighting against the coronavirus. It is a combination of a largely secular image of the motherland India and an image of the Hindu goddess Durga or Kali (another embodiment of the Mother Goddess) killing the virus-demon with a divine trident. She wears a mask on her face and gloves on all five pairs of hands, and holds a stethoscope, a syringe, and a first aid kit. A caption under the image says: "Bhārat Mātā will end the virus, but it is every Indian's duty to stay at home and follow the [sanitary] rules. Jai Hind! [Long live India or Hail India]." Its message is clear not only to Hindus; the complete artwork, published on social media, captured people's attention across India and abroad. The novelty of the work lies in the combination of strictly religious and nationalist themes, as the new goddess is wearing the colours of the Indian flag: orange, white, and green (Srinivas, 2020). Thus, the cultural code proposed by the artist has a chance to cross religious barriers. Despite this novel design, it is hard to say if it is going to be enthusiastically welcomed by followers of other religions, for example Muslims or Christians. Understanding a message is not equivalent necessarily to accepting its content, especially if it is embedded in another religion.

There are many different renditions of the goddess Durga fighting with the coronavirus. One intriguing example is an image depicting her in a lab coat (as a doctor goddess), wearing a face mask, with medical instruments in two of her hands and a trident in the other two, using the trident to pierce a virus-shaped demon.[7] The message for believers seems clear, although two different interpretations are possible. According to the first, Durga's actions are beneficial to her worshipers, as a doctor's actions would help their patients. The other interpretation that may be drawn, however, is that a doctor or a nurse acts like the goddess Durga herself, slaying the virus, represented as a mythical demon. The latter interpretation may be particularly significant given the reports about outbreaks of violent behaviour toward health professionals who are highly exposed to infection and, as a result, suspected of spreading the disease in their neighbourhoods (Pandey, 2020).

Restrictions affecting the organization of religious festivals and the frequency of visiting temples have made the pandemic a part of a new narrative. Warnings and orders to follow the sanitary procedures are now integrated into temple decorations, and a goddess statue (for example, in Kolkata) may wear a face mask, which has become a common artistic and educational practice. Such religious and artistic creativity in response to the pandemic risk is widely accepted among Hindus, which arises from an assumption that "God is present in different ways in the created word," and from a belief in numerous divine incarnations (avatars), whose stories are recounted in canonical texts. From this perspective, the coronavirus is not completely new, simply the latest incarnation of familiar misfortunes that have plagued humans, and depicting it as another adversary of a worshipped goddess serves to integrate the pandemic phenomenon into the familiar mythological paradigm. This, in turn, helps to adapt to new challenges and gradually reduces the fear of the unknown. As an extreme example of such incorporation, Indian confectioneries even go so far as to sell coronavirus-shaped candies and cookies.

The pandemic has also forced significant changes in religious customs. An illustrative example is one of India's grandest festivals celebrating the elephant-headed deity Ganesh, the god of wisdom and prosperity. In Mumbai, India's most populous metropolis with more than 20 million residents, a huge festival is held every year, during which devotees immerse idols of Ganesh in the waters of the Arabian Sea. Clearly, during the coronavirus pandemic, mass gatherings of this type would explode into superspreader events, so an alternative form of the celebration was proposed and accepted by Hindu priests and believers. Special mobile tanks full of sea water were mounted on decorated trucks and carried to each municipal ward, so that devotees could perform the traditional ritual. What is particularly fascinating in this example is that, instead of imposing an absolute ban on religious activities, which could dishearten devotees and lead to apathy or even aggression, creative religious and cultural substitutes were sought, which helped to sustain the idea of social cooperation and respect for millions of followers of Hinduism (Frayer and Pathak, 2020).

Be that as it may, we cannot ignore the fact that the pandemic crisis has also contributed to increased inter-religious tensions in India. Discrimination against Muslims by the Hindu majority has grown significantly since 2015 (Kłodkowski, 2019), and COVID-19 has expanded the areas of conflict. Already in April 2020, the Secretary General of the Organization of Islamic Cooperation voiced his deep concern caused by media reports about India's rising anti-Muslim sentiments and islamophobia, both in political circles and in the media, and protested against any condemnation of the Muslim minority for the spread of the coronavirus.[8] One pretext for these negative attitudes was a massive religious congregation organized in Delhi in March 2020 by Tablighti Jamaat, a transnational Muslim missionary organization, which turned out to be a COVID-19 superspreader event. Noticeably, examples of similar behaviours among other religious communities were not as highly publicized by traditional and social media. Asim Ali offers an emblematic example of "pandemic discrimination" in Kolya, a village in India's state of Karnataka. Here, posters were put up at the entrance to the village saying: "No Muslim trader is allowed into the village till the coronavirus has completely gone away. Signed: All Hindus, Kolya" (Ali, 2020). No data is available on the numbers of COVID-19 infections by religion (no such research has been conducted), so it would be difficult to support the claim that SARS-CoV-2 transmission is higher (or lower) in one religious group than in others. Publishing such data, however, would probably have catastrophic social consequences, leading to even greater conflict between Hindus and Muslims (Menon, 2020).

Nearly a year after the COVID-19 outbreak, India appeared to be in control of the pandemic and be in a position to curb its spread across the country. In January and February 2021, the daily number of confirmed cases oscillated between 10,000 and 15,000, but started surging in the latter half of March, exceeding 400,000 toward the end of April, which made India among one of the most affected countries in the world. The dramatic deterioration was also reflected in the number of COVID-19 deaths; as early as May more than 200,000 coronavirus deaths were reported, in total.[9] There were certainly several causes contributing to the sharp rise in the pandemic wave in India, but a major factor was definitely Kumbh Mela – a Hindu festival attended by millions of devout pilgrims. Probably the world's largest religious gathering, Kumbh Mela is celebrated in a cycle of 12 years, switching between four different pilgrimage sites.[10] The 2021 festival was to be held in Haridwar, by the sacred river Ganges, and was scheduled to begin in mid-January and finish at the end of April. Attempts to limit the number of pilgrims, to shorten the festival, and to impose strict sanitary rules did not have much tangible effect. Sanitary discipline could not be effectively maintained in the huge crowd of pilgrims.[11] Between January and April 2021 more than 9 million pilgrims arrived in Haridwar to immerse their bodies in the waters of the Ganges, with the largest number, about 6 million, coming in April, which coincided with

174 *Culture and Policy in Pandemics: Case Studies*

a dramatic growth in infections. In Haridwar itself, and later in the entire Uttarakhand state, the number of infections and deaths grew vertiginously.

The Indian example shows that by adopting proven principles of communication, messages conveying the risk of virus spread to the local culture can be highly effective. Nevertheless, for millions of believers the need for a religious experience, in this case, the desire to take part in the Kumbh Mela pilgrimage, is stronger than the fear of any pandemic risks officially announced by the government. Even though this observation is not true for all Hindus, of course, it is still a clear case of how culture and religion regulate human behaviour.

7.3 CONCLUDING REMARKS

Differences in communication do not mean that different cultures function as "closed monads" and that appropriate low-context messages from Europe or America should always, with no exceptions, be adjusted to the cultural environments of their recipients, especially high-context ones in Asia and the Middle East. Kishore Mahbubani identified seven "pillars of Western wisdom" that he believes have been adopted by many Asian cultures and adjusted to the local conditions. The list includes meritocracy, modern science and technology, pragmatism, and the rule of law, which have all engendered swift economic development and significant social modernization (Mahbubani, 2008). Mahbubani focuses primarily on countries of East and South East Asia, but these Western values have also diffused across other regions of the Asian continent and, at least to some extent, the Middle East and North Africa. The universal language of science, used to communicate the pandemic-related risks and the recommended precautions, would now be easily understood by experts and most educated members of the middle class throughout Asia. Nearly identical explanations of COVID-19 and its treatments are provided in official pronouncements in EU countries, Pakistan, South Korea, or Thailand. However, both the prolonged pandemic and the constantly growing numbers of infections and deaths raise questions that go beyond the domain of science and often touch on metaphysical issues. From this perspective, guidelines on everyday sanitary procedures can be seen as a "user manual" or technical instructions, whereas the religious narrative explains the deeper meaning of the measures, motivating believers to earnestly comply with the bans and requirements. This may be true both for uneducated people and for highly successful members of the middle class. This has already been well outlined by the above examples from Islam and Hinduism.

Finally, let us emphasize that reducing virus spread during a pandemic requires conformity to social norms that are strongly related to social and political identification. Unfortunately, about 1.8 billion people, that is, 26% of the world's population, live in fragile states, characterized not only by weak state institutions but also by low levels of legitimacy vis-à-vis their political authorities and social capital (Fund For Peace, 2019). Under these circumstances, it is not easy to utilize the potential of local residents to set up effective anti-pandemic strategies, when, all the while, strong feelings of anxiety, augmented by the weakness of the state, may easily trigger violent intergroup conflicts, which in turn increases migration pressure and, as a consequence, enables the virus to transmit itself uncontrollably to other regions of the world. These phenomena had already been remarked upon in 2014 during the Ebola epidemic in Guinea, Liberia, and Sierra Leone. At that time, the International Crisis Group reported that "the virus initially spread unchecked not only because of the weakness of epidemiological monitoring and inadequate health system capacity and response, but also because people were skeptical of what their governments were saying or asking them to do" (Crisis Group Africa Report N° 232, 2015).

In unstable states, communicating risk is extremely problematic and associated with the increased danger of producing mass panic responses or unchecked aggression. In the face of such challenges, responses from world leaders become absolutely vital. During a pandemic, the temptation to focus on their own backyard and stop or limit humanitarian aid, peace operations, and diplomatic initiatives may become overwhelming. At lower levels of government, unscrupulous local politicians can use a pandemic to their own ends, which will exacerbate internal or international crises and, at the same time, hinder health-promoting responses.

The COVID-19 pandemic, which hit equally hard across continents and cultures, confronted politicians and scientists alike with the challenge of communicating risk and informing the public about the strategies for battling the virus. Even though the disease itself and the fear of it have become universal, effective prevention seems to depend on the careful consideration of the context of people's behaviours and the specific local conditions, defined primarily by culture and religion. Therefore, a pandemic, which is by definition global and rapidly evolving, poses a special communication challenge. It requires an understanding of what is universal or common to all cultures, and, conversely, what is different and specific for each culture. Adopting both the universalist and intercultural perspectives will help develop guidelines that have a chance of being as effective as we all wish them to be.

Notes

1 As regards research on the relationship between belief in God and morality (i.e., on whether belief in God is seen as necessary to be moral in different cultures), the Global God Divide survey by the Pew Research Center (July 2020) found that the proportion of people supporting this relationship was the smallest in Western Europe: 15% in France, 9% in Sweden, and 22% in the Netherlands. Among post-communist countries, it was 50% in Ukraine and Bulgaria, 37% in Russia, 36% in Poland, and 45% in Slovakia, but only 14% in the Czech Republic. An outlier is Greece, which has a large number of residents supporting this link – 53%. By way of contrast, in selected Muslim countries – Indonesia, Turkey, and Tunisia – the proportions were 96%, 75%, and 84% respectively. Among Japanese and Korean Buddhists, it was 53% and 51% respectively.

One should bear in mind, of course, that Buddhists do not hold a belief in a personal god, so in their case, the relationship is more between metaphysical teachings and morality (Pew Research Center, 2020).

2 For example, countries such as Saudi Arabia, Afghanistan, Bahrain, Brunei, Egypt, Iran, Libya, Oman, Turkey, and Yemen are classified as "not free" by Freedom House, whereas Morocco, Bangladesh, and Pakistan are "partly free." In turn, Tunisia has been classified as "free," (Freedom House, 2020).

3 According to BBC Persia (*Coronavirus: Iran cover-up of deaths revealed by data leak*), the number of coronavirus deaths in Iran as of July 20, 2020, was three times higher than officially claimed by the Ministry of Health (42,000 and 14,405 respectively), whereas the number of people known to be infected was twice as high as official figures (451,024 and 278,827 respectively). The actual numbers of deaths and infected people were included in official government records (which were informally passed to BBC Persia) but were concealed from the public (BBC, 2020).

4 In today's Shia Islam, which dominates in Iran, one can talk about the clergy as a social class, distinguished from the rest of the society by their theological education, social status, hierarchy of titles, and even their clothes. The terms "clergy" and "clerics" are used here only with reference to Shia Islam.

5 Wifaq ul Madaris Al-Arabia is the largest federation of Islamic seminaries and madrasas in Pakistan, founded in 1959. It has its own autonomous curriculum, and is, in fact, unsupervised by the state.

6 https://twitter.com/suhailshaheen1/status/1239594471576256512.

7 A copy of the image is available on social media: https://www.dreamstime.com/print-image183264960 (accessed on September 29, 2020).

8 https://www.oic-oci.org/topic/?t_id=23342&t_ref=13984&lan=en (accessed on September 24, 2020).

9 All the data comes from COVID-19 Data Repository by the Center for Systems Science and Engineering (CSSE) at Johns Hopkins University, https://github.com/CSSEGISandData/COVID-19 (accessed on May 2, 2021).

10 The dates of Kumbh Mela celebrations are calculated based on the astrological positions of Jupiter, the sun, and the moon. The 12-year cycle applies to each pilgrimage site separately, which means, for example, that the celebration in Prayag (Allahabad) takes place three years after the Haridwar festival, and three years before the Ujjain and Nashik celebrations. In 2021, Kumbh Mela was to be celebrated in Haridwar.

11 Source: Hindustan Times. (2021). 9.1 million thronged Mahakumbh despite Covid-19 surge. (April 30). Govt data, https://www.hindustantimes.com/cities/dehradun-news/91-million-thronged-mahakumbh-despite-covid-19-surge-govt-data-101619729096750.html (accessed on May 1, 2021).

8 PUBLIC POLICY RESPONSES TO THE PANDEMIC
A COMPARATIVE PERSPECTIVE

Jarosław Górniak, Seweryn Krupnik,
and Maciej Koniewski

8.1 INTRODUCTION

Evidence-based or (less radically) *evidence-informed* public policy is postulated as the gold standard in the 21st century. The achievements of evidence-based medicine attest to the value of gaining a clear understanding of the causal mechanisms of relevant phenomena before applying any treatment. They also teach us that conclusions based on superficially observed relationships can be very deceptive and that we should always build on the solid foundations of the scientific method when collecting knowledge to inform decision-making processes.

In medicine, meeting the quality of evidence requirements is not easy, but when it comes to public policies, even greater difficulties pile up at every turn, as the public policy process involves making decisions that pertain to a large number of people. These decisions should be based on accurate assessments, including a good understanding of the decision-making processes and behaviours of those affected. In theory, they should be easier to make given policymakers' competence and better access to evidence. In practice, however, the call for public policy decisions to be evidence-based encounters several hurdles.

One of the most substantial challenges is the availability of evidence needed for decision making. Policymakers often put in requests for conclusions and recommendations that are needed in short order, whereas scientific procedures involve a lengthy process of collecting data and obtaining data from numerous studies. Another challenge involves the quality of data and the ability to evaluate the information gathered. Scientists and policymakers use different criteria for what can be regarded as "good enough" data and evidence. For example, anecdotal evidence is commonly used in policymakers' arguments but has little to no value for scientists.

Purely methodological challenges are also significant. When studying social processes, it is not easy to use controlled experiments and, at the same time, ensure high ecological validity, that is, high consistency between the effects obtained in a study and those occurring in real-life settings. Yet another hindrance is the shortage of in-depth, theory-informed evaluations of

DOI: 10.4324/9781003254133-11

public policies, which would provide a basis for repeating effective patterns of action and eliminating ineffective ones. However, issues with the quality and validity of scientific evidence are not the only obstacles to evidence-based policy making. Every public policy involves pure politics, and they are influenced by games of interests, power struggles, and strong ideological beliefs. Furthermore, the scale and range of public policies, as well as their complexity, usually exceed the level of social science findings.

Public policy decisions take account of values, interests, and beliefs. So how do findings from social and behavioural sciences fit within such decision making? We are talking here about evidence from causal, theoretically founded, and methodologically rigorous research. In social science, there are numerous normative, conceptual, and interpretation-oriented trends that contribute to the discourse about important aspects of political decisions. These are not to be overlooked or dismissed lightly. For the record, however, it is worth differentiating between the two approaches. In this context, let us repeat the question about the purpose of using scientific knowledge in public policy making. Despite the abovementioned limitations, we see its role as providing all the actors involved in policy making – public authorities, programme implementers, citizens, and external observers – with the best available knowledge about how the social world works, what makes people tick, and what influences their choices. This helps to improve the evaluation of the costs and benefits of each decision and to incorporate meaningful arguments into debates defined by differences in beliefs. This in turn may assist in laying a rational foundation for conflict resolution, enabling the parties to negotiate reasonable compromises without losing their ideological identity. This modest ambition inspired our work on the current review of behavioural and social science evidence.

The COVID-19 pandemic requires public authorities to act under uncertainty and to balance the disease-related risks to people's life and health with the consequences of restrictions imposed on social and economic life. Until effective drugs and a vaccine are widely available, both types of risks can be reduced by allowing the economy to function as freely as possible while maintaining a high level of social self-discipline in adhering to sanitary rules, supported by a selective use of necessary positive and negative stimuli. In recent times, we have experienced two markedly different stages in handling the COVID-19 epidemic.

Stage one, which began in mid-March and peaked in April 2020, after a short initial period of doubt and disbelief, was characterized by major restrictions on movement and social life as well as the closure of places that involve direct contact among large numbers of people (such as stores, churches, cultural institutions, schools, hotels, etc.), combined with a very high level of social self-discipline. In fact, there were very few rule violations, given the scale of restrictions and the number of those affected.

Stage two, coming out of lockdown, has been in progress since the end of May 2020, when governments announced step-by-step plans to reopen the economy and lift the restrictions. During stage two, the removal of formal restrictions was soon accompanied by a widespread decline in social self-discipline. Even when the number of cases started to grow again, self-discipline never returned to the levels observed during stage one.

Today, when the work on this chapter is coming to an end (October 2020), many countries have reported a new surge in infection numbers. Once again, their governments have to balance (i) the challenges related to the risks to people's life and health caused by the spread of the disease and to the consequences of restrictions imposed on social life with (ii) economic life. The coronavirus pandemic may stretch out to one or two more years, or even longer, depending on whether and when a truly effective vaccine or drug is developed and distributed worldwide. It is still uncertain whether herd immunity can be achieved against COVID-19. At the same time, the economy and administration ought to operate as normally as possible because the losses and risks (including risks to people's life and health) resulting from long-term social and economic lockdown may well be much more severe than the immediate health consequences of the pandemic. Public policies, including various pandemic-related regulations, should facilitate adaptation to a potentially prolonged pandemic. Such steps are already being taken. Specific solutions within the regulatory framework for the economy, the labour code, or public administration are beyond the scope of this publication. The review of social-behavioural research, discussed earlier in this book, focuses on the potential to influence people's behaviours in order to reduce the spread of the virus. Appropriate steps in this area are an essential component of a comprehensive policy response to COVID-19. Grappling with and persevering through a prolonged pandemic requires a combination of measures that enable efficient functioning of the economy and the state, not to mention the self-discipline of the citizenry in following sanitary rules and preventing the spread of the virus. While sophisticated public policies are needed in both areas, our discussion here will focus on the latter.

The outbreak of the SARS-CoV-2 pandemic posed a huge challenge to public authorities in countries around the world. The initial period of the fight against COVID-19 has already demonstrated the importance of having not only a solid research base with the capacity to develop tests, treatments, and vaccines in a sufficiently short time, but also a high-quality base for analyzing public policies.

The functions of public policy analysis include (Bardach and Patashnik, 2019):

- fast and accurate assessment of a problem and its causal mechanisms;
- initiating appropriate research processes and integrating the available knowledge about the nature, dynamics, and consequences of the problem;
- generating alternative solutions (variants);
- evaluating the potential effects of each variant, its costs and benefits;

180   *Culture and Policy in Pandemics: Case Studies*

- developing recommendations for policy makers;
- developing a plan for implementing the selected solution;
- evaluating the implementation processes and policy effects; and
- building a base of knowledge about intervention effectiveness and efficiency.

Public policy analysis centres should work closely with policy makers and, at the same time, systematically cooperate with scientists and experts, be able to mobilize them rapidly, and work with them productively in emergency situations, such as COVID-19. To this end, it is important to create working relationships, work out principles of cooperation, and develop databases of experts. In many countries, components of such relationships are present but there is no elaborate, integrated, and functional system. One consequence of the lack of such systemic solutions is the limited utilization of knowledge generated through the evaluation of public programmes and policies in decision-making processes. Another problem is the insufficient range and quality of data necessary for proper decision making. One of the key public policy dimensions is the ability to implement solutions. Public policies affect individuals included in numerous social groups and networks. Therefore, it is necessary to systematically glean evidence from social-behavioural research and transform it into a format useful in public policy design. This publication is a minor step toward this goal. Ideally, it could become a starting point for the systematic process of building a knowledge base for public policy making, inspired by decision makers' need for information.

8.2 INTERVENTIONS DESIGNED TO STOP THE PANDEMIC

Public intervention planning is always based on a number of assumptions, including ones about the behaviours of the people who will be affected by the intervention. These assumptions are given a reality-check during their implementation, which makes them similar to research hypotheses. Planning and reporting the results of hypothesis testing is central to all research endeavour. When it comes to public interventions, evaluation should play the same role.

These assumptions can be described on two dimensions. First, they can be broken into different aspects or components, such as the context, the target group, barriers, actions, and outcomes. Second, we can identify interventions based on a similar set of assumptions. A detailed review of classifications is provided in Olejniczak et al. (2020). In this chapter, we use Soman's (2017) classification, which includes the following categories: equipping people with resources that enable appropriate behaviour; banning undesired behaviour; and informing and encouraging people to promote the expected behaviour. Each intervention category is based on a different set of assumptions, which can then be linked to different sciences and practices: in this case, economic, legal, and marketing practices respectively.

When it comes to interventions designed to halt the pandemic, actions are planned and implemented in various contexts. These comprise demographic characteristics (population age structure, population density), geographic factors (temperature, humidity, insular location), economic and social factors (trust in public institutions, the level of civil society development), and political factors (the quality of leadership, elections), as well as the current pandemic situation around the world and in the country in question. Added to this is the country's potential to manage the pandemic. Table 8.1 describes interventions in terms of the remaining categories.

Providing appropriate resources for services engaged in the fight against the pandemic was one of the simplest and most publicized interventions (given such resources were available). In parallel to the state's responses, several private and civil-society interventions were initiated in many countries in order to better equip health services. Resources were also redirected to other areas. For example, public institutions responsible for funding research and development programmes mobilized special funds for the fight against the pandemic and its consequences. When resources were scarce, decision makers faced particularly thorny dilemmas about how they should be allocated (Emanuel et al., 2020).

Restrictions on movement and social contact were the most inconvenient measures in the eyes of citizens, and, at the same time, have a documented effect on containing the pandemic (Flaxman et al., 2020). Support for these measures varied across countries (Sabat et al., 2020). Given their high economic and social cost, states gradually eased such restrictions during stage two of the pandemic, and when the second wave began, they often reimposed bans with quite a delay.

Compared to other public policy areas, informing citizens effectively became particularly important during the pandemic. The outcomes of this intervention category are more difficult to measure than the other two. At the same time, the preceding chapters of this book have clearly demonstrated that the importance of appropriate communication efforts, informing the public both about the pandemic and about any government responses, can hardly be overestimated. Based on the research findings presented in this book, a number of recommendations can be offered to those responsible for designing such interventions (Box 8.1). These recommendations can increase people's motivation to engage in self-control and take precautions to reduce the risk of infection as well as strengthen their willingness to get vaccinated (when vaccines are available). They may also increase social control over relevant individual behaviours. Many of them constitute guidelines concerning the content of messages and how to communicate them to citizens. Notably, information is conveyed not only by intentional

Table 8.1 Different intervention categories and the related assumptions about target groups' behaviours.

Target group	Barriers	Interventions	Outcomes
		Equipping	
Primarily healthcare professionals, but also uniformed services and researchers.	Lack of resources (financial, human, technological, or know-how).	Providing resources, guidelines, and action plans. Specific actions: - supplying funds and equipment for healthcare facilities; creating additional, temporary hospitals; - resources for healthcare professionals, including Personal Protective Equipment (PPE); - extending decision makers' prerogatives (e.g., at the local level); - issuing guidelines for various categories of citizens and institutions (e.g., healthcare facilities, public services, schools, restaurants); - providing resources for a range of institutions (e.g., sanitizers, soap for schools); - providing easier access to health services (e.g., electronic prescriptions, telehealth); - developing infrastructure related to SARS-CoV-2 testing; - providing resources for services responsible for enforcing COVID-19 restrictions; - offering funds for research; - increasing the availability of flu and pneumococcal vaccines; - mobilizing additional workforce (e.g., healthcare workers); and - introducing temporary reductions of tax rates on some goods.	Higher effectiveness of target groups translates into limiting the spread of the pandemic.

Banning

All citizens, including those engaging in behaviours that may contribute to the spread of the virus: travelers, participants in gatherings (political, religious, etc.), students.	Individuals engaging in certain behaviours will not refrain from them voluntarily. Only officially imposed bans may curb the pandemic. The effectiveness of bans depends on the effectiveness of their administration and on sanctions for non-compliance.	Apart from (legal) action itself, awareness-raising, monitoring, and enforcing measures play a significant role. Specific actions: – limiting access to various institutions/facilities (e.g., physical therapy centres) and services; – imposing travel restrictions: shutting down airports, banning flights; – closing borders to all non-citizens or people from selected countries; – closing educational facilities (kindergartens, schools, universities); – closing businesses in some industries (e.g., restaurants, gyms); – banning the export of vital resources (e.g., ventilators); – limiting patient access to health services; – price-fixing; – imposing quarantines; and – setting size limits on gatherings.	Eliminating behaviours that foster the spread of the disease.

(Continued)

Target group	Barriers	Interventions	Outcomes
		Informing/Encouraging	
All citizens, including those who may be exposed to specific risks.	Lack of knowledge or motivation to engage in desired behaviours. The state and its institutions are one of many competitive sources of information. Other sources include the media (traditional and social), scientific authorities, and media experts.	Key characteristics of interventions for informing the public include usefulness, message accuracy and coherence, and reaching the target group. Specific actions: – implementing sets of recommended measures (e.g., encouraging working from home, avoiding handshakes, prescribing mask wearing, and social distancing); – creating new communication channels (e.g., websites, helplines, apps, social media, text messaging); – holding press conferences; – launching campaigns on relevant subjects (e.g. mental health in times of pandemic, protecting the elderly, being honest about one's symptoms when talking to healthcare workers); and – communicating with opinion leaders (e.g., religious authorities).	Behavioural change that helps to curb the pandemic.

Source: Own work; intervention categories based on Soman (2017) and Olejniczak et al. (2020). Specific actions come from a dataset of non-pharmaceutical interventions (NPIs) (Desvars-Larrive et al., 2020).

Public Policy Responses to the Pandemic 185

Box 8.1 Guidelines for informing/encouraging interventions based on social-behavioural research evidence.

1. **Avoid minimizing the consequences of becoming infected**, as this could result in excessively low levels of anxiety and, in turn, depleted motivation to comply with hygiene or sanitary recommendations.

2. On the other hand, **avoid causing extreme levels of fear associated with becoming infected**, which could lead to irrational behaviours and a limited ability to process factual information or instructions.

3. **Provide accessible, clear, and reliable information about the symptoms, course, and consequences of the disease** to prevent excessive mass-scale health anxiety, which could have a paralyzing social effect.

4. Inform the public broadly and accessibly about the means of reducing the risk of **contracting the disease** and infecting others. This should be accompanied by compelling examples and evidence supporting the effectiveness of these precautions as well as the consequences of not taking them. A belief in the effectiveness of certain behaviours is crucial for engaging in them. As discussed in this book, people are more likely to engage in behaviours that are well-known, commonly accepted, and proven to be effective. One should remember that, under threat, when experiencing anxiety and other negative emotions, **people have limited information-processing capacity, especially when there is a surfeit of information and it is in flux.** This may lead the public to disregard advice and recommendations.

5. **Facilitate people's engagement in health-promoting and helping behaviours**, such as sewing face masks, supporting healthcare workers, etc., which helps to reduce excessive anxiety and activates prosocial motivations. It is important to **identify potential barriers and support NGOs and voluntary groups' efforts** in this respect.

6. **Avoid deploying ethnocentric arguments or identifying outgroups as a risk factor**, as this may lead to very negative affective and behavioural consequences, including violence and acts of terrorism.

7. **Run a campaign to promote caring for the health and safety of others, especially the elderly and vulnerable, as an up-to-date, forward-looking, and respected attitude**. This should be done with the use of social media, trendsetters and influencers, content placement, and other trend- and attitude-promoting

strategies. Such interventions should be professionally developed by advertising and social communication practitioners and adapted to a diverse audience. Behaviours and statements standing in opposition to evidence-based principles should be condemned and deprecated (an example being the use of the German term *Covidioten*). **Socially shared standards will motivate people to engage in desired behaviours.**

8. It is important to **induce positive emotions even under threat**, as they promote cooperation, unlike negative emotions such as fear or disgust.

9. At the time of completing this book, a massive wave of positive emotions is evidently prompted by the lifting of COVID-19 restrictions. These **positive feelings make people filter out and ignore negative information, which in turn reduces preventive behaviours** at an individual level. As noted earlier in this book: "If anxiety is too low or absent (for example, as a result of certain brain dysfunctions), the individual's motivation to take protective measures (such as wearing a face mask or using hand sanitizer) will also be low, leading to an increased risk of infection, or even death."

10. It is important that vaccination promotion campaigns raise general awareness of the following:

    a. The probability of becoming infected is high in the given community.
    b. Everyone is at risk of getting COVID-19.
    c. The effects of the disease can be severe.

11. When designing public communications, **follow the guidelines for effective communication**, such as the ones offered below:

    a. Carefully develop and review – in cooperation with experts – the content that should be publicized to help people make the right decisions.
    b. The communicated content should concern not only the health risks, but also the economic situation, the related risks, and any knowledge beneficial to rational decision making. When under threat, people are more likely to make decisions focused on short-term benefits, which they may later come to regret. Substantive, expert knowledge about various scenarios and the consequences of different decisions should be available.
    c. Data on the epidemic situation should be provided in a comparative context, to make it clearer how figures should be interpreted in terms of risk assessment.

Public Policy Responses to the Pandemic   187

d. The long-term consequences of the pandemic should be communicated more clearly.

e. Research, research, and then research some more! Conduct systematic studies on people's beliefs about numerous aspects of pandemic-related risks and their own behaviour, as well as on the effects of information and regulations.

f. Ensure clear, understandable, **and stable communication**; to this end:

i. **Develop your message carefully** so that significant content does not need to be changed frequently.

ii. **Test!** Make sure key guidelines and their justifications are correctly recalled.

iii. **Respond to feedback** about information confusion and ignorance to prevent any overestimation of the risks as a result of misunderstanding, or conversely, any underestimation of the risks due to ignorance.

iv. **Use strategies that foster comprehension and recall**, such as limiting the number of significant elements in a message to three, using multimodal messages (e.g., a simple text message illustrated with images and sounds), using natural frequencies rather than probabilities expressed as percentages or fractions.

v. **Utilize knowledge about factors that increase the effectiveness of communication** (e.g., that the colour red attracts attention more than other colours, and improves the effectiveness of persuasive messages).

vi. Combine information about risks and their negative consequences with advice on how to handle those risks, and positive examples of effective responses.

vii. **Design messages so that they do not just focus on risks** but also create a positive, proactive orientation. Messages should be differentiated across target groups.

g. **Study** the effects of messages and **review** the agenda, form, and content of messages based on research evidence.

h. **Adhere to the principle that the communication source should be highly trusted**, bearing in mind that people will attribute more reliability to experts who support their own existing opinions, which may lead to biases and distortions. This should be taken into account in designing messages; to this end, **target groups' beliefs need to be well understood.**

i. Carefully **test and evaluate the effects of messages formulated by important decision makers and high-profile**

figures (in partnership with professional researchers) and give them appropriate feedback about these effects, especially in terms of increased and reduced anxiety. Both excessive anxiety reduction and the related tendency to neglect precautions, and conversely, escalating anxiety levels **that** limit the capacity to think rationally, are undesirable.

j.   If the abovementioned guidelines are **to** be successfully applied, a professional government agency should be established that will cooperate with the research base to manage public communications during a crisis.

12. Social identity or group identification is crucial for people's health, perceived control, and self-efficacy. Social divides should be narrowed, as their escalation makes it impossible to utilize the effects of identification with a group that distinguishes itself positively from the others. Perceived membership in an inferior group has several negative consequences; in particular, it makes people unlikely to work for the common good. Low social identification may also lead to conspiracy thinking. Political differences are an important factor underlying social divides. Given that group norms and sources of authority vary between different parts of society, it is important to seek agreement with local opinion leaders on how to promote norms affecting people's health and life. Communal orientation helps to survive a crisis and fosters behaviours that serve to protect others and improve their wellbeing, both in terms of health and with regard to the economic conditions. Sharp political divisions associated with other types of divides (e.g., elites – society; the privileged – victims of discrimination; patriots – traitors, etc.) are damaging to community and, as a result, reduce the ability to successfully overcome the consequences of the pandemic.

13. In public policy making, it is important to remain particularly sensitive to the potential emergence of **a belief that a certain group's situation (as a whole) has deteriorated unfairly, and to the resulting angry feelings**. This increases the likelihood of social protests and other collective actions. **It is important to monitor public opinion concerning those elements, identify their causes, and respond adequately.**

14. It may be helpful to refer to general moral norms, as research has demonstrated that behaviours driven by moral beliefs are more lasting and less dependent on contextual factors, such as easy access to protective equipment or the likelihood of being punished for inappropriate behaviour. That said, simple strategies should not be neglected either (e.g., easily accessible sanitizers or visual reminders about the rules of behaviour). Moral norms can be invoked either directly or indirectly, for example by content placement in popular

TV shows. Behaviour consistent with moral norms should be a standard for evaluating someone as an upstanding citizen acting in the interests of the community.

15. **Effective leadership is crucial during a pandemic crisis**. Those performing leadership roles have to remember that these can only be successfully fulfilled if:

    a. People feel the leader works **in the interest of the whole community**, and not just for their favourites.
    b. **The leader explains** and clarifies, **helping** people to make sense of what is going on.

16. Trust in the government and in state institutions is a key factor in terms of compliance with COVID-19 rules and restrictions.

    a. News reports about unfair conduct, both in the public sphere (e.g., corruption, nepotism) and in a person's private life (e.g., sex **scandals**) have a particularly damaging effect on trust.
    b. The development of trust depends on evaluations of performance and the quality of procedures, as well as the extent to which they are complied with, particularly with respect to fairness and impartiality.
    c. **Perceived procedural fairness has a stronger effect on cooperation than the fear of sanctions**. This should be taken into consideration as a horizontal principle in public policy making.

17. **Citizen participation in decision making** is an important factor that increases legitimacy and fosters compliance. Therefore, it is desirable to incorporate consultation and participation mechanisms into policy making.

18. Trust in people and institutions, and social capital, that is, social networks and ties that can be expected to provide support and cooperation, are of vital importance in managing a pandemic and its social and economic consequences. Social capital is built through group or social activities. It is important to support the development of this key social asset through the provision of an appropriate institutional framework as well as informational resources and financial support.

messages, but also by a wide range of features characterizing government responses and decisions.

When faced with a grave and sudden threat, states relied primarily on proven and relatively straightforward solutions. There was no time for any of the recently popular, more sophisticated interventions based on changing the choice architecture, such as nudging (Thaler and Sunstein, 2008).

190   *Culture and Policy in Pandemics: Case Studies*

The pandemic interventions, however, were unique in their wide impact and accumulation within a short period of time.

Research activity is based on data collected systematically and with strict methodological rigour. If the subjects to be analyzed are public policies aimed at managing a pandemic, information about interventions that have already been implemented must be gathered initially. An analysis of the systematized data will provide a basis for drawing conclusions, which could guide further public policies. Given its unprecedented scale, the COVID-19 pandemic is a new and unique phenomenon, and governments have responded to it with measures that may have unpredictable effects. Data on public interventions being collected today offers us a chance to learn from others' failures and successes, and will enable better decision making in the future. So, what is it that social sciences can offer to decision makers today to diminish the level of uncertainty they have to deal with in a novel situation such as the current pandemic? What tools are available to help them design better and more thorough interventions?

The research community has been working on the development of data-sets compiling information about public policy responses to the COVID-19 pandemic around the world (Daly et al., 2020). In this chapter, we would like to explore a dataset on non-pharmaceutical interventions (NPIs), published in *Nature* (https://github.com/amel-github/covid19-interventionmeasures, Desvars-Larrive et al., 2020). Our analyses are based on the dataset accessed on October 7, 2020. We will discuss an example of how this information can be used, highlight traps you may encounter when interpreting data, and show how to assess the quality of data before using it to inform public policy decisions. Our analyses will demonstrate how the OECD countries differed with regard to the scope and timing of interventions.

8.3 KEY DECISIONS TO BE MADE PRIOR TO ANALYZING DATA

The current analysis seeks to answer the question of whether the OECD member countries differed in terms of restrictions imposed during the first wave of the pandemic. Can those countries be grouped by the types and timing of implemented interventions? Were some of those countries more successful than others in minimizing the epidemic growth rates? Several analytical decisions have to be made, however, prior to performing the analyses. Knowledge about the choices that were made and the alternatives that were considered is also crucial to a decision maker who would like to use the analyses to inform public policy making. Decisions made during data selection, preparation, and processing play a key role in offering accurate interpretations of the results of the analyses.

The first decision to be made involves defining the subjects of the analysis, that is, choosing the countries to be compared. Policy makers should be interested in comparisons with other countries that are strikingly similar to their country, rather than, for instance, with the Diamond Princess cruise ship, which has been included in the dataset along with 56 countries. Comparisons may be limited, for example, to the Schengen Area. Alternatively, countries may be selected according to the development or governance indicators proposed by The World Bank. For the purposes of our example, we narrowed our analysis to the OECD countries available in the dataset, which form a comparable and stable group of developed and democratic nations. We only used interventions coded at the national level; however, interventions coded at the regional level are also available in the dataset. It should be noted here that this selection method has its downsides – some interventions will not appear on the national level, especially in countries which comprise autonomous regions, which have been implementing their own regional policies to combat the pandemic (e.g., Spain, Germany, and Switzerland).

Second, it is necessary to define the thematic scope of the analysis, that is, which crisis management strategies will be included. The authors of the dataset proposed a hierarchical four-level classification scheme of public interventions undertaken by various countries to manage the spread of COVID-19. There are many possible approaches to defining the thematic scope of an analysis. One possibility is to use the pre-defined codes suggested by the authors of the dataset. Another approach is to develop one's own classification based on the lowest coding level available (i.e., L4). Since many intervention categories coded at the second (L2) and third (L3) levels are quite heterogeneous, and evaluating the content based on a single category label could be misleading, we chose only ten intervention types for our analyses. These are the following, at level L2: *airport restrictions* (e.g., closing airports, cancellation of domestic and international flights, landing bans on aircrafts from high risk areas), *border restrictions* (e.g., border control, entry ban for non-citizens, conditional entry for citizens), *closures of educational institutions* (in most cases complete closure, rarely partial closure), *mass gathering cancellations* (which included closure of non-essential public places, work places, conferences, meetings, trade fairs, cultural places and events, places of worship, bans on sport, recreation, and other indoor activities), *national lockdowns, small gathering cancellations* (e.g., the closure of shops selling non-essentials, restaurants/bars/cafes, mandatory home office use), *public transport restrictions, quarantine* (contact persons, incoming residents and travellers, suspected cases), *individual movement restrictions* (non-essential trips and movement forbidden); and at level L3: the *mandatory use of masks*.

In the third step, the time span should be well-defined. We focused only on interventions undertaken in response to the first wave of COVID-19. Hence, we skipped "returning to normal life" interventions and second-wave policies.

Fourth, the indicators on the basis of which countries are compared should be defined. In their "country-cluster analysis of the government control strategies" (Desvars-Larrive et al., 2020), the authors of the dataset defined (a) responsiveness (the time of launch of an intervention, i.e., "early measures" meaning those launched between the day when 10 cases were reported and the day when 200 cases were reported, and "late responses" defined as those introduced after the point at which 200 cases were reported) and (b) aggressiveness (i.e., the number of mandatory government interventions). We have not taken the number of interventions to be a valid indicator. What does it

192 *Culture and Policy in Pandemics: Case Studies*

mean that a country introduced numerous interventions? Is it a sign of poor planning or a lack of strategic thinking? Or does it suggest that responses to the pandemic were fine-tuned and interventions were adjusted to make the most of them? Hence, we decided not to use "aggressiveness" in our analyses but just focus on timing, (i.e., when the first intervention of a given type was introduced relative to the first reported case in a country). We defined "early measures" as those implemented within the first two weeks after the first case had been reported in a country. We defined "late responses" as those launched in the third week or later after the first case had been reported. Please bear in mind that different definitions might lead to different conclusions. Hence, the interpretation of the results is always bounded by the definitions of indicators. The authors of this chapter and Desvars-Larrive et al. (2020) both used the COVID-19 Data Repository by the JHU CSSE (https://github.com/CSSEGISandData/COVID-19) for dates and numbers of reported cases.

Policy makers typically expect this type of analysis to let them know what works or which interventions are money well spent. To answer these questions, it is necessary to define a "success criterion," which is the fifth crucial step prior to data analysis. One could use a simple categorization of countries based on their performance in combatting the pandemic, for example, the categories of green, yellow, and red countries, just as managers track the performance of their companies on dashboards (e.g., https://www.endcoronavirus.org/countries). However, some might find this categorization unsuitable, or it may turn out that the methodology behind it has not been published or is incomplete. Therefore, we chose a different, straightforward measure of success. Using the JHU CSSE data, we calculated the geometrical mean of daily changes in new cases during six months from the day when the first 100 cases were reported in each country. The geometrical mean of daily changes in new cases ranged between 1.6% and 6.2% for the OECD countries included in the dataset (all OECD members are represented in the dataset except for Australia, Chile, Colombia, Ireland, Israel, Latvia, Luxembourg, and Turkey). We later grouped the countries into four categories based on quartiles, as presented in Table 8.2, meaning, for instance, that the best performing countries were in the first quartile.

In the sixth step, it is important to establish what methodology was used for collecting the data that we intend to analyze. Ideally, data should be collected automatically, for example using such techniques as text mining or data

Table 8.2 OECD countries included in the dataset by Desvars-Larrive et al. (2020), grouped in quartiles based on the geometrical mean of daily changes in new cases during six months from the day when the first 100 COVID-19 cases were reported in each country

---

Q1: New Zealand, Iceland, Estonia, Slovenia, Lithuania, Finland, Slovakia, Greece
Q2: Denmark, Norway, South Korea, Hungary, Czech Rep., Austria, Switzerland
Q3: Japan, Portugal, Sweden, Netherlands, Poland, Belgium, Canada
Q4: Italy, Germany, France, UK, Spain, Mexico, USA

---

scraping. Automated data collection enables more accurate testing, full transparency, and replicability. However, the data on NPIs (Desvars-Larrive et al. 2020) that we use here was collected manually by students, researchers, and volunteers in various countries. Usually, study designers do their best to standardize the data collection procedure, if their data is to be used for statistical analyses. This was certainly true in this case. However, when data is collected manually and by numerous people, the risk of error is always present. This should be kept in mind when analyzing and interpreting the results. Most errors (if there are any) can only be identified during data analysis or even later, when interpreting the results. For example, while writing these words, the author is watching a street in Barcelona, where everyone is wearing a mask. In most autonomous regions of Spain mandatory mask wearing has been in force since July 2020, but this fact has not been entered in the dataset, neither at the regional level nor nationally. Similar errors or gaps may exist in the dataset.

8.4 RESULTS

We performed a multiple correspondence analysis (MCA) and a cluster analysis (CA) to explore possible clusters of countries according to different patterns of interventions and their timing. For analyses, we used R packages "FactoMineR" and "factoextra." As shown in Figure 8.1, several country clusters could be identified. Please note that the clustering proposed here is based purely on exploratory data analysis and is just one of many possibilities.

Sweden, Canada, Japan, South Korea, and Mexico did not implement many measures, and even the few ones put in place were introduced at quite a late stage. What differentiates these countries from other OECD members is the lack of restrictions on small gatherings and individual movement, as well as a delay in introducing airport restrictions. Educational institutions also remained open in these countries.

France, Italy, and the UK, as well as Belgium, Denmark, Finland, Germany, Iceland, Norway, and Spain, either delayed the introduction of many restrictions or did not impose them at all. This group of countries was characterized by late cancellation of small and mass gatherings, late closure of educational institutions, and the delayed introduction of restrictions on individual movement. Furthermore, no strict airport restrictions or flight cancellations were imposed.

Austria, Lithuania, New Zealand, and the US were also relatively sluggish in their response to the pandemic. Almost 8 out of the 10 measures included in our analyses were implemented in the third week or later after the first case had been reported. What was characteristic of this group of countries was the late introduction of small gathering cancellations and national lockdowns.

The Czech Republic, Greece, Hungary, Poland, Portugal, Slovakia, and Slovenia were all early-responding countries. However, they had more time than others because their first cases were recorded later than elsewhere, that is, in late February or early March. What differentiated these countries from other OECD members was the early introduction of airport and border

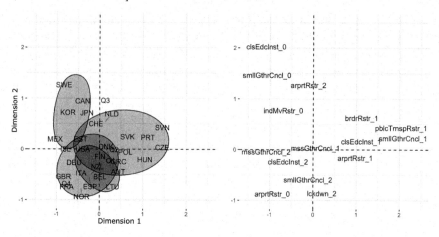

Figure 8.1 Country clusters (left panel) and intervention categories (right panel).
Notes: The right plot shows 15 (out of 30) categories contributing the most to dimensions 1 and 2. Dimensions 1 and 2 explain 73.5% (Benzécri's method) of variance in strategies undertaken by the OECD member countries to manage the COVID-19 pandemic. "0" = no intervention, "1" = early intervention, "2" = late intervention; Q1–Q4 quartiles based on the geometrical mean of daily changes in new cases during six months from the day when the first 100 cases were diagnosed in each country; arprtRstr = Airport restrictions; brdrRstr = Border restrictions; clsEdcInst = Closure of educational institutions; mssGthrCncl = Mass gathering cancellation; lckdwn = National lockdown; smllGthrCncl = Small gathering cancellation; pblcTrnspRstr = Public transport restrictions; qrntn = Quarantine; indMvRstr = Individual movement restrictions; mndtryMsks = Mandatory use of masks.

restrictions, early closure of educational institutions, and early restrictions on small and mass gatherings. Estonia, the Netherlands, and Switzerland also belong to this group, but they do not quite match the cluster's profile. Their distinctive feature was the lack of a national lockdown.

Which intervention patterns or strategies have proven most successful in managing the spread of COVID-19? Some studies suggest the important role of a quick and decisive response at an early stage of the pandemic (Capano et al., 2020). The examples of some countries in the last cluster (such as Poland or Portugal) show, however, that these benefits may decline over time. Furthermore, at the time of completing the work on this publication (the end of October 2020), the remaining countries in this group (the Czech Republic, Greece, Hungary, Slovakia, and Slovenia) are beginning to report massive increases in new cases. There is no statistically significant relationship between the mean daily change in new COVID-19 cases (keeping this value low serves as a success criterion) and the pattern of public policy responses to the pandemic (reflected in cluster membership). Therefore, the conclusion is rather disquieting: No matter what countries did, in the long run, the virus was unstoppable, until mass vaccination programs were launched.

Nevertheless, some conclusions can be drawn based on the analysis of individual countries. Our results point to the importance of external factors that are beyond policy makers' control. Some of the countries that were perceived as best prepared before the outbreak of COVID-19 (such as the UK or the US) are among those most affected by the pandemic (Abbey et al., 2020). On the other hand, factors that appear significant for the best performing countries include the ability to isolate themselves more easily from other countries' residents (e.g., insular or relatively small countries). This is clearly illustrated by the presence of New Zealand and Iceland among the countries that have managed the pandemic best.

Apart from looking for similarities in patterns of interventions introduced in response to the pandemic, we were also interested in the extent to which countries copied each other's strategies, not only in terms of their scope but also in terms of timing. As shown in Figure 8.2, most countries implemented their first strategies in week 11 of 2020, that is, March 9–15.

That move was probably linked to the pressure that was exerted when the WHO declared the COVID-19 outbreak a pandemic on March 11, 2020.

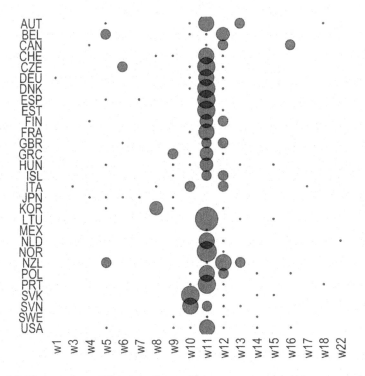

Figure 8.2 The numbers of interventions within ten categories (Airport restrictions, Border restrictions, Closure of educational institutions, Mass gathering cancellation, National lockdown, Small gathering cancellation, Public transport restrictions, Quarantine, Individual movement restrictions, Mandatory use of masks) introduced by the OECD countries in the following weeks of 2020.

Apparently, the initial restrictions were imposed not so much because the first COVID-19 cases had been identified, but rather due to the international pressure and reports of other countries' responses. Among the OECD countries, the first cases were reported in Japan, South Korea, the United States, and France (January 22–24, 2020). The majority of restrictions in those countries were imposed late, if they were introduced at all, except for mandatory quarantine in Japan, South Korea, and, in the US, restrictions on people coming in from high-risk areas, suspected cases, and contact persons. Japan was also relatively quick to introduce border restrictions. A few weeks before COVID-19 was declared a pandemic, multiple interventions (or intervention packages) had only just been introduced by Belgium, New Zealand, and the Czech Republic. Another thought-provoking conclusion that can be drawn from Figure 8.2 is that some countries introduced most of the analyzed intervention types all at once (e.g., Lithuania and Norway), whereas others implemented them incrementally over time (e.g., Japan and Hungary).

8.5 CONCLUSIONS

The purpose of this chapter was to present the variety of country-by-country responses to the COVID-19 pandemic and to demonstrate the potential of systematized datasets on public interventions in supporting the development of public policy responses to an epidemic crisis. The discussion was based on evidence from other sciences, presented in the preceding chapters.

It was not our priority to develop a model that would explain the effects of public interventions on curbing the pandemic, but rather to identify different patterns detectable among the OECD countries' responses to COVID-19. Additionally, our analyses provided a background for presenting several traps that are easy to fall prey to when too little attention is paid to data quality assessment, when your information objectives are ill-defined, and when the inherent limitations of both the data itself and the adopted indicators are not recognized.

The analyses reported in this chapter are inconclusive, but they suggest that, regardless of the scope and "aggressiveness" of the interventions introduced, virtually all countries have to endure seasonal epidemic peaks. The inconclusiveness of the analyses presented here points to the essential role of contextual factors, which lead to differences in both policy makers' responses and their outcomes. Suggested lists of such factors and examples of more in-depth analyses are available in the literature (Balmford et al., 2020; Bloukh et al., 2020; Capano et al., 2020; Priyadarsini and Suresh, 2020).

References

Abbey, E. J., Khalifa, B. A. A., Oduwole, M. O. et al. (2020) The Global Health Security Index is not predictive of coronavirus pandemic responses among Organization for Economic Cooperation and Development countries. *PLoS ONE*, 15(10), e0239398. https://doi.org/10.1371/journal.pone.0239398

Al Eid, N. A. & Arnout, B. A. (2020). Crisis and disaster management in the light of the Islamic approach: COVID-19 pandemic crisis as a model (a qualitative study using the grounded theory). *Journal of Public Affairs*, e2217. https://doi.org/10.1002/pa.2217

Ali, A. (2020). Covid an excuse to push Indian Muslims out of informal sector jobs. Apartheid the next step. (9 April). *The Print*. https://theprint.in/opinion/covid-an-excuse-to-push-indian-muslims-out-of-informal-sector-jobs-apartheid-the-next-step/398236/

Al-Tamimi, A. J. (2020). Islamic State Editorial on the Coronavirus Pandemic, http://www.aymennjawad.org/2020/03/islamic-state-editorial-on-the-coronavirus

Balmford, B., Annan, J. D., Hargreaves, J. C., Altoè, M., & Bateman, I. J. (2020). Cross-country comparisons of Covid-19: policy, politics and the price of life. *Environmental and Resource Economics*, 76, 525–551. https://doi.org/10.1007/s10640-020-00466-5

Bardach, E., & Patashnik, E. M. (2019). *A Practical Guide for Policy Analysis: The Eightfold Path to More Effective Problem Solving* (5th ed.). Thousand Oaks: CQ Press.

BBC (2020). Coronavirus: Iran cover-up of deaths revealed by data leak. (3 August). https://www.bbc.com/news/world-middle-east-53598965 (accessed on September 26, 2020).

Bloukh, S. H., Edis, Z., Shaikh, A. A., & Pathan, H. M. (2020) A look behind the scenes at COVID-19: National strategies of infection control and their impact on mortality. *International Journal of Environmental Research and Public Health*, 17, 5616.

Boussel, P. (2020). Covid-19, jihadism and the challenge of a pandemic. *Foundation for Strategic Research*. https://www.frstrategie.org/en/publications/notes/covid-19-jihadism-and-challenge-pandemic-2020

Bozorgmehr, N. (2020). How Iran's clergy fought back against coronavirus. (17 June). *Financial Times*. https://www.ft.com/content/8e9b50bb-ebf7-4702-9894-1f2081ae869a

Capano, G., Howlett, M., Jarvis, D. S. L , Ramesh, M., & Goyal, N. (2020). Mobilizing policy (in)capacity to fight COVID-19: Understanding variations in state responses, *Policy and Society*, 39(3), 285–308. https://doi.org/10.1080/14494035.2020.1787628

198 *Culture and Policy in Pandemics: Case Studies*

Crisis Group Africa Report N° 232 (28 October 2015). The Politics Behind the Ebola Crisis. https://www.crisisgroup.org/africa/west-africa/politics-behind-ebola-crisis

Daly, M., Ebbinghaus, B., Lehner, L., Naczyk, M., & Vlandas, T. (2020). *Oxford Supertracker: The Global Directory for COVID Policy Trackers and Surveys*. Department of Social Policy and Intervention.

Desvars-Larrive, A., Dervic, E., Haug, N. et al. (2020). A structured open dataset of government interventions in response to COVID-19. *Scientific Data*, 7, 285. https://doi.org/10.1038/s41597-020-00609-9

Dong, E., Du, H., & Gardner, L. (2020). An interactive web-based dashboard to track COVID-19 in real time. *The Lancet*, 20(5), 533–534. https://doi.org/10.1016/S1473-3099(20)30120-1

Emanuel, E. J., Persad, G., Upshur, R. et al. (2020). Fair allocation of scarce medical resources in the time of Covid-19. *The New England Journal of Medicine*, 382, 2049–2055. https://doi.org/10.1056/NEJMsb2005114

Flaxman, S., Mishra, S., Gandy, A. et al. (2020) Estimating the effects of non-pharmaceutical interventions on COVID-19 in Europe. *Nature*, 584, 257–261. https://doi.org/10.1038/s41586-020-2405-7

Frayer, L., & Pathak, S. (2020). Hindus Work Around Coronavirus To Celebrate God Ganesh, Remover Of Obstacles. (August 27). *NPR*. https://www.npr.org/sections/coronavirus-live-updates/2020/08/27/906719241/hindus-find-ways-around-coronavirus-to-celebrate-god-ganesh-remover-of-obstacles [Accessed November 25, 2020]

Freedom House. (2020). Countries and Territories: Global Freedom Scores. https://freedomhouse.org/countries/freedom-world/scores (accessed on September 26, 2020).

Fund For Peace. (2019). Fragile States Index. https://fundforpeace.org/2019/04/10/fragile-states-index-2019/

Hackett, C. (2017). By 2050, India to have world's largest populations of Hindus and Muslims. (April 21, 2015). Pew Research Center. https://www.pewresearch.org/fact-tank/2015/04/21/by-2050-india-to-have-worlds-largest-populations-of-hindus-and-muslims/ [Accessed November 30, 2021]

Hall, E. T. (1990). *The Hidden Dimension*. New York: Anchor Books Edition.

Hashim, A. (2020). In Pakistan, mosques become coronavirus battleground issue. (6 May). *Aljazeera*. https://www.aljazeera.com/news/2020/05/06/in-pakistan-mosques-become-coronavirus-battleground-issue/

Hofstede, G. (2004). *Cultures and Organizations. Software of the Mind: Intercultural Cooperation and Its Importance for Survival*. New York: McGraw-Hill.

Islamic Relief Worldwide. (2020). Guidance on safe religious practice for Muslim communities during the coronavirus pandemic. https://www.islamic-relief.org/islamic-relief-launches-guidance-on-safe-religious-practice-during-the-coronavirus-pandemic/

Kapur, R., & Saxena, C. (2020). The Taliban makes the most of Covid-19 crisis in Afghanistan. (April 27). *The Interpreter*. https://www.lowyinstitute.org/the-interpreter/taliban-makes-most-covid-19-crisis-afghanistan [Accessed June 25, 2020]

Kłodkowski, P. (2015). *Homo Mysticus of Hinduism and Islam. Mystical Bhakti Movement and Sufism*. Warszawa: Dialog.

References 199

Kłodkowski, P. (2019). Socialism, secularism, free market economy and Hindutva: The Indian narrative on the state and its ideology in a historical perspective. *International Affairs*, 4, 91–113.

Lipka, M. (2017). Muslims and Islam: Key findings in the U.S. and around the world. (August 9). Pew Research Center. https://www.pewresearch.org/fact-tank/2017/08/09/muslims-and-islam-key-findings-in-the-u-s-and-around-the-world/ [Accessed November 30, 2021]

Mahbubani, K. (2008). *The New Asian Hemisphere. The Irresistible Shift of Global Power to the East*. New York, Public Affairs.

Menon, A. (2020). Covid-19 surge across India. (April 8). *The Quint*. https://www.thequint.com/news/india/coronavirus-muslims-attacked-covid19-karnataka-haryana

O'Donnell, L., & Khan, M. (2020). Factional Struggles Emerge in Virus-Afflicted Taliban Top Ranks, Foreign Policy. (9 June). https://foreignpolicy.com/2020/06/09/coronavirus-pandemic-taliban-afghanistan-peace-talks/

Olejniczak, K., Śliwowski P., & Leeuw, F. (2020). Comparing behavioral assumptions of policy tools: Framework for policy designers. *Journal of Comparative Policy Analysis: Research and Practice*, 22(6), 498–520. https://doi.org/10.1080/13876988.2020.1808465

Pandey, V. (2020). Coronavirus: India doctors 'spat at and attacked'. (3 April). *BBC*. https://www.bbc.com/news/world-asia-india-52151141#:~:text=Several%20healthcare%20workers%20in%20India,vulgar%20language%20towards%20female%20nurses

Pew Research Center. (2020). Most in Western Europe say belief in God not needed to be moral. (July 17). https://www.pewresearch.org/global/2020/07/20/the-global-god-divide/pg_2020-07-20_global-religion_0-03/ (accessed on September 29, 2020).

Priyadarsini, S. L., & Suresh, M. (2020) Factors influencing the epidemiological characteristics of pandemic COVID 19: A TISM approach. *International Journal of Healthcare Management*, 13(2), 89–98. https://doi.org/10.1080/20479700.2020.1755804

Sabat, I., Neuman-Böhme, S., Varghese, N. E. et al. (2020). United but divided: Policy responses and people's perceptions in the EU during the COVID-19 outbreak. *Health Policy*, 124(9), 909–918. https://doi.org/10.1016/j.healthpol.2020.06.009

Soman, D. (2017). *The Last Mile. Creating Social and Economic Value from Behavioral Insights*. Toronto: University of Toronto Press.

Srinivas, T. (2020). India's goddesses of contagion provide protection in the pandemic – just don't make them angry. *The Conversation*. https://theconversation.com/indias-goddesses-of-contagion-provide-protection-in-the-pandemic-just-dont-make-them-angry-139745 [Accessed September 20, 2020]

Takeyh, R. (2020). Iran's Perplexing Pandemic Response. *Council on Foreign Relations*. (August 15). https://www.cfr.org/in-brief/irans-perplexing-pandemic-response

Thaler, R., & Sunstein, C. (2008). *Nudge: Improving Decisions about Health, Wealth, and Happiness*. New Haven, CT: Yale University Press.

Tharoor, S. (2007). Indian identity is forged in diversity. Every one of us is in a minority. (August 14). *The Guardian*. https://www.theguardian.com/commentisfree/2007/aug/15/comment.india [Accessed November 20, 2020)

Tharoor, S. (2018). *Why I am a Hindu*. New Delhi: Aleph.

Index

Note: **Bold** page numbers refer to tables, *Italic* page numbers refer to figures and page numbers followed by "n" refer to end notes.

5G towers, and COVID-19 disinformation 86, 87

above average effect 49
affect heuristic 95–96, 107
Afghanistan, Taliban's management of COVID-19 pandemic 169–170
age, and decision making/risk taking 39–40, 100
aggressive behaviour 9–11, 23, 25, 52, 97; *see also* violence
A/H1N1 virus *see* H1N1 (subtype of influenza A virus)
AIDS 154; goddess AIDSAmma (India) 171
Al Eid, N. A. 165–166
Al-Azhar University (Cairo), Supreme Ulema Council 163–164, 167
Albertson, B. 75
Ali, A. 173
Al-Qaida, response to COVID-19 pandemic 168–169, 170
anger 21, 23, 60, 97
anti-vaccine movement 46–47
anxiety: anxiety disorders 52; anxiety levels and compliance 10, 16; anxiety sensitivity and vulnerable groups 14; anxiety susceptibility, varied levels of and tailoring of support 16–17; crisis-related anxiety, universality of 6; death anxiety 11–14; and decision-making 39, 98; and depression/stress 15–16; health anxiety 10–11, 23, 47, 98; and information processing capacity 20–21, 24, 98; and negative memories, retrieval of 20; pandemic-related

anxiety 3–4, 8–9, 24, 36; and preventive behaviours 97; and risk perception/taking 22, 24–25, 36, 98, 99; social anxiety 9, 23; and social media 85; *see also* depression; fear; stress; threats; uncertainty
Ardern, J. 56
Argentina, COVID-19 disinformation 86
Arndt, J. 12
Arnout, B. A. 165–166
Asians, violent attacks against during COVID-19 pandemic 51
Australia: conspiracy theories and lack of trust in governmental COVID-19 policies 59; COVID-19 disinformation 86; SARS-CoV-2 genome, sharing of first sequences 154
authoritarian: governments in Muslim countries 166, 168; policies as result of overestimated pandemic-related risks 25
avian influenza (bird flu) 75

Bangladesh, COVID-19 pandemic 169
Bardach, E. 179–180
Barlas, S. 41–42
Beattie, J. 41–42
beauty products, increased sales during COVID-19 pandemic 18
behavioural economics 54
behavioural immune system 22
Besta, T. 60
bird flu (avian influenza) 75
Boko Haram, response to COVID-19 pandemic 168, 169
Bostrom, A. 94–95

202   *Index*

Boussel, P. 168
British Board of Scholars and Imams 164
Bruine de Bruin, W. 94–95
Buddhism, cultural *vs.* religious
   differences 162, 163
Bush, G. W. 73
Butt, A. 167

calculative trust (rational trust) 66–67, 72
Calderwood, C. 56
Capraro, V. 54
care facilities, residents' pandemic-related
   stress 14
Catena, A. 36
CDC (Centers for Disease Control and
   Prevention, US) 47, 86
Charité Hospital (Berlin), SARS-CoV-2
   test 154
Cheng, S.-T. 28
China: COVID-19 outbreak in Wuhan
   153, 154; COVID-19 response, not
   followed by Europe/US 50; cultural
   vs. religious differences 163; flood
   risk perception and institutional trust
   72; proxemics and social distancing
   161; scapegoated by other countries
   ("Wuhan virus") 51; Uighur
   Muslims 168
Christianity, cultural *vs.* religious
   differences 162
Cialdini, R. B. 54
civil obedience: and trust 7–8; *see also*
   compliance
Clark, D. 56
Clark, M. S. 57
climate change (environmental) risks
   35, 96
cognition: cognitive factors and
   compliance 19; cognitive mechanisms
   to cope with threats 23–25; motivated
   cognition 24; optimism as cognitive
   system key function 25–26; risk
   assessment and cognitive biases
   24–25, 32–33, 99; risk perception,
   cognitive-emotional model of 34–37,
   38, 99–100; and unknown risk 34–35,
   99; *see also* information processing;
   memory; social capital
cognitive behavioural therapy (CBT) 23
'cognitive miser' metaphor 54
cognitive psychology 23–24, 32, 33
collective action, 51, 61–62
collectivist cultures 57

communal orientation 57, 58, 101–102
communication: and alleviating fears
   and anxiety 17; and cultural/religious
   differences 161, 163, 174–175; and
   emotions 21–22; guidelines based
   on social-behavioural research
   evidence 180–181, 185–189; and
   universal language of science 174; *see
   also* disinformation (fake news); risk
   communication
community resilience 84, 106
compassion 13, 52, 57, 58, 102
compliance: and anger from others 21,
   97; and anxiety levels 10, 16; cognitive
   factors 19; contributing factors 53; and
   distrust in healthcare system (Poland)
   7–8; and healthcare institutions, trust
   in 76; and information processing
   capacity, limitations of 24; and
   institutional trust/legitimacy 65–66,
   71, 75–76, 104–105; maneuvering
   one's way around restrictions 66;
   non-compliance, pragmatic reasons for
   8; non-compliance and complicated
   rules/regulations 25; non-compliance
   and existential threat 52; non-
   compliance and polarization 59–60;
   non-compliance and underestimation
   of risks 24–25; non-compliance as
   norm 102; non-compliance groups
   4; and political beliefs 59–60; and
   procedural fairness 71; and social
   capital 77–79, 82, 106; and social
   inequalities 63; and "social proof"
   (influence of authority) 19; and
   subjective beliefs about disease 19;
   and trust 3, 53, 77–78; and unrealistic
   optimism 30; *see also* preventive
   behaviours
confirmation bias 44–45, 103–104
conspiracy theories 28, 47, 58–59, 87, 91,
   96, 103; Muslim world 166, 168–169;
   Poland 156, 159
cooperation: collectivist *vs.* individualistic
   cultures 57; communal orientation
   57, 58, 101–102; and emotions 22, 98;
   exchange (market pricing) orientation
   57–58, 102; financial cooperation 57,
   101; methods/strategies to promote
   56–57; and social inequalities 102;
   and stress 22, 98; *see also* community
   resilience; compliance; solidarity
"coronaracism" notion 86

Index   203

coronavirus pandemics *see* COVID-19 (SARS-CoV-2) pandemic; SARS-CoV pandemic (2003)

corruption 69, 71–72

COVID-19 (SARS-CoV-2) pandemic: brief summary of research findings 153–154; China's role 50, 51, 153, 154; comparisons between countries 50; COVID-19/SARS-CoV-2 names 153; declared a pandemic by WHO 155, 195–196; Delta variant 159; disinformation 86–87, 88; disinformation, measures to combat 89–91; likely to persist for years 160; new variants 153–154; pluridisciplinarity and book's objectives 5, 6; psychological and social factors 3, 4–5; PubMed database publications 153; SARS-CoV-2 genome, sharing of first sequences 154; state of pandemic (May-July 2020) 5–6; testing kits 87, 90; tests, types of 153, 154; vaccines 3, 5, 46; *see also* compliance; COVID-19 intervention measures dataset analysis (J. Górniak, S. Krupnik, M. Koniewski); cultural differences and pandemic (P. Kłodkowski and A. Siewierska-Chmaj); Hinduism and COVID-19 pandemic in India (P. Kłodkowski and A. Siewierska-Chmaj); Muslims and COVID-19 pandemic (P. Kłodkowski and A. Siewierska-Chmaj); Poland and COVID-19 epidemic (Jerzy Duszyński); preventive behaviours; public policy responses to pandemic (J. Górniak, S. Krupnik, M. Koniewski); vaccines

COVID-19 Data Repository (JHU CSSE) 176n9, 192

COVID-19 intervention measures dataset analysis (J. Górniak, S. Krupnik, M. Koniewski): analysis of differences between OECD countries' restrictions (first wave) 190, 196; choosing countries for comparison 190–191; choosing intervention types 191; defining data collection procedure 192–193; defining indicators 191–192; defining success criterion 192; defining time span 191; OECD countries grouped in quartiles 192, **192**; results: cluster analysis 193–194, *194*; importance of external factors beyond

control 194–195; timing of first strategies and international pressure 195–196, *195*; unstoppability of virus regardless of interventions 194, 196

crisis management 4, 5–6; Islamic model of 165–166

crowds, psychology of 62–63

cultural differences and pandemic (P. Kłodkowski and A. Siewierska-Chmaj): cultural/religious differences and communication 161, 163, 174–175; cultural/religious differences and fatality rates variations 161; relationship between culture and religion 161–163; universal language of science 174; *see also* Hinduism and COVID-19 pandemic in India (P. Kłodkowski and A. Siewierska-Chmaj); Muslims and COVID-19 pandemic (P. Kłodkowski and A. Siewierska-Chmaj)

cyberchondria 10, 98

Cyprus, economic crisis and social trust 80

Czarnek, G. 40, 59–60, 85, 96n1

Czech Republic, Christianity and cultural *vs.* religious differences 162

data presentation, and natural frequencies 34, 93, 99, 108

Davidai, S. 64

DDM (distancing, disinfection, masks) rule 158, 160

death anxiety 11–14

decision aversion 43, 101

decision making: and age 39–40, 100; and anxiety 39, 98; confirmation bias 44–45, 103–104; and dearth of information 3, 43; egocentric advice discounting 44; and expert advice 43–46, 103–104; and "human-as problem" perspective 7; motivated reasoning 44, 45, 104; and motivation 40–41, 100; multi-attribute utility theory 39; and personality/temperament 40; preference potentiation 22, 98; and public policy analysis 180; and risk 38–41; and sex (gender) 39, 40, 41, 100; trade-off decision making 41–43, 100–101; trade-offs and decision aversion/rationalizations 43, 101; *see also* risk; risk communication; risk perception/taking

204 Index

Delta variant 159
Denmark: COVID-19 pandemic and institutional/political trust 73; Mette Frederiksen's leadership during COVID-19 pandemic 55
depression 4, 9, 15–16, 25, 80
Desvars-Larrive, A. 190, 191, 192, 193
digital literacy skills 91
disgust 21–22, 24, 51–52, 97, 98
disinfection *see* DDM (distancing, disinfection, masks) rule; hand washing/sanitizer use
DisinfoLab 90
disinformation (fake news): anxiety-inducing social media 85; COVID-19 disinformation 85–87, 88; fast spreading of false news 87–88; measures against COVID-19 disinformation 89–91; media literacy and cognitive immunity to fake news 91–92; and optimists *vs.* pessimists 28; *see also* fact checking
distance learning 4, 79, 155
distancing, disinfection, masks (DDM) rule 158, 160
domestic violence 4, 17, 80, 156
dread *see* anxiety; fear
"dread risk" 34–35, 99
dual coding principle 92
Durante, F. 64
Durga or Kali (Hindu Mother Goddess) 171, 172
Duszyński, J. 14, 48n1; *see also* Poland and COVID-19 epidemic (Jerzy Duszyński)

Ebola virus epidemic (2014-15) 9, 86, 168, 175
economy: economic assistance, trust in and risk perception 72; economic crisis and institutional/political trust 73–74; economic crisis and social trust 80, 83; expert advice and confirmation bias 44–45; financial cooperation 57, 101; financial support and social capital 79, 82; financial/economic literacy 37, 91, 95–96, 107; and lockdowns 42, 101, 155; pandemic and supply hoarding 37, 52, 86; and pandemic-related anxiety 3–4, 9; pandemic-related complicated legal regulations 25; pandemic-related recession 158; pandemic-related recession, World Bank's forecast

5; pandemic-related situation and optimists 27–28; pandemic's long-term effects, difficult to predict 43; personal (egotropic) *vs.* sociotropic economic perceptions 68; *see also* public policy responses to pandemic (J. Górniak, S. Krupnik, M. Koniewski); social inequalities
education: distance learning 4, 79, 155; home schooling 16; and lockdowns 155; and pandemic-related anxiety 3–4
egocentric advice discounting 44
egotropic (personal) perceptions, *vs.* sociotropic perceptions 68
elevation 57, 102; moral elevation 52
emotional intelligence 20
emotions: affect heuristic 95–96, 107; anger 21, 23, 60, 97; communicative function of 21–22; compassion 13, 52, 57, 58, 102; and cooperation 22, 98; disgust 21–22, 24, 51–52, 97, 98; and "dread risk" 34–35, 99; elevation 52, 57, 102; emotional contagion 23, 97; and evolution, emotional network shaped by 20; and false *vs.* accurate information 87; and information processing 20–21, 24, 98; love 57, 102; moral emotions 51–52; moral outrage 42, 87, 101; multiple functions of 97; and polarization 59; and risk communication 93; risk perception, cognitive-emotional model of 34–37, 38, 99–100; and risk taking 22, 99; self-regulatory functions of 21; social effects of 22; and threats 20–23; and trade-offs in decision making 41, 100–101; and trust 22, 98; and working memory capacity 25; *see also* anxiety; fear
environmental (climate change) risks 35, 96
epistemic motivation 40
Epton, T. 38
European Centre for Disease Prevention and Control (ECDPC) 86
European Social Survey (2006-12) 83
European Union: COVID-19 pandemic, unprepared for 51; COVID-19 disinformation 86, 91; DisinfoLab 90; EUvsDiSiNFO 90; social trust and economic crisis 83; trust in EU institutions and economic crisis 74
evaluation-based trust 67, 70, 104

evidence-based 6, 154, 177–178
evolution, emotional network shaped by 20
exchange (market pricing) orientation 57–58, 102
existential threat 51, 52
experts: databases of for public policy analysis 180; perceived as "the elite" 45; trust issues 43–46, 103–104

Facebook 85, 86, 89–90
fact checking 88, 89, 91, 92
factcheck.org website 91
fake news *see* disinformation (fake news)
FakerFact websites 91
fear: of becoming infected 6, 14; copying strategies 17, 18; of economic recession 4; and emotional contagion 23, 97; and information processing capacity 20–21, 24, 98; key issue during pandemic 9, 16, 22; and negative memories, retrieval of 20; and social mobilization 61; *see also* anxiety; threats; uncertainty
Ferrer, R. A. 37
financial issues *see* economy
Finland, Sanny Martin's leadership during COVID-19 pandemic 55
Fiske, A. P. 57, 58
fit principle 60
Fragale, A. R. 88
France: Christianity and cultural *vs.* religious differences 162; COVID-19 vaccine take up (July 2021) 159; domestic violence special code messages 80; proxemics and social distancing 161; terrorist attacks (2015) 73
Frederiksen, M. 55
free riding 78, 106, 160
Freedom House 166

Gadarian, S. K. 75
Gailliot, M. T. 13
Ganesh (Hindu god) 172
Garcia-Retamero, R. 36
Gasiorowska, A. 45, 58
gender (sex), and decision making/risk taking 39, 40, 41, 100
Germany: comparison of Poland's and Germany's COVID-19 daily confirmed cases and deaths (2020-21) *157*; COVID-19 disinformation 86; COVID-19 first wave 156, 158;

COVID-19 second wave 158; SARS-CoV-2 test from Charité Hospital 154; trust in government 7
Gigerenzer, G. 32–33, 34, 93
Gilovich, T. 64
global identity 61–62
goal pursuit: and anger 21, 23, 97; and optimism 25–26, 27
Goldenberg, J. L. 12
Google 89–90
Gordon-Hecker, T. 43
Górniak, J. *see* COVID-19 intervention measures dataset analysis (J. Górniak, S. Krupnik, M. Koniewski); public policy responses to pandemic (J. Górniak, S. Krupnik, M. Koniewski)
governments: breaking their own pandemic-related rules 7, 56; competing for resources during pandemic 51; high status groups' pressure on governments during pandemic 50; "human-as problem" perspective 7; inadequacies of and hunting for scapegoats 51; trust in 7, 56, 59, 67–70, 73, 75, 78; *see also* institutional trust; leaders; politics
Grant, A. M. 58
Greece: economic crisis (2009) 74; economic crisis and social trust 80; vaccine hesitancy 48
Greenberg, J. 13
group perspective: conspiracy theories and polarization 58–60; cooperation and communal *vs.* individualistic orientations 56–58; in-groups and outgroups 49, 51, 52, 60, 63; groups and social identity 49–50, 51; high *vs.* low status groups 50–51; identity construction process 50–51; influencing groups 53–56; "nation" category in crisis situation 51; role of existential threat 51, 52; role of moral emotions 51–52; role of political leaders/governments 51; shared social identity and risk perception/taking 52; social identity and engagement 61; social inequalities, perception of 63–64; social unrest, protests and collective behaviour 60–63
Guinea, Ebola epidemic (2014) 175

H1N1 (subtype of influenza A virus) 30, 75, 81

206 *Index*

habituation 101

Hall, E. T. 161

hand washing/sanitizer use: and anger against rule-breakers 21, 97; and anxiety 21; DDM (distancing, disinfection, masks) rule 158, 160; guidance from Islamic Relief Worldwide 165; guidance from Taliban in Afghanistan 169; hand sanitizers ads banned on social media 90; and normative influence 53–54; and nudging 55; and optimism 27, 31; and positive illusions (unrealistic optimism) 30; and risk perception 31, 37, 97; and social networks 81

Harris, P. R. 38

Haslam, S. A. 7, 51, 59

health: and optimism 27; and positive illusions (unrealistic optimism) 29–30; and social capital 80–82, 84, 105; somatic health 16, 20, 25, 26; telehealth 14

health anxiety 10–11, 23, 47, 98

health information: and social media 85–86; *see also* risk communication

healthcare professionals: anti-vaccine sentiment 47; lack of trust in (Poland) 159; pandemic-related stress 14; violence against 14, 172

healthcare systems: COVID-19 pandemic, impact on (Poland) 155; distrust in and compliance (Poland) 7–8; trust in and compliance 76

Heath, C. 88

Hedman, E. 10

herd immunity issue 42, 78, 179

high-risk groups: need to tailor support to 16–17; pandemic-related stress 14

Hinduism, number of Hindu believers worldwide 163

Hinduism and COVID-19 pandemic in India (P. Kłodkowski and A. Siewierska-Chmaj): cultural *vs.* religious differences 162; female deities used in awareness-raising campaigns 171; folk and philosophical versions of Hinduism 170–171; Ganesh festival adapted to pandemic conditions 172–173; goddess Mariamman 171; goddess Shitala 171; Kumbh Mela festival and dramatic growth of infections 173–174; Mother Goddess (Durga or Kali) 171, 172; Mother-India (religious and nationalist image) 171–172; "pandemic

discrimination" against Muslims 173; pandemic statistics (2021) 173; sales of coronavirus-shaped candies/cookies 172; sanitary procedures integrated into temple decorations 172; sanitary rules grounded in Hinduism 170

Hirsch, C. R. 23

HIV (Human Immunodeficiency Virus) 154; *see also* AIDS

hoarding (of supplies) 37, 52, 86

Hofstede, G. 161

Holmes, E. A. 23

home schooling 16; *see also* distance learning

homophily 77

Hong Kong, SARS pandemic (2003) 86

Hsee, C. K. 36, 57

Human Immunodeficiency Virus (HIV) 154; *see also* AIDS

"human-as-solution", *vs.* "human-as-problem" 7–8

Hurricane Katrina disaster (US, 2005) 69, 74, 76

identity: global identity 61–62; social identity 49–50, 51, 52, 54, 61, 62

identity-based trust 67, 104

ideology 102–103, 178; *see also* conspiracy theories; polarization; politics

Iglič, H. 83

ignorance: and preventive behaviours 103; *see also* disinformation (fake news)

immunization *see* vaccines

India: caste system 64; Delta variant of SARS-CoV-2 virus 159; proxemics and social distancing 161; violence against health workers 172; *see also* Hinduism and COVID-19 pandemic in India (P. Kłodkowski and A. Siewierska-Chmaj)

individual perspective: "human-as-solution" *vs.* "human-as-problem" 7–8; *see also* anxiety; decision making; optimism; risk; risk communication; risk perception/taking; threats; trust; uncertainty

individualistic cultures 57; *see also* exchange (market pricing) orientation

Indonesia, economic crisis (1990s) and social capital 83

inequalities *see* social inequalities

influencing: informational influence 53; normative influence 53–54; nudging 54–55, 189; role of leaders 55–56

influenza: avian influenza (bird flu) 75;
  H1N1 (subtype of influenza A virus)
  30, 75, 81
"infodemic" notion 85, 154
information overload 25
information processing: and emotions
  20–21, 24, 98; and epistemic
  motivation 40; and political beliefs
  69; selective information processing
  20–21, 24, 39, 44, 69, 98, 104
informational influence 53
Instagram 89, 90
institutional trust: defining 65; evaluation-
  based trust 67, 70, 104; identity-based
  trust 67, 104; impact of economic
  crises on 73–74; impact of military/
  terrorist crises on 73, 105; impact
  of natural disasters on 74; impact of
  pandemics on 75, 105; legitimacy, trust
  and compliance 65–66, 71, 75–76,
  104–105; local (frontline) institutions,
  trust in 67, 70, 104, 105; political
  institutions, trust in 67–70, 73–74,
  104, 105; procedural fairness 70–72,
  104–105; public institutions, trust
  in 70; rational (or calculative) trust
  66–67, 72; relational trust 66–67, 72;
  risk perception and institutional trust
  72–73, 74, 75, 76, 105; see also trust
International Crisis Group 175
International Fact-Checking Network
  (IFCN) 89
internet: assessing information 43–44;
  cyberchondria 10, 98; sustaining social
  capital during natural disasters 83–84,
  106; see also social media
Iraq, Islam and cultural vs. religious
  differences 162
Iran, COVID-19 pandemic, management
  of 166–167
Ireland, economic crisis and social trust 80
Islam: Islamic model of crisis
  management 165–166; see also
  Muslims; Muslims and COVID-19
  pandemic (P. Kłodkowski and A.
  Siewierska-Chmaj)
Islamic Relief Worldwide, "Guidance
  on safe religious practice for Muslim
  communities during the coronavirus
  pandemic" 164–165
Islamic State (IS), response to COVID-19
  pandemic 168–169, 170
isolation: forced isolation 27, 28, 57, 66;
  isolation rules 18, 25, 97; self-isolation

21, 45, 55, 94, 99, 164, 165; see also
  quarantine
Italy: COVID-19 vaccine take up
  (July 2021) 159; San Siro match and
  COVID-19 epidemic in Bergamo,
  Lombardy 158; violent attacks
  on Asians during COVID-19
  pandemic 51

Jagiellonian University, Institute of
  Psychology's pandemic-related advice
  website 14
Jalandhari, Hanif 167
JHU CSSE see Johns Hopkins University
  (JHU), Center for Systems Science and
  Engineering (CSSE)
job loss: anxiety/stress caused by 16;
  coping strategies 17; and financial
  cooperation 57; and support
  network 28
Johns Hopkins University (JHU), Center
  for Systems Science and Engineering
  (CSSE), COVID-19 Data Repository
  176n9, 192
Jonas, E. 13
Jordan, Islam and cultural vs. religious
  differences 162
Josef, A. K. 40

Kaczyński, J. 56
Kaczyński, L. 56
Kali or Durga (Hindu Mother Goddess)
  171, 172
Kapur, R. 169
Keltner, D. 36
Khan, I. 167
Kim, H. K. 30
Kłodkowski, P. see cultural differences
  and pandemic (P. Kłodkowski and A.
  Siewierska-Chmaj); Hinduism and
  COVID-19 pandemic in India (P.
  Kłodkowski and A. Siewierska-Chmaj);
  Muslims and COVID-19 pandemic (P.
  Kłodkowski and A. Siewierska-Chmaj)
knowledge, and risk perception 36, 37
Koniewski, M. see COVID-19
  intervention measures dataset analysis
  (J. Górniak, S. Krupnik, M. Koniewski);
  public policy responses to pandemic (J.
  Górniak, S. Krupnik, M. Koniewski)
Kossowska, M.a: co-author of Part 1
  chapters 3, 7, 49, 65, 85, 97; co-editor
  of Part 2 chapters 151; political beliefs
  and biased perceptions of reality

208 *Index*

59–60; positive effects of uncertainty 13; trust in experts and scientists 45
Kruglanski, A. W. 44
Krupnik, S. *see* COVID-19 intervention measures dataset analysis (J. Górniak, S. Krupnik, M. Koniewski); public policy responses to pandemic (J. Górniak, S. Krupnik, M. Koniewski)
Kumari, S. 171
Kumbh Mela festival (India, 2021) 173–174

Lai, J. C. L. 28
Lauriola, M. 40
Le Bon, G. 62
leaders: attempts at unity-building activities during COVID-19 pandemic 51; community building in time of crisis 55; effective influence of, conditions for 55–56; female leaders during COVID-19 pandemic 55, 56; religious leaders 52; *see also* governments; politics
legitimacy: institutional legitimacy and procedural fairness 71; institutional trust-based legitimacy and compliance 65–66, 71, 75–76, 104–105; police legitimacy 66; vaccine legitimacy 47
Leiser, D. 95
Lerner, J. S. 36
Letki, N.: co-author of Part 1 chapters 3, 7, 49, 65, 85, 97; co-editor of Part 2 chapters 151
Leuker, C. 42
Lewandowski, R.t and Lewandowski, A. 52
LGBTQI+ persons, impact of pandemic on (Polish case) 156
Liberia, Ebola epidemic (2014) 175
Lighthall, N. R. 39
Linden, S. van der 91
LinkedIn 89
literacy: digital literacy 91; economic/financial literacy 37, 91, 95–96, 107; media literacy 91
lockdowns: deciding on timing 7; domestic violence and lack of institutional support 80; economic effects of 42, 101, 155; educational effects of 155; lifting of and decline in social discipline 178–179; losses and risks resulting from 179; in Poland 5, 155, 156; uncertainty/anxiety about effectiveness of 9; violations of rules and existential threat 52

love 57, 102
Lubell, M. 75–76
Lusardi, A. 37

Madrid (Spain), 2004 terrorist attacks 73
Mahbubani, Kishore 174
Margolis, J. D. 58
Mariamman (Hindu goddess) 171
market pricing (exchange) orientation 57–58, 102
Martin, S. 55
mask wearing: in Afghanistan 169; and anger against rule-breakers 21, 97; and anxiety 9, 21; and community building/good leadership 55; DDM (distancing, disinfection, masks) rule 158, 160; and disinformation 86; effectiveness of, insufficient evidence for 9; and health anxiety 10; and Hindu goddess statues 172; in Iran 166; and optimism 27, 31; and risk perception 31, 37, 97; and social capital 77; social media's banning of ads 89, 90; and social networks 81; in Spain 193; uncertainty and sewing masks 17
mass gatherings: nudging to avoid 55; and risk taking 52
measles, 2019 outbreaks 46
measles, mumps, and rubella (MMR) vaccine issue 46, 47, 48
media: and health anxiety, images contributing to 23; and "human-as problem" perspective 7; media literacy skills 91; message framing 94; messaging, conflicting and inconsistent 103; political stance and readers' selective information processing 69; reports about attacks against suspected COVID-19 sufferers 23; reports on political standards and institutional trust 69–70; second-hand knowledge from and institutional trust 67–68, 104; trust, lack of trust in (Poland) 159; trust in under military/terrorist crisis 73; *see also* disinformation (fake news); internet; social media
memory: anxiety/fear and retrieval of negative memories 20; emotions and working memory capacity 25
mental health: and emotional processing 20; neglect of groups with during pandemic 4; and social media 85; *see also* anxiety; depression; stress
messaging *see* media; risk communication

military crisis, impact on institutional/ political trust 73, 105
Mills, J. R. 57
minorities 14, 86, 156
misinformation *see* disinformation (fake news)
Mitchell, O. S. 37
MMR (measles, mumps, and rubella) vaccine issue 46, 47, 48
molecular tests 153
Molinsky, A. L. 58
moral emotions 51–52; "moral elevation" concept 52
moral nudges 54–55
moral outrage 42, 87, 101
motivated cognition 24
motivated reasoning 44, 45, 104
motivation: and behaviour change 54; and decision making/risk taking 40–41, 100; epistemic motivation 40; and "human-as-solution" perspective 8; and preventive behaviours 19, 31, 37–38; *see also* nudging
Mousavi Tabrizi, H. 166–167
Muhammad, Prophet 164, 166, 168
multi-attribute utility theory 39
Murphy, D. 9
Muslims: number of Muslim believers worldwide 163; "pandemic discrimination" against in India 173
Muslims and COVID-19 pandemic (P. Kłodkowski and A. Siewierska-Chmaj): Afghanistan/Taliban 169–170; Boko Haram 168, 169; Iran 166–167; Islamic State/Al-Qaida 168–169, 170; Pakistan 167–168, 169; Saudi Arabia 167; conspiracy theories 166, 168–169; cultural *vs.* religious differences 161–163; fatwa from Supreme Ulema Council (banning collective prayers) 163–164, 167; Guidance from Islamic Relief Worldwide 164–165; guidance on burials/cremation 164, 165; guidance on closing mosques 164; guidance on hand sanitizers 165; guidance on self-isolation 164, 165; Islamic model of crisis management 165–166; justifications for sanitary rules grounded in Islam 170; local religious leaders' rejection of government decisions 167; "obligation" rather than "recommendations" 164; radical Islam's response 168–170; Shia Muslims (or Shiites) 163, 166–167; Sunnis Muslims 163, 164; warnings

against spreading unconfirmed news 164
Myanmar, Buddhism and cultural *vs.* religious differences 162

Namaki, S. 166
"nation" concept, in crisis situation 51
natural disasters: and community resilience 84; and institutional trust 74; and risk perception 74, 75, 79; and social trust 79, 83–84, 106; *see also* Hurricane Katrina disaster (US, 2005)
natural frequencies, and probability data presentation 34, 93, 99, 108
Nature: dataset on non-pharmaceutical interventions (NPIs) 190; *see also* COVID-19 intervention measures dataset analysis (J. Górniak, S. Krupnik, M. Koniewski)
Nazis 43
Nes, L. S. 27
Netherlands: Christianity and cultural *vs.* religious differences 162; COVID-19 disinformation 86; institutional trust and flood risk perception 72; institutional trust and H1N1 pandemic (2009) 75
New York City (US): disinformation about SARS outbreak in Chinatown 86; Hart Island COVID-19 victim mass graves 168; September 11, 2001 terrorist attacks 13, 73
New Zealand: COVID-19 rules broken by Health Minister 56; Jacinda Ardern's leadership during COVID-19 pandemic 56
Ngan, H. F. 30
Niederdeppe, J. 30
Nigeria, vaccine hesitancy 48
Nordic countries: Christianity and cultural *vs.* religious differences 162; proxemics and social distancing 161
normative influence 53–54
Norway, Erny Solberg's leadership during COVID-19 pandemic 55
nudging 54–55, 189; moral nudges 54–55; in pandemic situation 55
numeracy 37

OECD: 2020 report on COVID-19 disinformation 85, 86, 88, 89–90; *see also* COVID-19 intervention measures dataset analysis (J. Górniak, S. Krupnik, M. Koniewski)
Olejniczak, K. 180

210 *Index*

online platforms *see* internet; social media
optimism: cognitive system key function 25–26; defining 26; and goal pursuit 25–26, 27; and health 27; rational behaviour during pandemic 27–28, 30–31; unrealistic optimism (positive illusions) 25, 28–30, 31; unrealistic optimism during pandemic 30, 31, 103

Pakistan: COVID-19 pandemic, management of 167–168, 169; Islam and cultural *vs.* religious differences 162
panic: collective/mass panic responses 23, 97, 175; panic stories 28; "panic" term and message framing 94
panic attacks 4
party identification 60
party identity protective cognition 60
Patashnik, E. M. 179–180
PCR (polymerase chain reaction) technique 154
Pennycook, G. 92
personal (egotropic) perceptions, *vs.* sociotropic perceptions 68
personal protective equipment *see* PPE (personal protective equipment)
pessimism 26–27, 28; *see also* optimism
Peters, E. 10
Petrova, D. 36
phobias 9; social phobia 23
physical attractiveness, and behavioural immune system 22
Pinterest 89
Pligt, J. van der 36
Poland: COVID-19 Advisory Team to the President of the Polish Academy of Sciences 14, 160n1; COVID-19 as political issue 59–60; COVID-19 pandemic, state of in July 2020 5; entrepreneurs protest during pandemic 61, 63; healthcare system, distrust in and compliance 7–8; Kaczyński's access to closed cemetery 56; mask-wearing, inconsistent official recommendations on 9; nudging and religion 55; Polish Tatars 162; political identity and collective action 61; scientists/experts, trust in 45; *see also* Poland and COVID-19 epidemic (Jerzy Duszyński)
Poland and COVID-19 epidemic (Jerzy Duszyński): brief overview of global

research findings 153–154; cases and deaths, number of (July 2021) 155; comparison of Poland's and Germany's daily confirmed cases and deaths (2020-21) *157*; comparison with Germany 156, *157*, 158; comparison with Italy and Spain 158; conspiracy theories 156, 159; effectiveness of measures and public's changing attitudes 156, 158, 159; first lockdown 155, 156; first wave 154–155, 156, 158; fourth wave and Delta variant 159; healthcare professionals, lack of trust in 159; impact of epidemic on economy 158; impact of epidemic on LGBTQI+ persons 156; impact of epidemic on minorities 156; impact of epidemic on young people 155–156; impact of epidemy on healthcare system 155; impact of lockdowns on economy 155; impact of lockdowns on education 155; lessons to be learnt (institutions and solidarity) 160; politicians/media, lack of trust in 159; second wave 156, 158; third wave 156, 158, 159; vaccine take up (July 2021) 159
polarization 59–60, 68–69, 91, 103; affective polarization 59
police: police legitimacy 66; police violence 63, 66
politics: polarization 59–60, 68–69, 91, 103; political false news, spreading of 87; political identity and behaviour 54; political identity and collective action 61; protests (social unrest) 60–63, 66; rally-round-the-flag effect 73, 105; trust in political institutions 67–70, 73–74, 104, 105; trust in politicians, lack of (Poland) 159; *see also* governments; leaders; public policy responses to pandemic (J. Górniak, S. Krupnik, M. Koniewski)
polymerase chain reaction (PCR) technique 154
positive illusions (unrealistic optimism) 25, 28–31, 103
post-traumatic stress 23
poverty *see* social inequalities
PPE (personal protective equipment): ads banned on social media platforms 90; shortages of 14
preference potentiation 22, 98

prejudice 11, 14, 22
preventive behaviours: and ignorance 103; and motivation 19, 31, 37–38; and normative influence 53–54; and nudging 55; and risk overestimation 36; and risk perception 31, 37–38, 39–40, 97, 100; and social networks 81; *see also* compliance; COVID-19 intervention measures dataset analysis (J. Górniak, S. Krupnik, M. Koniewski); hand washing/sanitizer use; isolation; lockdowns; mask wearing; public policy responses to pandemic (J. Górniak, S. Krupnik, M. Koniewski); quarantine; social distancing; vaccines
probability data presentation, and natural frequencies 34, 93, 99, 108
procedural fairness 70–72, 104–105
processing fluency 87
protective behaviours *see* preventive behaviours
protests (social unrest) 60–63, 66
proxemics 161
psychoeducation 13–14, 17
psychometric paradigm, and risk perception 34–36, 99
public policy responses to pandemic (J. Górniak, S. Krupnik, M. Koniewski): COVID-19 lockdown, lifting of and decline in social discipline 178–179; evidence-based approach and ideology 177–178; functions of public policy analysis 179–180; interventions aimed at stopping pandemic 180–181, 189–190; interventions and target groups' behaviours 180–181, **182–184**; pandemic-related communication, guidelines based on social-behavioural research evidence 180–181, 185–189; policies for potentially prolonged pandemic 179; resource allocation/ redirecting 181; restrictions on movement and social contact 181; *see also* COVID-19 intervention measures dataset analysis (J. Górniak, S. Krupnik, M. Koniewski)
PubMed database, COVID-19/ SARS-CoV-2 publications, number of 153

Qom Seminary 166
quarantine 17, 18, 83, 86, 94, 169; *see also* isolation

rally-round-the-flag effect 73, 105
rational behaviour: 'human beings as irrational' perspective 54; and optimism *vs.* pessimism 27–28; resistance to evidence-based rationality 154
rational trust (calculative trust) 66–67, 72
rationalizations 43, 101
reciprocity, and cognitive social capital 76, 77–78, 106
red (colour), use of in messages 93, 108
Red Cross 169
Reddit 85, 86, 89
Reicher, S. D. 62
relational trust 66–67, 72
religion: and nudge techniques 55; religious leaders 52; religious/ cultural differences during pandemic 161–163, 174–175; *see also* Buddhism; Christianity; Hinduism; Hinduism and COVID-19 pandemic in India (P. Kłodkowski and A. Siewierska-Chmaj); Muslims; Muslims and COVID-19 pandemic (P. Kłodkowski and A. Siewierska-Chmaj)
remote interventions 14
remote work 4, 16
resilience: to anxiety/stress 15; community resilience 84, 106
restrictions *see* compliance; COVID-19 intervention measures dataset analysis (J. Górniak, S. Krupnik, M. Koniewski); preventive behaviours; public policy responses to pandemic (J. Górniak, S. Krupnik, M. Koniewski)
risk: decision making under risk 38–41; diversity of risks during pandemic 98–99; dread risk *vs.* unknown risk 34–35, 99; risk assessment and cognitive biases 24–25, 32–33, 99; risk assessment and methods to communicate data 33–34, 99; risk reduction strategies 18; risk-as-feelings hypothesis 22; *see also* risk communication; risk perception/ taking
risk communication: aim of process 92, 106–107; colour red 93, 108; message clarity 92–93, 107–108; message framing 93–94; probability data presentation and natural frequencies 34, 93, 99, 108; risk avoidance and self-efficacy 93, 108; risk communication

212 *Index*

four-step model 94–96, 107; *see also* communication; disinformation (fake news)

risk perception/taking: about analysing risk perception 31–32; and affect heuristic 95–96, 107; and age 39–40, 100; and anxiety 22, 24–25, 36, 98, 99; cognitive-emotional model of risk perception 34–37, 38, 99–100; and emotions 22, 99; and institutional trust 72–73, 74, 75, 76, 105; and knowledge 36, 37; and mass gatherings 52; and motivation 40–41, 100; and preventive behaviours 31, 37–38, 39–40, 97, 100; and sex (gender) 39, 40, 41, 100; and shared social identity 52; and social networks 82; and social trust 78–79; and temperament/personality 40, 100; and unrealistic optimism 25, 29, 103; and vaccine take up 38, 100

role models, moral role models 52

Roozenbeek, J. 91

Rottenstreich, Y. 36

Routledge, C. 12

"sacred values" concept 42, 101

safety measures *see* preventive behaviours

SAGE, Working Group on Vaccine Hesitancy 48

sanitizer use *see* hand washing/sanitizer use

SARS-CoV pandemic (2003) 9, 86, 154

SARS-CoV-2 pandemic *see* COVID-19 (SARS-CoV-2) pandemic

Saudi Arabia: COVID-19 pandemic, management of 167; Islam and cultural *vs.* religious differences 162, 163

Saxena, Chayaniki 169

scapegoating 51

Scholz, J. T. 75–76

science/scientists: COVID-19 research findings 153–154; evidence-based 6, 154, 177–178; general public's exposure to scientific process 154; insufficient knowledge 9; scientific method 177; trust in scientists 7, 45, 56; universal language of science 174; *see also* experts

Scotland, COVID-19 rules broken by Chief Medical Officer 56

Segerstrom, S. C. 27

self-efficacy 16, 38, 49, 93, 100, 108

self-esteem: and death anxiety 11, 12–13; and depression 15–16; and motivated

reasoning 45, 104; and optimism 31; and social identity 49

self-isolation *see* isolation

Self-Regulatory Model 18–19

September 11, 2001 terrorist attacks (US) 13, 73

serological tests 153

sex (gender), and decision making/risk taking 39, 40, 41, 100

Shaheen, Suhail 170

Sheeran, P. 38

Shekau, Aboubakar 168

Shemesh, Y. S. 95

Shia Muslims (or Shiites) 163, 166–167

Shin, J. 88

Shitala (Hindu goddess) 171

Sierra Leone, Ebola epidemic (2014) 175

Siewierska-Chmaj, Anna *see* cultural differences and pandemic (P. Kłodkowski and A. Siewierska-Chmaj); Hinduism and COVID-19 pandemic in India (P. Kłodkowski and A. Siewierska-Chmaj); Muslims and COVID-19 pandemic (P. Kłodkowski and A. Siewierska-Chmaj)

Snapchat 89

Snopes website 91

Sobkow, A. 10

social anxiety 9, 23

social capital: behavioural (formal/informal social networks) 76–77, 78–79; bonding social capital 76–77, 84; bridging social capital 76–77, 84; cognitive (trust and reciprocity) 76, 77–78, 106; and community resilience 84, 106; and compliance 77–79, 82, 106; and crisis 83–84, 106; and free riding 78, 106; and health 80–82, 84, 105; and social inequalities 77, 81, 82–83, 84, 105; social trust 76, 78–79, 80; as source of support and resources 79, 105; and wellbeing 79–80, 84, 105

social distancing: and coping strategies against uncertainty 18; DDM (distancing, disinfection, masks) rule 158, 160; and disinformation 86; guidance from Taliban in Afghanistan 169; in Iran 166; mandatory *vs.* recommended 19; and media's "human-as-problem" approach 7; and normative influence 53–54; and nudging 55; and optimism 27, 31; and proxemics 161; and risk perception 31; uncertainty/anxiety about effectiveness of 9

Index 213

social identity 49–50, 51, 52, 54, 61, 62
social inequalities: and cooperation 102; as long-term effects of COVID-19 pandemic 63, 84; perception of inequalities 63–64; poor hardest hit by crises/COVID-19 pandemic 8, 63; and social capital 77, 82–83, 84, 105; and social capital-health relationship 81; and virus transmission 82–83
social media: algorithms 88, 90, 91; anti-vaccine movement 47; anxiety-inducing 85; banning of COVID-19 related product ads 90; collective panic responses 23; coping strategies against uncertainty 18; COVID-19 disinformation 86–87; COVID-19 disinformation, measures to combat 89–91; digital literacy skills 91; fast spreading of false news 87–88; health information, main source of 85–86; message framing 94; Muslim leaders' use of for COVID-19 guidance 165, 169; selective information processing and politics 69; self-esteem and peer groups 13; *see also* internet
social mobility 64, 79
social mobilization 60, 61
social networks 57, 76–77, 78–79, 80, 81–82, 83, 84, 105
social norms 53–54; dynamic norms 54; norm internalization 55
social phobia 23
"social proof" (influence of authority) 19
social trust 56, 76, 78, 80, 81, 83, 84, 106
social unrest (protests) 60–63, 66
social-behavioural research 179, 180–181, 185–189
societal level *see* institutional trust; social capital
sociotropic perceptions, *vs.* personal (egotropic) perceptions 68
Solberg, E. 55
solidarity 8, 60, 61, 64, 160; *see also* community resilience; compliance; cooperation
Soman, D. 180
somatic health 16, 20, 25, 26
South Africa, protests against forced isolation facilities (2007) 66
South Korea: COVID-19 disinformation 86; cultural *vs.* religious differences 163
Spain: COVID-19 disinformation 86; COVID-19 pandemic 158; COVID-19 vaccine take up (July 2021) 159;

domestic violence special code messages 80; economic crisis and social trust 80; mask wearing 193; terrorist attacks in Madrid (2004) 73
Sri Lanka, Buddhism and cultural *vs.* religious differences 162
Srinivas, Tulasi 171
the state *see* governments; institutional trust; leaders
status groups, high *vs.* low status 50–51
Stockholm University, pandemic-related advice to staff members 14
Stoffels, P. 46
stress: and community resilience 84; and cooperation 22, 98; and depression 15–16; and information overload 25; pandemic-related stress 13–15; post-traumatic stress 23; and risk taking 39, 40, 100; and self-efficacy 16; *see also* anxiety; depression
suicide, depression-related 15, 25
Sunni Muslims 163, 164
supply hoarding 37, 52, 86
Supreme Ulema Council (Al-Azhar University, Cairo), fatwa banning collective prayers during COVID-19 pandemic 163–164, 167
Sweden: COVID-19 pandemic and institutional trust 73; COVID-19 pandemic and social trust 83; trust in scientists 7
Szwed, P. 46, 48n5, 59–60

Tablighti Jamaat (transnational Muslim missionary organization) 173
Tajfel, H. 50
Tatars, Islam and cultural *vs.* religious differences 162
Taylor, S. 10, 11
Tech Transparency Project 90
Tedros Adhanom Ghebreyesus 85
telehealth 14
telepsychology 14
terrorism: 2001, September 11 attacks in US 13, 73; 2004 attacks in Madrid 73; 2015 attacks in France 73; impact on institutional/political trust 73
tests for COVID-19: molecular tests 153; PCR (polymerase chain reaction) technique 154; serological tests 153; testing kits 87, 90
Thailand, Buddhism and cultural *vs.* religious differences 162
Thorson, K. 88

threats: cognitive mechanisms 23–25; and decision-making 39; and depression 15–16; emotional mechanisms 20–23; and emotions 22–23; existential threat 51, 52; and informational influence 53; and self-efficacy 16; stress caused by 15; survival strategies and increased feeling of threat 8; threat severity/reduction and anxiety 20, 21; universality of psychological mechanisms 9; *see also* anxiety; risk; risk communication; risk perception/taking; uncertainty

TikTok 89

tokenism 101

trade-off decision making 41–43, 100–101

trust: and civil obedience 7; and cognitive social capital 76, 77–78, 106; and compliance 3, 53, 77–78; and emotions 22, 98; in experts 43–46, 103–104; in government 7, 56, 59, 67–70, 73, 75, 78; intergroup trust and social inequalities 63; multidimensional phenomenon 65; and polarization 59; Polish case 159; in scientists 7, 45, 56; social trust 56, 76, 78, 80, 81, 83, 84, 106; *see also* institutional trust

Tunisia, Islam and cultural *vs.* religious differences 163

Turkey, Islam and cultural *vs.* religious differences 162

Twitter 85, 89–90, 170

Tze-Ngai Vong, L. 30

Uighurs 168

uncertainty: and cooperation/communal orientation 57; coping strategies 17–18; death-related uncertainty 12, 13–14; and decision-making 3; and epistemic motivation 40; and exchange (market pricing) orientation 58, 102; and information seeking limited by memory capacity 25; and informational influence 53; and optimism 26, 31; and pandemic-related anxiety 3–4, 8–9, 24; and risk perception 36; and social inequalities 64; and social mobilization 61; and social support 28; and stress 15; universality of crisis-related uncertainty 6; universality of uncertainty-related psychological mechanisms 9; varied tolerance of uncertainty and tailoring of

recommendations 16; *see also* anxiety; risk; risk communication; risk perception/taking; threats

unemployment *see* job loss

United Kingdom (UK): Christianity and cultural *vs.* religious differences 162; conspiracy theories and lack of trust in governmental COVID-19 policies 59; COVID-19 disinformation 86; COVID-19 vaccine take up (July 2021) 159; Delta variant of SARS-CoV-2 virus 159; economic crisis and social trust 80, 83; MMR (measles, mumps, and rubella) vaccine issue 48

United States (US): CDC (Centers for Disease Control and Prevention) 47, 86; climate change risks, perception of 96; conspiracy theories and lack of trust in governmental COVID-19 policies 59; COVID-19 disinformation 86; COVID-19 YouGov poll 96; Hurricane Katrina disaster (2005) 69, 74, 76; individualism and financial cooperation 57; political identity and collective action 61; politicization of institutional policies 69; proxemics and social distancing 161; Republicans' reduced adherence to COVID-19 restrictions 60; scientists perceived as liberals 45; September 11, 2001 terrorist attacks 13, 73; social mobility, perceptions of 64; violent attacks on Asians during COVID-19 pandemic 51; *see also* New York City (US)

vaccines: anti-vaccine movement 46–47; COVID-19 vaccines, news of in 2020 summer 5; COVID-19 vaccines, numbers of 46; COVID-19 vaccines, ongoing research 3; limited effectiveness of 160; MMR (measles, mumps, and rubella) vaccine issue 46, 47, 48; optimism and pro-vaccine stance 28; positive illusions (unrealistic optimism) and anti-vaccine stance 30; risk perception and vaccine take up 38, 100; social capital and vaccine take up 80–81; social trust and vaccine take up 81; trust in government and vaccine take up 75; trust in scientists and vaccine take up 45; vaccine hesitancy 47–48; vaccine legitimacy 47; vaccine safety 47; vaccine take up in Poland, France, UK, Spain, Italy (July 2021) 159

Vail, K. 13
Vietnam, cultural *vs.* religious
   differences 163
violence: aimed at Asians during
   COVID-19 pandemic 51; aimed at
   health professionals 14, 172; aimed at
   known/suspected COVID-19 sufferers
   10, 23; aimed at minorities 86, 156;
   and anxiety 9, 10; and crowds 62–63;
   domestic violence 4, 17, 80, 156; police
   violence 63, 66; and social inequalities
   63; *see also* aggressive behaviour
volunteering, as coping strategy 17
vulnerable groups *see* high-risk groups;
   LGBTQI+ persons; minorities

Wakefield, A. 47
"we are in it together" feeling 55
Weber, E. U. 57
wellbeing, and social capital 79–80,
   84, 105
WhatsApp 165, 169
Wichary, S.: co-author of Part 1 chapters
   3, 7, 49, 65, 85, 97; co-editor of Part 2
   chapters 151
work *see* job loss; remote work
World Bank, forecast of COVD-19
   pandemic-related recession 5
World Health Organization (WHO):
   COVID-19 cases, biggest daily

increase in (18 July 2020) 5; COVID-
19 outbreak declared a pandemic
155, 195–196; COVID-19/SARS-
CoV-2 names 153; dissemination
of information 86, 89, 90; Islamic
Relief Worldwide's guidance based
on opinions of 164; MMR (measles,
mumps, and rubella) vaccine crisis
(2019) 46; risk reduction strategies
18; Taliban's lifting of ban on WHO
activity in Afghanistan 169–170; "we're
fighting an infodemic" (Feb. 2020
conference) 85

xenophobia 51
Xie, W. 19

YouGov poll 96, 159
young people: impact of pandemic/home
   confinement on 155–156; pandemic-
   related stress 14, 155; risk taking 40;
   unrealistic optimism 29–30
YouTube 85–86, 89, 90

Zaleskiewicz, T.: co-author of Part 1
   chapters 3, 7, 49, 65, 85, 97; co-editor
   of Part 2 chapters 151; exchange
   (market pricing) orientation 58;
   motivated reasoning 45
Zika pandemic 86

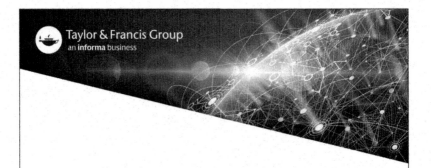